Public Health and the Modernization of China, 1865–2015

This book, based on extensive original research, traces the development of China's public health system, showing how advances in public health have been an integral part of China's rise. It outlines the phenomenal improvements in public health, for example the increase in life expectancy from 38 in 1949 to 73 in 2010; relates developments in public health to prevailing political ideologies; and discusses how the drivers of health improvements were, unlike in the West, modern medical professionals and intellectuals who understood that, whatever the prevailing ideology, China needs to be a strong country. The book explores how public health concepts, policies, programmes, institutions and practices changed and developed through social and political upheavals, war, and famine, and argues that this perspective of China's development is refreshingly different from China's development viewed purely in political terms.

Liping Bu is a Professor of History at Alma College, Michigan, USA.

Routledge Studies in the Modern History of Asia

113 Science, Technology, and Medicine in the Modern Japanese Empire
Edited by David G. Wittner and Philip C. Brown

114 Street Performers and Society in Urban Japan, 1600–1900
Gerald Groemer

115 Suicide in Twentieth Century Japan
Francesca Di Marco

116 Treaty Ports in Modern China
Law, Land and Power
Edited by Robert Bickers and Isabella Jackson

117 Kyoto Visual Culture in the Early Edo and Meiji Periods
The Arts of Reinvention
Edited by Morgan Pitelka and Alice Y. Tseng

118 Health Policy and Disease in Colonial and Post-Colonial Hong Kong, 1841–2003
Ka-che Yip, Philip Yuen-sang Leung, and Timothy Man-Kong Wong

119 Britain's Imperial Retreat from China, 1900–1931
Phoebe Chow

120 Constitution Making in Asia
Decolonisation and State-Building in the Aftermath of the British Empire
H. Kumarasingham

121 Neutrality in Southeast Asia
Concepts and Contexts
Nicholas Tarling

122 Britain's Retreat from Empire in East Asia, 1905–1980
Edited by Antony Best

123 The Dismantling of Japan's Empire in East Asia
Deimperialization, Postwar Legitimation and Imperial Afterlife
Edited by Barak Kushner and Sherzod Muminov

124 Public Health and the Modernization of China, 1865–2015
Liping Bu

Public Health and the Modernization of China, 1865–2015

Liping Bu

Routledge
Taylor & Francis Group
LONDON AND NEW YORK

First published 2017
by Routledge
4 Park Square, Milton Park, Abingdon, Oxon OX14 4RN

and by Routledge
605 Third Avenue, New York, NY 10017

Routledge is an imprint of the Taylor & Francis Group, an informa business

British Library Cataloguing in Publication Data
A catalogue record for this book is available from the British Library

Library of Congress Cataloging in Publication Data
Names: Bu, Liping, 1960- author.
Title: Public health and the modernization of China, 1910-2015 / Liping Bu.
Other titles: Routledge studies in the modern history of Asia (2005) ; 124.
Description: Abingdon, Oxon ; New York, NY : Routledge, 2017. | Series: Routledge studies in the modern history of Asia ; 124 | Includes bibliographical references and index.
Identifiers: LCCN 2016040347| ISBN 9781138845817 (hardback) | ISBN 9781315727912 (ebook)
Subjects: | MESH: Public Health—history | Health Policy—history | Health Planning—history | History, 20th Century | History, 21st Century | China
Classification: LCC RA395.C53 | NLM WA 11 JC6 | DDC 362.10951—dc23
LC record available at https://lccn.loc.gov/2016040347

ISBN: 978-1-138-84581-7 (hbk)
ISBN: 978-1-315-72791-2 (ebk)

Typeset in Times New Roman
by Swales & Willis Ltd, Exeter, Devon, UK

In memory of my parents

Contents

Illustrations

Figures

Tables

Acknowledgements

This book has been a long time in the making. It started in 2001 when I was examining the YMCA archives at the University of Minnesota on a possible topic of physical education and national strength in early twentieth-century China. I had just completed a monograph, *Making the World Like Us: Education, Cultural Expansion, and the American Century*, and wanted to continue the research on American educational influence abroad. I was surprised to find, with great excitement, that the YMCA had engaged in active public health education in China, which had not been closely examined by scholars. In the following decade, I read and examined documents on public health at various libraries and archival centers in China, the United States, and the United Kingdom. I was fortunate that many local archives were opened up to the public in China and various grants enabled me to carry out the research.

In 2006, an Andrew Mellon fellowship at Needham Research Institute allowed me to do systematic reading and research on medicine and public health during my sabbatical at Cambridge University. I took the opportunity to broaden my knowledge by attending classes and lectures in the Department of History and Philosophy of Science at Cambridge. I am grateful to Professors Sir Geoffrey Lloyd and Christopher Cullen for letting me sit in their classes. The weekly reading seminar at Needham Research Institute was the best of its kind, where scholars shared their readings of original texts by translating, interpreting, discussing, and debating the accurate meaning of the original texts in translation. How do you translate *daoyin* (道引, a kind of Chinese yoga exercise) into English when there is no cultural equivalent to convey its meaning to a Western audience? The seminar deepened my appreciation of the practice of close reading of original texts in research and the emphasis of language and cultural proficiency in intercultural studies. Colleagues and friends at the NRI reading seminar will notice its sustained influence on me when they read the introduction paragraph of this book. With fond memories and deep appreciation, I thank John Moffett, Susan Bennett, and Christopher Cullen of the Needham Research Institute, and fellow researchers for the wonderful experience of shared intellectual pursuit and productive research.

The "Symposium on Global Health Histories" at the Natcher Conference Center on the campus of the National Institutes of Health in November 2005 was a turning point in the extension of my research into the second half of the twentieth century. The conference not only introduced me to the professional network of public health scholars but also to the new archival collection of Chinese public health at the National Library of Medicine. The health posters of the collection offered extraordinary visual and textual information on Chinese public health campaigns from the 1930s to the 1980s. I was fortunate to have the opportunity to work on the splendid health posters over several summers, during which I examined the data and gradually reshaped the design of my research and writing of China's public health movement and modernization. The visual images provided unique values of information as historical data. I am most grateful to Drs. Elizabeth Fee and Paul Theerman for the opportunity to work on the collection at the History of Medicine Division. The research also provided me delightful opportunities to collaborate with Liz Fee on several public health essays. I recall these wonderful productive summers with gratitude to Liz for the joyful writing of essays, and to the staff at the History of Medicine Division for their collegial support and friendship.

At the National Library of Medicine, I had the pleasant opportunities to attend formal lectures on the history of medicine and engage in casual lunch conversations with medical scientists on the campus of NIH. At one of the lunch conversations, a young medical scientist surprised me with the comment that "Chinese medicine (中医) has no science." The implication was Chinese medicine had little value. When I told him that he sounded like those who wanted to abolish Chinese medicine in the 1920s, he conceded "maybe [it has] 30 percent of science." Non-Western medicine is still considered non-scientific by many in the scientific profession. Perhaps, a good educational effort is a way to reduce the bias of conventional impressions. In that regard, I was fortunate working with some staff members at the History of Medicine Division to curate several digital and physical exhibits on Chinese anti-disease health movements at the National Library of Medicine. I also created a higher education digital module on Chinese health campaigns in the twentieth century, which can be accessed at the National Library of Medicine. I hope these educational materials will help people better understand public health and Chinese medicine.

Local archives in China, especially the municipal archives of Beijing, Shanghai, and Nanjing, proved essential for my research. I am grateful for the professional assistance I received at the Chinese archival institutions and libraries. In particular, I thank the staff at Beijing Municipal Archives for their assistance with my research needs and their kindness of ordering lunch for researchers.

Over the years, I have shared my research with Chinese scholars and graduate students on various occasions. With deep appreciation of their support and for the opportunities, I thank Professor Zhang Daqing at Peking University, Professor Zhang Xianwen at Nanjing University, Professor Yu Xinzhong at Nankai University, and Professor Gao Xi at Fudan University.

The research of the book project also brought me in contact with many scholars in the unique field of history of medicine and public health at professional conferences in the United States, China, United Kingdom, and France. I had the good fortune of organizing several collaborative projects with scholars of different countries, including the "International Workshop on Public Health" at North Tarrytown in 2009, and the two volumes on *Science, Public Health and the State in Modern Asia* (2012) and *Public Health and National Reconstruction in Post-War Asia: International Influences, Local Transformation* (2014). Thanks to Darwin Stapleton, Jack Meyers, James Allen Smith and Camilla Harris at Rockefeller Archive Center for their support. Thanks to Darwin Stapleton and Ka-che Yip for sharing the editing work, and to each of the chapter contributors for sharing their latest research in the books on Asian public health.

When the China Medical Board was preparing book projects for its centennial celebration, I was honored to participate in the conferences in Boston and Beijing that led to the book, *Medical Transitions in Twentieth-Century China*. The conferences provided broad perspectives and stimulating intellectual discussions on the medical and public health development in the past century. I am grateful to Mary Bullock and Lincoln Chen at China Medical Board for the opportunities.

This book project has been supported by funding from various sources over the years. An Andrew Mellon Research Fellowship allowed me to do research at the Needham Research Institute, Cambridge, UK. A grant from the National Library of Medicine (G13LM009601-02) made it possible for me to receive valuable released time from teaching to work on this book. Grants-in-aid from the Rockefeller Archive Center supported my archival research at the Center. Alma College supported this project with annual faculty small grants and professional development funds. I acknowledge with great appreciation the various funding support. The content of this book, however, is solely my own responsibility and does not represent the views of any of the funding sources.

Portions of the text were published in journal articles and book chapters. I am grateful for the permissions of publishers from Peter Lang, University of Minnesota University Press, and Indiana University Press.

Many other people have given support and encouragement over the years. While I cannot list them all here, I'd like to thank Thomas Rosenbaum, Dagmar Getz, Ryan Bean, Bridie Andrews, Marta Hanson, Socrates Litsios, Nicole Elizabeth Barnes, Thomas Dubois, Zhen Cheng, Fang Xiaoping, Jiang Yuhong, Zhang Xia, Alyssa Walters, Gloria Tseng, Ba Ba Zhang, Ginny Roth, Doug Atkins, Lorreta Tang, Jacque-Lynn Shulman, Lois Cohen, and Susan Speaker. Thanks also to Michael Selmon the provost, colleagues, and library staff at Alma College.

Special thanks to Peter Sowden at Routledge. His encouragement and interest help to sustain the progress of this book project. Thanks to Laura Christopher and her team for their detailed attention and excellent work in the production of this book. Thanks to Ting Baker, whose copy-editing skills improved the quality of the book.

Abbreviations

CCP	Chinese Communist Party
CEPB/NEPC	Central Epidemic Prevention Bureau/National Epidemic Prevention Bureau
CFHS	Central Field Health Station
CMA	Chinese Medical Association
CMB	China Medical Board
CMMA	China Medical Missionary Association
GMD	Guomindang, Nationalist Party
IHB/IHD	International Health Board/International Health Division
JPHA	Jiangsu Public Health Association
LNHO	League of Nations Health Organization
MEM	Mass Education Movement
NHA	National Health Administration
NMAC	National Medical Association of China
NRCMS	New Rural Cooperative Medical System
PUMC	Peking Union Medical College
RAC	Rockefeller Archives Center
RF	Rockefeller Foundation
SMC	Shanghai Medical College
YMCA	Young Men's Christian Association

Primary sources

Archives

Annual and Quarterly Reports of Field Secretaries of the YMCA, Kautz Family YMCA Archives, University of Minnesota, St. Paul, Minnesota, USA.

Beijing Metropolitan Police Archives, Beijing Municipal Archives, Beijing, China.

Beiping Education Bureau and School Health Archives, Beijing Municipal Archives, Beijing.

Beiping Health Bureau Archives, Beijing Municipal Archives, Beijing.

Beiping Social Bureau Archives, Beijing Municipal Archives, Beijing.

Beiyang Government Archives, the Second Historical Archives of China, Nanjing, China.

Biographical Files, Kautz Family YMCA Archives, University of Minnesota Libraries, St. Paul, Minnesota.

China Medical Board Inc. Archives, the Rockefeller Archive Center, North Tarrytown, New York, USA.

Chinese Collections, Cambridge University Library, Cambridge, UK.

Chinese Public Health Collection, National Library of Medicine, National Institutes of Health, Bethesda, Maryland, USA.

East Asian History of Science Library, Needham Research Institute, Cambridge, UK.

Health Ministry of the Nationalist Government Archives, the Second Historical Archives of China, Nanjing.

Health Station, PUMC Archives, Beijing Xiehe Medical University, Beijing, China.

International Health Board/Division Archives, Rockefeller Archive Center, North Tarrytown, New York.

James Earl Russell Papers, Teachers College Special Collections, Columbia University, New York, USA.

John B. Grant, Public Health Department, PUMC Archives, Beijing Xiehe Medical University, Beijing.

Letters and Correspondence of YMCA Field Secretaries, Kautz Family YMCA Archives, University of Minnesota, St. Paul, Minnesota.

Minguo wenxian [Literature on the Republic of China], Nanjing Library, Nanjing, China.

Liu Ruiheng Papers, PUMC Archives, Beijing Xiehe Medical University, Beijing.

Medical and Public Health of China, the National Archives, Kew, Surrey, UK.

Nanjing Municipal Government Archives, the Second Historical Archives of China, Nanjing.

Paul Monroe Papers, Teachers College Special Collections, Columbia University, New York.

Police Department Archives, the First Historical Archives of China, Beijing.

Public Health Archives, Nanjing Municipal Archives, Nanjing.

Public Health, Tianjin Municipal Archives, Tianjin, China.

Public Health Practice in Counties and Village Towns, Jiangsu Provincial Archives, Nanjing.

Public Health, Shanghai Municipal Council, Shanghai Municipal Archives, Shanghai.

Rockefeller Foundation Archives, the Rockefeller Archive Center, North Tarrytown, New York.

Shanghai Municipal Council Minutes, Shanghai Municipal Archives, Shanghai.

Shanghai Sanitation and Hygiene, Shanghai Municipal Archives, Shanghai.

Special Municipality of Beiping Archives, Beijing Municipal Archives, Beijing.

The Executive Yuan of the Republic of China Archives, the Second Historical Archives of China, Nanjing.

The Reminiscences of Dr. John B. Grant, Columbia University Oral History Project, Columbia University, New York, USA.

Reports, journals, yearbooks, and newspapers

Annual Report of the Central Epidemic Prevention Bureau, Beijing

Annual Report of the Health Organization of the League of Nations

Annual Report of the Rockefeller Foundation

Boston Evening Transcript

Chinese Medical Journal

Dagongbao

Dongfang zazhi [Eastern Miscellany]

Fanglao tongxun [Anti-Tuberculosis Newsletter]

Hankou ribao

Huadong weisheng [East China Health]

Kexue [Science]

Milbank Memorial Fund Quarterly Bulletin

Peking Gazette

Quarterly Bulletin of the Health Organization of the League of Nations

Renmin ribao

Report of the National Quarantine Service, Shanghai

Shengjing shibao

The China Medical Journal

The National Medical Journal of China

The New York Times

The World's Work

Xin Zhongguo funü [Women of New China]

Xin zhongyiyao [New Chinese Medicine]

Xinhua yuebao

Xin qingnian [La Jeunesse, The New Youth]

Zhongguo yaoxue zazhi [Chinese Journal of Pharmacy]

Zhonghua yishi zazhi [Chinese Journal of Medical History]

Zhonghua yixue zazhi (Chinese and English versions)

Collections of documents

Beijing shi zhongyao wenxian xuanbian (1952) [Selection of Important Documents of Beijing Municipality, 1952]. Zhongguo dang'an chubanshe, 2002.

Collection of Historical Documents of the Public Health Department of Shanghai Municipal Council, multi volumes, Shanghai Municipal Archives.

Dangdai Zhongguo de weisheng shiye [Health of Contemporary China]. Beijing: Zhongguo shehui kexue chubanshe, 1986.

Dangdai Zhongguo weisheng dashi ji (1949–1990) [Major Events of Health Work in Contemporary China, 1949–1990]. Renmin weisheng chubanshe, 1993.

Jianguo yilai Mao Zedong wengao [Manuscripts of Mao Zedong since the Founding of the People's Republic of China]. Zhongyang wenxian chubanshe, 2000.

Jianguo yilai zhongyao wenxian xuanbian [Selection of Important Documents since the Founding of the People's Republic of China]. Zhongyang wenxian chubanshe, 1993.

Mao Zedong shuxin xuanji [Selection of Mao Zedong's Correspondence and Letters]. Zhongyang wenxian chubanshe, 2003.

National Health Statistics. Beijing: Ministry of Health, 2002.

Selected Works of Mao Tse-tung. Peking: Foreign Language Press, 1967.

Weishengbu jicheng weisheng he fuyou baojian si [Bureau of Basic Health and Maternal and Children's Health of the Health Ministry], *Nongcun weisheng wenjian huibian (1951–2000)* [Collection of Documents on Rural Health Work, 1951–2000]. Zhonghua renmin gongheguo weishengbu, 2001.

Xin Zhongguo yufang yixue lishi ziliao xuanbian (1) [Selection of Historical Documents on Preventive Medicine of New China, vol. 1]. Beijing: Renmin junyi chubanshe, 1986.

Zhongguo nueji de fangzhi yu yanjiu bianweihui [Editorial Committee on Malaria Prevention and Research in China], *Zhongguo nueji de fangzhi yu yanjiu* [Malaria Prevention and Research in China]. Beijing: Remin weisheng chubanshe, 1991.

Zhongguo weisheng nianjian [Health Yearbook of the People's Republic of China]. Beijing: Renmin weisheng chubanshe, 1997.

Zhongguo weisheng tongji nianqian [Annual Medical and Health Statistics of China]. Beijing: Zhongguo xiehe yike daxue chubanshe, 2009.

Zhongyi gongzuo wenjian huibian (1949–1983) [Collection of Documents on Chinese Medicine Work, 1949–1983]. Zhonghua renmin gongheguo weishengbu, 1985.

Zhongyi gongzuo ziliao huibian [Collection of Documentary Materials on Chinese Medicine Work]. Zhonghua renmin gongheguo weishengbu, 1956.

Introduction

Modernization and public health

> The science of hygiene is originated in Europe. Westerners claim that the more civilized a country and the more important a nation, then the more sophisticated their laws of hygiene are; of the opposite is a weak country and an inferior people.[1]

Thus began the article "On Hygiene" in the popular Chinese magazine, *Dongfang zazhi* (东方杂志, *Eastern Miscellany*), in 1905. The author discussed the importance of hygiene and modern medicine in relation to China's future, and made the argument that hygiene, on a small scale, affected the health of individuals and families, but on a large scale, defined the fate of a country and its people. He put hygiene squarely in the equation of the advancement of a country and the quality of a people. In the article, the author lamented the decline of Chinese medical development and the sanitary neglect by the people and the officialdom, which, in his opinion, led to the status of a weak China. This point of argument was common among Chinese modernizers who regarded hygiene and modern medicine essential elements of a strong and modern China. After the 1895 Sino-Japanese War, China was portrayed as "the sick man of Asia," a humiliating metaphor previously used to describe the declined Ottoman empire.[2] Writings of Western missionaries and newspapermen also popularized that China was a filthy and disease-ridden backward country that needed Western "progressive" forces to transform it. Chinese modernizers including intellectuals, officials and urban merchants, out of admiration of the advancement and power of the West and concerns over China's plight in the struggle against foreign dominance, understood hygiene and public health in light of national strength. They urged the Chinese government to emulate the West to create a clean and healthy nation to join the modern world. Scholars have examined the subject of hygiene and public health from different perspectives. Ruth Rogaski analyzes that hygienic modernity had deeper implications of racial prejudice and social and cultural biases.[3] Hu Cheng points out that foreigners and Chinese had different narratives of the "unsanitary" China, which showed that perceptions of foreigners were closely tied to their attitude of Western cultural superiority whereas Chinese views were intertwined with China's struggle to modernize and maintain national sovereignty.[4]

The idea of a clean and healthy nation gained significant social and cultural meanings in the late nineteenth and early twentieth centuries when the West was energized by the social reforms of hygiene and sanitary movement. Cleanliness defined the advancement of a civilized nation and the virtues of modern citizens in terms of good morals, physical health, and cultured manners. The opposite indicated the backwardness of a weak uncivilized country and the lack of moral virtues of individuals. In dissecting the power of the concept of civilization in modern history, Brett Bowden exposes it as a stage-managed account of history that legitimizes imperialism, uniformity, and conformity to Western standards.[5] He argues that the idea of civilization has been deployed to dichotomize peoples, cultures, and histories to justify all manner of interventions, aggressive colonization, and sociopolitical engineering in the history of the West. Nonetheless, cleanliness became a hallmark of modern citizens and "civilized" societies, while uncleanliness and high death rates characterized "uncivilized" societies. China, India, and Egypt—countries of distinct ancient civilizations—were defined as uncivilized in contrast to the "civilized world" of the West. Newspapers and popular magazines helped spread the image of these countries as unclean and uncivilized societies in the public mind to construct the divide of the advanced West and the backward non-West. Chinese elite and modernizers, who bought into but were anxious to change the dichotomy, used the power of media to disseminate information of hygiene and public health and compel Chinese people to take action and clean up the image of an unsanitary China.[6] The discourse of cleanliness was integral to the repertoire of modernity and national rejuvenation throughout twentieth-century China. It projected the prospect of a nation and people emerging from the old society of dark and sickly ignorance into the bright and healthy enlightenment of human advancement.

Chinese hygiene and public health movement started differently from the Western movement in terms of circumstances, motivations and purposes. Europe and America began the sanitary and public health movement as social reforms to address the problems of filth, poverty and epidemic diseases brought on by industrialization, with the purpose of achieving economic efficiency and productivity and humanitarian improvement of the working poor. Voluntary associations of concerned citizens played important pioneering roles in getting the local and national governments involved to take on the responsibility of sanitation administration and public health in Western nations.[7] Chinese promotion of sanitation and public health was initiated by intellectuals and modern medical professionals who sought to modernize China to transform old institutions and to change people's social and political thinking and behavior. They were not motivated by the concerns of economic loss of diseased people to national power as the West did, but by the concerns of China's decline and inability to keep its sovereignty in encountering the aggressive foreign powers. Public health advocates promoted modern medicine and public health as a spearhead to change China from a weak traditional society into a strong modern nation.

The history of Chinese public health modernization was intertwined with the major events of China's political, cultural and social developments. The public health movement promoted science as the central force of modernization to transform China. Emphasis on science helped shape the rhetoric of the Chinese public health movement and facilitated the dissemination of scientific knowledge of disease and modern medicine. Moreover, public health and scientific knowledge were promoted in relation to the political, social and cultural needs of reforms and revolutions that had been led by various groups who held different ideological convictions. In the endeavor to make China modern and strong over the long decades of the twentieth century, different political beliefs and competing visions of a modern China only enriched the various modes or paradigms of modernity to be applied to the reconstruction of China from the late Qing to the current era of reforms. The paradigm of modernity during the Republican era (民国时期) was informed by anti-imperialist nationalism and Social Darwinian concepts of competition and adaptation. Modernization meant imitation of Western institutions and emphasis on science as the core value of culture. The socialist paradigm of the People's Republic of China (PRC) was guided by a clear theoretical framework with the Soviet experience initially used as the model of state-building and national development before a Chinese model of socialist modernization was created in the Mao era. The post-Mao economic reforms emphasized the four modernizations as the paradigm of modernity by shifting to a system of market economy to achieve national prosperity and power.

The late Qing government adopted the "New Policy" (新政) of reforms to modernize the polity in 1901 under both domestic and foreign pressures. Institutional modernization included the establishment of the first public health agency of China, the Beiyang Sanitary Service, in 1902. Social Darwinian thought dominated the intellectual persuasion of the urgent needs to reform the system and to change the culture. The tensions within the society and Qing's inability to effectively carry out reforms led to its fall in the 1911 revolution, which ended the two-thousand-year-old dynastic system and created a republic political system. The revolutionary acceleration of institutional change of modernization saw the introduction of more public health measures and the support of popular health education, the most significant of which was the legislation on notifiable diseases by the government and the health education campaign by social and professional organizations. The Beiyang government (北洋政府) of the early Republic projected its progressive image by promoting sanitation and public health in a changing society, but the commitment to building a modern health system did not come until the establishment of the Nationalist government in Nanjing in 1927. The Nationalist government created a Ministry of Health in 1928 in accordance with the organizational standards of modern nations and propagated Sun Yat-sen's three people's principles as the paradigm of modernization.[8] A close examination of government propaganda materials reveal, however, that a strong anti-imperialist nationalistic argument informed by both Social Darwinian concepts and modern science was popularized in the health education and national development campaigns. Moreover, modern medical professional elite, rather than the political leaders, worked as the true driving force of the institutionalization of a health administrative system in the Nationalist era, opting to follow the state medicine model to solve China's huge health challenges. When the PRC was established in 1949, a socialist paradigm of modernization was applied to reconstructing China and building a people's healthcare system with the provision of free healthcare to the vast urban and rural population. The system, however, was fundamentally changed with economic reforms since the 1980s. The introduction of market forces to the economy helped create enormous wealth for the nation, but the market reform of the health system resulted in unaffordability and inaccessibility of healthcare, seriously eroding the vision of a fair and just society that the government set out to build. The current government is committed to deepening the health system reform and continues to search for a health system that will be affordable and accessible with provision of primary healthcare to everyone.

This book on public health provides a focal point to examine the long process of modernization of China from the late Qing to the current era of reforms in a global context. It investigates not only domestic political, social and cultural transformations but also China's relations with the larger world. Buzan and Lawson recently made the argument that industrialization, modern state-building, ideologies of nationalism, socialism and racism, and the destabilization of balance of power fundamentally contributed to the global transformation in the nineteenth and twentieth centuries.[9] Such an argument can be readily applied to the transformation of China as a case study, as these elements influenced China's modernizations and its interactions with other countries and international organizations. The hygiene and public health modernization, which was part and parcel of modern state-building and national development, was a politicized endeavor that intertwined with Chinese reforms and revolutions in a broad sense. It encompasses the change of people's mentality and behavior and the reconstruction of institutions and political systems of a modern state. From Social Darwinian views and the discourse of "the sick man of Asia" through the revolutions to the rise of China again, national health has been the image and the substance of the modern transformation of China.

My examination of public health modernization concentrates on disease-prevention, healthcare, reforms and revolutions, and modern reconstruction of China. It does not deal with anti-opium and anti-smoking movements, which are important subjects of public health that merit separate treatments.[10] In this book, I use the plural form of "Western and Chinese medicines" to mean not only different drugs but also different systems of medicine. The term "Western medicine" (*xiyi*, 西医) has been used interchangeably with "modern medicine," "new medicine," and "scientific medicine" in modern China, and this particular feature is reflected in the writing of this book. Similarly, the Chinese term "*weishing*, 卫生" is used broadly to convey the meanings of hygiene, sanitation, and health. The word "health" has been used in Chinese documents as "*jiankang*, 健康," "*weishging*, 卫生," and "*baojian*, 保健" at different historical times and different contexts, as school health has been translated as "*xuexiao jiankang*, 学校健康," and "*xuexiao weishing*, 学校卫生," and people's health has been translated as "*renmin jiankang*, 人民健康," "*renmin weisheng*, 人民卫生," and "*renmin baojian*, 保健." The term "public health" is usually translated as "*gonggong weisheng*, 公共卫生" or "*weisheng*, 卫生." A few themes have emerged to illuminate the interplays of different parallels of events in this extensive study of public health and the modernization of China.

International and transnational influence

Westerners considered Chinese cities salubrious and Chinese people healthy in comparison with those in Europe and America in the mid-nineteenth century when China had fewer of the epidemics that plagued Western industrial cities. The picture changed after industrial factories were increasingly built in treaty port cities after 1860s. Western nations had opened up Chinese ports for trades and factories with wars and unequal treaties since China lost the war over British opium traffic in1842.[11] Urban squalor, slums, poverty and disease had grown along with modern industries, as factories expanded into farming lands and shanty towns emerged near the factories. Western missionaries were known as the first critics of Chinese unsanitary conditions but they were less known for being amazed at the hygienic habits of Chinese people who had the tradition of using boiled water and having public bathhouses. Missionaries carried to China the modern ideas of sanitation and disease prevention that were developing in their home countries in the nineteenth century. They promoted and practiced modern medicine to open up China for evangelization, and initiated hygiene education and disease prevention in places where they exercised broad influence. In propagating Christianity and Western culture, they promoted Western medicine as the scientific medicine and criticized Chinese medicine as unscientific superstition to negate the value and relevance of traditional culture in modernity. Since knowledge of hygiene and disease prevention was part of modern medicine, the dissemination of health knowledge further helped legitimize Western medicine as the true knowledge to challenge Chinese medical knowledge. The popular health education campaigns in the 1910s brought modern hygiene and disease prevention to a wide range of Chinese social classes and places as they were held in major cities across China. The campaigns were organized and conducted in collaboration with local governments by medical missionaries, the YMCAs, and Western-trained Chinese doctors of modern medicine. These three groups formed the Joint Council on Public Health Education in 1916 (renamed Council on Health Education in 1920) to lead the week-long health education campaigns in different provinces to promote Western medicine and public health. Missionaries' interest in health education was initially driven by their zeal to evangelize China but their enthusiasm tapered off when the campaigns took on a new life as a health education movement. Chinese local governments sponsored the campaigns with financial and human resources while the Council provided the technical expertise and educational materials. In each city where the campaign took place, students, teachers, officials, missionaries and YMCA secretaries were mobilized to help organize and lead the health lectures and the explanation of health exhibits, which attracted people of all walks of life. Tens of thousands of urban residents, men and women, attended the health education campaigns as major events in their cities. Visual materials and illustrations, such as pictures, posters, charts and diagrams, helped disseminate information about the cause of disease, flies as the agents to spread disease, and the importance of hygiene and health in relation to individual well-being and national strength. The health education campaigns helped raise public awareness, particularly those in cities, about the individual's ability to prevent disease and keep healthy. Moreover, the campaigns sometimes conducted smallpox vaccination and contributed to the development of a modern public health discourse in Chinese society before the training of public health professionals was established at medical schools. The key leader of the campaigns, William Wesley Peter (known as W. W. Peter), who was a YMCA secretary with unique talents of health showmanship, urged Chinese participants to think of education, laws, and statistics as the main building blocks to the foundation of public health in China. The Council bequeathed a large collection of visual health education materials and a rich legacy of methods to popularize health knowledge. For his significant beneficiary contribution to China, Peter was recognized by the Chinese government with a 5th class medal of the Order of Golden Grain (*wudeng jiahe zhang*, 五等嘉禾章).[12] John D. Rockefeller, Jr. received the same type of medal for his contribution to China by building the Peking Union Medical College (PUMC).[13]

The Rockefeller philanthropy came to China immediately after the 1911 revolution, with investigations of the health and medical conditions of China. When the Rockefeller Foundation (RF) was formed in 1914, it envisioned modernizing China with medical science by establishing a world-class medical college, Peking Union Medical College, to spearhead the modern medical enterprise in China. For that purpose, the RF created a China Medical Board (CMB) to take charge of PUMC and related matters. PUMC was built upon the medical school that Anglo-American missionaries had created and run for over a decade. Rarely did a transfer of the ownership of a medical school from the missionary to the philanthropist impact the future of an entire nation's medical and health profession in such a degree as the PUMC, for the college produced a small but influential group of elite medical professionals who eventually dominated Chinese medical education and health administration. The thrust of the Rockefeller medical enterprise signified the beginning of an end of the missionary-dominated modern medical education and the rise of secular education of medical science in China. It ultimately helped shape the creation of China's national health system, with John B. Grant and the PUMC circle playing the key role in the Nationalist government. The CMB and PUMC epitomized RF's influence in China, just as Standard Oil and YMCA embodied the American influence in China, in the first half of the twentieth century.[14]

The RF introduced modern medical science and public health knowledge to the training of Chinese medical students while using China as a medical laboratory to study diseases and health problems. With medical reform taking place at home in the United States, the RF found the power of medical science an ideal tool to advance mankind in a global scheme of transforming traditional "backward" societies via sanitation and disease control. Medical colleges and institutions and health programs were established in different countries across the globe, under the direction and supervision of the International Health Board (IHB, which became the International Health Division in 1927, IHD).[15] In order to publicize modern medicine and recruit students to study it, CMB enlisted the help of W. W. Peter and the Council on Health Education to a campaign to promote modern medicine among students to encourage them to take modern medicine as life work. In the meantime, medical scientists of the RF, who had low regard for the standard of medical education at missionary schools, tried to set up as rigorous a standard as the best American medical college would expect for the faculty and students at PUMC. They even made English the language of instruction, all in the name of upholding scientific standards. The PUMC produced a total of 321 medical doctors from 1921 to 1943 (World War II disrupted its operation), and graduated 279 nurses from 1924 to 1950.[16] Many of this small elite group became key leaders of the Nationalist health administration system and at medical institutions of research and education. With the production of such a small number of medical professionals, the RF's China medical enterprise barely made a difference in bringing the benefits of modern medical science to ordinary Chinese people. The RF's major influence in China lay in its contribution to medical education and the leadership of a modern health administration system, thanks particularly to the pivotal role played by John B. Grant.

Grant worked in China for 17 years from 1921 to 1938 as head of the Hygiene and Public Health Department at PUMC and the China representative of the IHB/IHD of the RF. His profound interest in and commitment to public health, facilitated by his extensive network and close relations with Chinese medical and political leaders, led to his exceptionally fruitful career in training public health leaders and shaping the development of a national health system in China during the tumultuous years of political instability and uncertainty. It is not an exaggeration that Grant, to a great extent, provided the continuity of guidance in public health professionalization and modernization from the Beiyang decade to the Nanjing era. He served, by invitation, as the advisor to the Chinese government in all matters pertaining to health, while he worked at PUMC. Grant's major contributions were not just his creation of public health programs and his influence in the development of a national health administrative system of the Nationalist government. More importantly, his teaching and promotion of the ideas of state medicine, social medicine and preventive medicine left indelible imprints in the Chinese health profession. His ideas and methods of public health education have exerted a long-term influence in China under different political systems.

Grant also played an important role in advising and facilitating the involvement of the League of Nations Health Organization (LNHO) in the modernization of China's health system and national development. From the initial negotiations to establish a National Quarantine Service in the 1920s to the building of a national health administrative system in the 1930s, the LNHO provided China not only assistance of professional expertise and the training of personnel but also the support of financial resources. The League of Nations' involvement even expanded beyond the health field to various aspects of economic planning and construction of China before it was disrupted by the outbreak of World War II.[17] Throughout, Grant and the RF worked with the League's representatives to influence China's national health programs and to provide parallel assistance of training and financial support, even though the LNHO leaders tried to distance themselves from the RF to retain more independent approaches to China's health modernization. The League's involvement positively influenced, to a certain extent, China's successful negotiations with foreign powers over its maritime sovereignty and the institutional building of a state medicine system.

While the Nationalist government was assisted mostly by the RF and the LNHO in its health modernization, the CCP government received international aid from different supporters in its health development. During the Yanan era, international health teams and individuals came from different countries to help the CCP in the anti-fascist movement of World War II. They brought not only advanced medical equipment but more importantly the badly needed medical expertise, which significantly helped improve the battle field medical service and the training of CCP medical personnel. With the victory of CCP over the Nationalists in the civil war (1946–1949) and the establishment of the PRC in 1949, the Soviet Union became a key influence in China's health reconstruction as well as national development in a broad sense. The Cold War had shaped the world into a bi-polar international order and China's participation in the Korean War made the United States an impossible model of development. The Soviet emphasis on preventive medicine, which had attracted the attention of Chinese health professionals in the 1930s–1940s, was now promoted by Chinese political and health leaders across the country. Although the emphasis on prevention had long been the health policy of the CCP, prevention of disease was incorporated into national defense in the new Patriotic Health Movement in the early 1950s as measures to defeat the alleged American germ-warfare during the Korean War. The Chinese health movement was a politically mobilized patriotic mass movement for disease prevention, national defense, economic productivity, and socialist reconstruction.

Economic reforms of the past three decades fully integrated China into the world, where major international organizations, such as the World Health Organization (WHO), World Back, International Monetary Fund (IMF) and United Nations organizations, worked with the Chinese government in the restructuring of the economy, health, and other aspects of social development. In regard to the health sector reforms, American influence was significant in shaping a new health insurance system to replace the socialist people's healthcare. But the American model has not been working well in China, and the government introduced a new plan of health system reform in 2009 with the intention to build a health system with provision of primary healthcare to everyone. The search is still going on for a healthcare system suitable for the socioeconomic conditions of the Chinese market economy, as the government deepens the reform of the health system.

Chinese modernizers, modern medicine, and public health

Edmund S. K. Fung argues that the interactions of three major trends of intellectual orientations, namely liberalism, conservatism, and socialism, underpinned the cultural and political modernity of China.[18] Marketization of the economy is apparently economic liberalism that underlies the current construction of Chinese modernity. Of all the different political and intellectual persuasions of twentieth-century China, there was a shared common goal of building a strong modern state with national unity. The semi-colonial status of China at the end of the nineteenth century resulted from constant foreign encroachment and the continuous decline of the Qing empire. The contrast of clean streets and bright tall buildings in the foreign settlements to the filthy and muddy streets and shanty towns in the Chinese sections in many treaty ports stimulated Chinese modernizers to seek fundamental reforms by learning from the West. The late Qing reformists, such as Yan Fu and Liang Qichao, noticed that Western nations all emphasized physical education of the people and promoted public health. They advocated physical fitness of the masses as one of the fundamental means to regain China's national strength. To the reformists, the hope of national revival lay in the training of Chinese people into new citizens of strong moral virtues, intelligence and physical fitness capable of defending their country and competing with other nations. Their thinking was profoundly influenced by Social Darwinian interpretation of a world of competing nations where the strong and superior (优) would survive and the weak and inferior (劣) would be weeded out. The meaning of "competition" and "evolution" was understood on both personal and national levels when foreign powers were carving up China into their spheres of influence. The individual to the national body was cast in the relation of the cell to a social organism in an evolutionary process of "survival of the fittest."[19]

Medicine was supposed to save people's lives and better the society, and medical modernization was thought an essential step towards reviving China. Sun Yat-sen and Lu Xun, for instance, both started their career by studying modern medicine, though each in their own ways realized that a fundamental change of China needed something more revolutionary than what modern medicine could offer. The issue of medicine and public health was played out in the larger context of political and social revolutions of China. Hence, modern public health was intertwined with Chinese nationalist struggle against foreign imperialist dominance and the transformation of the traditional Chinese society into a modern nation. Western medicine offered the science of prevention, and germ theory provided the powerful explanation that pinpointed the cause of disease; whereas Chinese medicine lacked the quality of modern medicine to zero in on one single cause of disease, but used instead a holistic approach of diagnosis. Because of this fundamental difference, modern medical professionals and modernizers attacked Chinese medicine as lacking scientific foundation and therefore labeling it useless superstition. The tensions between Chinese medicine and Western medicine were not merely medical competition but political and cultural contentions as well. This book shows that Chinese medicine faced the crisis of being eliminated by the modern authorities three times in 1914, 1929, and the early 1950s respectively, all in the name of modernization and science. The modern transformation of Chinese medicine illustrates the history of Chinese modernization and vice versa. In their recent books on the modernization of Chinese medicine, Sean Hsiang-Lin Lei investigates the tension and divide of Chinese and Western medicines and shows how practitioners of Chinese medicine turned the challenges into a modernizing force to transform themselves into an organized modern profession, whereas Bridie Andrews concentrates on the adaptation and accommodation of both Western and Chinese medicines.[20] Their scholarship further illuminates that medical developments were tied directly to the particular cultural settings and transformative modernization of China.

Modernizers of early twentieth-century China, including professionals of modern medicine, intellectuals, journalists, urban merchants and government officials, promoted Western medicine and public health with the political rhetoric of national strength and social progress. Vital statistics on national death rates provided them with the convincing data that public health was a critical element of modernity and nation strength, as advanced nations like the United States and Britain had low death rates, whereas weak nations like India and China had high death rates. The Western argument of economic gain in good health had little appealing power to the Chinese when their country was being dismembered by foreign powers. The first and utmost concern of the Chinese was the fate of their country in the face of foreign powers' scramble, and their attention to medicine and public health was stimulated by the larger political issues of national sovereignty. Of the first resolutions of the National Medical Association of China (NMAC, 中华医学会) upon its creation in 1915, was the request for the Chinese government to set up a modern Public Health Service to take care of national health, as did all advanced nations. The NMAC defined its mission as serving the nationalist effort to modernize and strengthen China by advocating modern medical science and arousing public interest in public health and preventive medicine. The Chinese medical association has been champion of public health throughout the twentieth century, which differed from their counterpart in America.[21] It played an active role in the early public health education campaigns and emphasized national health and national strength as the theme of health education.[22] Dissemination of public health information also served to promote science and Western medicine in Chinese society where people relied on Chinese medicine and had little knowledge of Western medicine. The medical field became a contesting ground of different political forces that pitted progress and modernity against backwardness and tradition. Progress and national strength were constant themes in the promotion of Western medicine as the scientific true knowledge in contrast to the attacks on Chinese medicine as unscientific superstition and backward tradition. In the early twentieth century, science attracted Chinese intelligentsia with significant meanings of cultural modernity in their search for a new national identity and order. When Western ideas and scientism increasingly shaped Chinese intellectual and political thinking, support of modern medicine and public health meant politically progressive and intellectually modern.

Chinese intellectuals launched frontal attacks on traditional culture while embracing science as the new culture during the New Culture and the May Fourth Movements. Science gained the cultural authority to define the truth not only in the medical field but also in every aspect of social, political and economic life. In the iconoclastic revolutionary transition from the traditional cultural mold to the new age of science, concepts of science and modernity became the driving force to orient Chinese intellectual pursuit and political revolution.[23] Intellectual modernizers considered the contention between Chinese and Western medicines not a question of medical profession but a political fight between the old and the new, the backward and the progressive, and the traditional and the modern. Chinese medicine was considered the symbol of old culture while Western medicine the practice of science and measure of modernity. The attacks on Chinese medicine and tradition influenced the young students in their critical view of Chinese medicine as things of the past. Attempts to promote Chinese medicine were identified with warlords' political militarism to return China to the past and to obstruct the revolutionary endeavor of the Nationalist Party (GMD, Guomindang). The new "cultural authority" of science was reshaping China's intellectual thinking, social values and political ideologies.[24] Science even became an "ideological identity' of the revolutionaries against the conservatives, permeating the medical front as well as the political and social and cultural domains.[25]

Both the Nationalist Party and the Chinese Communist Party (CCP, Gongchandang) embraced science as the foundation of their ideologies and promoted science in their revolutionary visions for a new society. Modern medicine and hygiene and public health were important parts of the revolutionary goals of the two political parties, but their divergent political beliefs guided their respective revolutions and state-building through different routes of national mobilization and reconstruction. The Nationalists established a government in Nanjing and continued the promotion of national health for a strong China by undertaking systematic modernization of medicine and health institutions. Significant accomplishments were the creation of a national health administrative system with the policy of state medicine and the establishment of medical training and research facilities. The Ministry of Health of the Nationalist government attempted the extreme action of abolishing Chinese medicine once for all, which intensified the confrontation between Chinese medicine and Western medicine but stimulated practitioners of Chinese medicine to unite and fight with new energy and modern political tactics. Jiang Jieshi, leader of the Nationalist Party and government, did not take serious interest in health modernization but emphasized personal hygiene and civilized behavior in the New Life Movement to shape the modernization of Chinese society. The Nationalist government focused on institutional building as the center of health modernization, and neglected to undertake land reforms to address the major socio-economic problems of poverty and subsistence living that were fundamental to public health.

The CCP launched health movements in their revolutionary bases in rural China, and emphasized disease prevention as an important aspect to preserve revolutionary force and better people's lives. The CCP health programs were guided by their socialist political ideology and vision of an equal society. To improve people's health conditions was one significant goal of the overall social reforms, as the revolution aimed to transform not only the socio-economic institutions but also the thinking and attitude of people from the old feudal and superstitious mode to the modern and scientific outlook of socialism. Hygiene and public health were advocated as important components of the revolutionary cause and were integrated in the activities of socioeconomic development in the CCP regions. Mao Zedong, leader of the CCP revolution, took a great interest in medicine and public health and wrote frequently to promote the importance of public health and the development of a new CCP-led society. In contrast to the Nationalists, the CCP made use and encouraged the integration of Chinese medicine and Western medicine in its revolutionary transformation of China. Prevention of disease and the unity of Chinese and Western medicines were key elements of the national health principles of the People's Republic of China in the creation of a people's healthcare system. The integration of Western and Chinese medicines was not without opposition from the health leaders in the early 1950s but the intervention of political leaders in the modernization of Chinese medicine with scientific knowledge led to the unique accomplishments of creating a new medicine called the integrative medicine (中西医结合), which co-exists with Western medicine (*xiyi*, 西医) and Chinese medicine (*zhongyi*, 中医) to benefit Chinese people today. The PRC made the extraordinary achievement of providing free healthcare to the large Chinese population with low costs in the 1950s–1970s. Dozens of major epidemic diseases, such as smallpox, plague, cholera, typhus, typhoid, polio, kala-azar, filariasis, schistosomiasis, tuberculosis and malaria, were either eradicated or brought under basic control. With accessible healthcare and improved living standards, people's health significantly improved with life expectancy increased from 38 in 1949 to 65 in 1975. China was considered a model for the developing world with the creation of a low-cost healthcare system.

The post-Mao economic reforms fundamentally shifted the foundation of economic structure through privatization and marketization. As a result, the people's healthcare that had been built upon the socialist collective economic system collapsed and the country experienced a healthcare crisis, with some old epidemic diseases re-emerging as health threats and high medical costs sending families into poverty. After the use of market forces to reform the health sector failed, the government introduced a comprehensive health system reform plan in 2009 and is continuing to deepen the health system reform. It's a challenging but imperative task for current Chinese modernizers to make the health system reform successful when they deliver the promise of a good life in a fair and just society under a new modernization paradigm.

Government policies and health institutions

Public health has been a vital component of the institutional building of a modern state and a transformative force to change people's attitude, values, and behavior.

The demand for the Chinese government to establish a modern sanitary administration initially came from foreign powers during the negotiations of returning of cities to China in the wake of suppression of the Boxer Uprising. The Beiyang Sanitary Service (北洋防疫处) was established in 1902 under the pressure of foreign powers and China's struggle to modernize and remain sovereign. This initiation of creating a government public health institution differentiated China from the West in the endeavor of public health administration, and underscored the issues of national sovereignty and struggle against foreign dominance in China's public health modernization. Within China, foreign powers enjoyed the authority of controlling public health at treaty ports in addition to many other privileges under the unequal treaty system.[26] Public health issues were often dealt with by the Ministry of Foreign Affairs rather than the Ministry of Interior of the late Qing government. As public health administration became a gauge to measure progress and modernization efforts at the turn of the twentieth century, both central and local governments set up public health institutions to project their progressive and modern image. Sometimes, local government went a step ahead of the central government in sponsoring and enforcing public health programs, especially in cities where Western influence was strong. The late Qing's decision to establish the Beiyang Sanitary Service came as part of the modernization programs of "New Policy." Yuan Shi-kai played a leading role in the modernization programs, despite his controversial place in modern Chinese history. He experimented with creating a variety of modern institutions, such as those of sanitation, police, education and the military, before the Qing court took steps in this direction. When he was Viceroy of Zhili, Yuan even set up the first women's medical department in Tianjin to take charge of a government-run women's medical school with a hospital. When a plague epidemic broke out in northeast China in 1910, the fight to control the plague was complicated by international intrigues of the powers to undermine Chinese sovereignty. When the Chinese medical scientist Wu Liande became the leader of the new North Manchurian Plague Prevention Service in 1911, China asserted its ability in modern administration of epidemic control and its sovereignty on the international stage.

The demise of the Qing dynasty signified not only the political transition from the dynastic imperial system to a modern polity of republic but also the creation of a new knowledge system of medicine and public health based on science. As president of the new Republic, Yuan Shikai favored modern medicine at the expense of Chinese medicine to publicize his government's political progressiveness and himself a committed modernizer of China. Presidential orders and government regulations were issued regarding the standards of food hygiene, sanitation, public safety, and the practice of midwifery. Yuan's support for modern medicine even led to the first attempt to abolish Chinese medicine in 1914. When the government promulgated "Regulations on the Prevention of Infectious Diseases" and the "Regulations on Medical and Pharmaceutical Examinations" in 1916, it took on the modern responsibility of fighting epidemics and standardizing medical practice. Given the chaotic and weak government of the early Republic, these regulations were not effectively enforced, but they set up the legal obligations of the government to public health.

The call for the state to take responsibility of national health grew when medical scientists and intellectuals actively voiced their opinions to shape government policies from their professional positions in modern public health institutions, such as the North Manchurian Plague Prevention Service, and the Central Epidemic Prevention Bureau. In the decades of the 1920s–1940s, scientific and medical professionals played a crucial role in the building of health institutions of a modern state. As science held unique significance for Chinese modernization, the promotion of Western medicine as the scientific medicine made it *the* choice for Chinese medical modernization, while Chinese medicine was excluded from the construction of a modern health system under the Nationalist government. The Nationalist elite with Western medical training formed the key force of health modernizers who worked with the League of Nations Health Organization (LNHO) and the Rockefeller Foundation in building an institutional structure of a centralized health administration based on modern medicine. In an attempt to make a clean slate for health modernization, the Nationalist medical elite decided to abolish Chinese medicine in 1929, only to be challenged by the unity of the Chinese medical world. The "old-style" Chinese medicine men were quite modern in their fight for Chinese medicine as they organized popular protests and political lobbying and gave the medicine a new name, "national medicine 国医." In the end, the Nationalist medical elite managed to exclude Chinese medicine from playing a role in the construction of a modern health system, despite their failure to abolish it. Working with the LNHO, the Nationalist health leaders decided on state medicine as the model for China, but they diverged in interpreting the meaning of state medicine when designing its delivery. While those who were doing the fieldwork of public health advocated health service to all people, the health bureaucrats concentrated on the institution building of a central health administration. The primary emphasis on institutional building could be attributed to factors such as bureaucratic convenience, limited manpower to provide medical and health service, and the lack of political commitment to a national health service. The Nationalist health modernizers, nevertheless, created an impressive modern national health administration system with research and training. Using health stations as pilot programs to conduct studies of sanitation and health, they gathered data of vital statistics and health, which lent the modern state the authority to exercise regulations of the health behavior of the public in the name of modernity and progress.[27] The Nationalist health system had segments of central and local health institutions, where the central institutions were systematically developed with international assistance, and the local institutions developed under the supervision of provincial governments without uniformity of standards. The Nationalist health modernizers were least successful in rural health construction, even though they had laid out detailed plans of a *xian* (county) centered rural health system. According to their plan, each *xiancheng* (county town) would have a center hospital to perform the simple health work of epidemic prevention, basic medical service, midwifery, health education and anti-opium smoking. The health work of a county center hospital would extend into villages with each rural district having a health station, and each village town a sub-station, and each village a health worker. These beautiful ideas of a three-tiered rural health structure, however, remained largely on paper under the Nationalist rule but were put into practice by the CCP government.

The Chinese Communist movement was located in rural areas in the 1920s–1940s, where the CCP health workers had limited medical resources but created a variety of health programs and services to meet the needs of the CCP military and local population. The CCP health policy emphasized prevention and the use of both Western and Chinese medicines. Health programs were integrated into the social reforms movements in their revolutionary bases where activities of literacy, land reform, women's liberation, and dissemination of revolutionary ideas were incorporated in the mobilization of peasants to participate in sanitation and health movements to prevent diseases. The CCP leaders valued Chinese medicine and encouraged the mutual learning of Western and Chinese medicines. In Yanan, medical doctors established the Society of National Medicine Studies (国医研究会) and the Association of Chinese and Western Medical Research (中西医药研究会). Health institutions were built, which included hospitals, medical schools, Chinese health and medical clinics, and people's health cooperatives for treatment and prevention. The CCP even tried to build a rural health system, quite similar to the Nationalist plan but on a modest scale, with a health station at each county (*xian*, 县), a health worker at a rural district, and a health committee in a village, making a three-tiered rural health network.

After the People's Republic of China was established in 1949, the central government formulated a national health policy with four key principles based on the CCP revolutionary vision and practice during the war time: (1) serving the needs of workers, peasants and soldiers, (2) prevention as the first priority, (3) uniting Chinese and Western medicines, and (4) combining health work with mass movement. In delivering the revolutionary health policy and commitment to people's healthcare, the government built diverse national systems of hospitals, clinics, health stations, maternal and child health stations, and health and epidemic prevention stations. Rapid expansion of medical education based on the Soviet model produced large numbers of medical and health professionals to meet the urgent needs of a large population. The three-tiered rural health system was made to work with the training of millions of part-time health workers called "barefoot doctors" to serve their fellow villagers with Western and Chinese medicines. Free healthcare at low costs was provided through two types of economic relations: employees of government and state enterprises (全民所有制人员) enjoyed healthcare at public expenses, while employees of collective enterprises (集体所有制人员) including small businesses and rural communes enjoyed healthcare at collective expenses.

Economic reforms since 1978 introduced private practice of medicine into the society. Private hospitals were established in cities and county towns to compete with public hospitals. Rural health workers including barefoot doctors were transformed into village doctors who conducted private medical practice at their own clinics with fees charged for service. The creation of private medical practice and institutions is supposed to encourage better quality and accessibility through market forces of competition, but the reality was far from the theoretical proposition, where high medical costs and low quality of service remain the two major complaints about the current health system. Enforcement of standardization and quality of operation badly need to be improved.

Health education and propaganda

Previous discussion has made clear that health modernization was integral to the political and social reforms and revolutions over the century-long struggle of China. Early propagation of health and cleanliness was promoted by local elites in treaty ports. The Chinese elite expounded cleanliness to excoriate their fellow countrymen to take action to improve themselves in the face of foreign criticism of unsanitary China. Chinese reformist and revolutionary intellectuals, influenced by the ideas of Social Darwinism and modern hygiene, wrote extensively to promote physical health and hygiene for the sake of reviving the nation. A major health education campaign was carried out in the 1910s when local government worked with the Council on Health Education to disseminate modern health knowledge and disease prevention. A large collection of health education material was created for the campaigns, which included health literature and visual material, such as bulletins, leaflets, posters, lecture charts, books, lantern slides, films, and exhibit items of the "health shows." Although there was little explicit explanation of the science of germ theory in the campaign, the idea of disease transmission via agents like flies was popularly demonstrated and displayed. Health programs, such as anti-tuberculosis and anti-cholera campaigns, better baby weeks, vision conservation, smallpox vaccination and health examination in schools, were carried out in urban cities.[28] National health essay contests were also organized among students to discuss national health and national strength. The methods and material of early popular health education of the Council on Health Education laid the ground work for health education and propaganda of the Nationalists and the Communists in the following decades.

The dissemination of public health and modern medicine promoted the direct link between personal health, public good, and national strength. It attracted various social groups and helped raise people's consciousness of sanitation, disease prevention, and the importance of public health in the overall modernization effort of building a strong nation. Newspapers and popular magazines frequently reported and commented on medicine and public health, broadly influencing public information of disease prevention, particularly during the outbreaks of epidemics. *Dagongbao* (*Ta Kung Pao*, 大公报) and *Shenbao* (申报), two major newspapers in China, published medical weeklys (医学周刊) to disseminate medical knowledge and hygiene, contributing to public interaction with the latest health and medical development. The government began popular education about disease transmission after the 1910 outbreak of a pneumonic plague epidemic in northeast China. A large quantity of anti-plague placards and pamphlets and public health notices was printed and distributed to instruct people on the methods of preventing plague from entering their communities and villages. The written educational material, however, accomplished little, due to the high illiteracy of people. In the meantime, media reports of the deadly plague epidemic caused widespread fear but stimulated calls for sanitation and prevention across the country. Monetary rewards were offered for catching mice, which were thought the culprits, only to find that Siberian marmots had transmitted the plague, possibly to bring revenge on humans who had been killing them for their highly desired fur.

The plague fight motivated more intellectuals and medical scientists to advocate public health education and broader social reforms. They felt the urgent need to educate the public about the scientific knowledge of medicine and modern preventive methods and blamed the ignorance (愚昧) and superstition (迷信) of people for not following anti-plague measures of disinfection and isolation. Medical scientists delivered public lectures on personal hygiene and disease prevention and wrote about these subjects in newspapers and popular magazines. Their explanation of the precise causation of disease popularized germ theory and modern medicine and made disease prevention a modern behavior of social progress. Popular education on germ theory and the new terminology associated with science took a prominent place in the New Culture and the May Fourth Movements when vernacular (*baihua*, 白话) writing was promoted to convey new ideas to the masses. Cities saw the rise of popular education institutes and health organizations where public lectures and exhibits were held to demonstrate new ideas and concepts. Health circulars and notices emphasized the danger of *chuanran* (传染, transmission) of diseases via germs, which were explained as tiny bugs. Public health bulletins explained the necessity of isolation and quarantine when family members were found infected because of *chuanran*. Scientific terms, such as germ, virus, microbe, pest, microscope, and contagious disease were popularized in vernacular health circulars and notices. Through newspapers, public lectures, health bulletins and vernacular circulars, concepts of germs and disease transmission were repeatedly conveyed to the public for the purpose of disease prevention and health protection.

The Nationalist government carried out extensive health education and propaganda with the clear guidance of GMD party ideology and modernization programs.[29] Health propaganda evoked Sun Yat-sen's three people's principles as the political rhetoric.[30] The Health Bureau of Nanjing claimed, in its publication, *Hygiene of the Capital* (首都卫生), that the state had the moral responsibility to protect the health of people in four basic areas of needs—food, clothing, shelter, and transportation (衣食住行). The Propaganda Department of the GMD Central Executive Committee compiled and published a "Propaganda Guide for the Health Movement" [卫生运动宣传纲要] in 1929, which promoted health movement as the movement of national independence, the movement of national salvation, and the movement of liberation. The guide informed people that national competition for existence had entered the most urgent moment and there were six key elements of competition: physique, intelligence, bravery, vigilance, tenacity, and unity. It instructed that the health movement must be popularized among the masses and conducted scientifically.[31] The GMD health advocates expounded that the foundation of national health depended on people's understanding that health was intertwined with the weal and woe of the Chinese nation and race.

In line with Sun Yat-sen's vision of different stages of national construction, the GMD propagandists planned three stages of propaganda (宣传), training (训练), and awakening (唤醒) for the long-term effect of health education for the ordinary people. A wide variety of methods was used in propaganda work but mainly divided into written and oral categories. Written material included health leaflets and booklets, posters, slogans and charts of vital statistics, while oral activities featured indoor lectures by celebrities and health professionals, traveling outdoor lectures by government officials and professional groups, and the use of slangs and songs for women and children. Health exhibits of popular education included various kinds of health pictures, posters, slogans, images of microbes, charts of diseases and vital statistics, and model devices of pathology. Radio talks on health were created to reach broader audience and were given by medical professionals. Short courses on health rules were offered to people of different trades, particularly those of restaurants, teahouses, bathhouses, barber shops, theaters and hotels, whose work directly impacted public health. Teachers were trained to give lessons on hygiene and public health, and to facilitate school health services. In the work of awakening, government-sponsored cleanliness campaigns took the center-stage of health propaganda in cities, where government officials led the city-wide cleanliness campaigns with meetings, parades and slogans to remove refuse and dirt on the streets. Disinfections, anti-pest movements against mosquitos, flies, fleas and rats were also carried out in urban districts and schools. Smallpox vaccinations were provided during health campaigns. The Nationalist health campaigns happened primarily in major cities, although a few county towns held sporadic campaigns of cleanliness in response to government calls.

While the Nationalist health propaganda attracted and educated mostly urban middle classes, the Communists worked with peasants to integrate health programs into the overall social reforms and revolution in their controlled areas. The CCP health propaganda addressed poverty, sanitation, literacy, women's equality, nutrition and farming production with the advocacy of hygienic and sanitary practice as revolutionary activities to transform traditional institutions and old habits and norms. The CCP adopted "prevention first" policy and encouraged all possible means to educate and mobilize the soldiers and the masses to get rid of major epidemic diseases. The CCP soldiers carried out hygiene-week programs with locals to do general cleaning while disseminating health and revolutionary information. The CCP's "Guide of the Health Movement" in 1933 promulgated that filth and disease were part of the problems of people's sufferings that had to be solved. It called on local governments and mass organizations to lead the people to fight against filth, disease, and old ideas and habits of superstition. Methods of disease-reporting and isolation and disinfection were developed, and popular health contests were held among the masses. The CCP used familiar forms of folk entertainment, such as folk dances and songs, and short skits and shows, to convey messages against superstition, witch doctors, and unhygienic behavior. Health talks and exhibits on hygiene and disease prevention were held during festivals and temple fairs where more people were present. Mass mobilization and participation characterized the CCP hygiene campaigns and public health propaganda and education.

The CCP continued mass health movements across the country after the establishment of the PRC. Health propaganda emphasized health improvement as an integral experience of the overall socialist reconstruction to transform Chinese society. The Patriotic Health Movement mobilized people to take active roles to fight diseases while disseminating new government policies, social values and scientific information of health to change people's attitudes and behavior. Chinese medicine, after a brief marginalization in the early 1950s, was highly promoted with national pride as a valuable medical system, quite different from the Nationalist era. In urban cities, health campaigns carried out vaccinations and general sanitation and cleanliness in city districts, schools and work units; whereas in rural China, health campaigns combined preventive vaccinations and sanitary activities with land reclamation and irrigation construction. Visual materials of posters and pictorials were widely used to popularize scientific knowledge of disease through health education and literacy movement in the 1950s–1970s. Health campaigns also promoted hygienic behavior as expected virtues of socialist citizens and good health as essential for economic production and national defense.

The promotion of four modernizations in the era of economic reforms has shifted public health and disease prevention from mass mobilization to reliance on medical science and technologies such as vaccines and medication. The de-collectivization of economy and decentralization of the health system have left health education greatly to the care of individual consumers who take particular caution against health threats of environmental hazards and industrialized food. The long-term effect of public health education has not been lost, especially among the retired and elderly, for they go out and exercise in parks and at public squares out of their own will and initiative.

Summary of chapters

The chapters are organized chronologically, but each chapter unfolds with thematic discussions of key topics situated in larger social, political and cultural contexts. International and transnational interactions constitute a significant feature of China's public health movements and modernization. Chapter 1 explores Chinese understanding of public health as national power in the modern world. It examines the change of landscape from a traditional agrarian society to modern factories in treaty ports, where the formerly salubrious cities were eroded by environmental degradation, pollution, slums, disease and filth of a typical industrializing urban setting. Modern facilities such as electricity, running water, sewage system, indoor plumbing, garbage collection and tall buildings with conspicuous wealth in foreign settlements contrasted sharply with poverty, crowdedness, filth, illness and disease, slums and cheap labor in the Chinese sections in the treaty ports. The divide of hygiene and modernity was not only expressed in the treaty port cities but also in the dealings of Chinese government with foreign powers. After the suppression of the Boxer Uprising, foreign powers set up provisional governments in major cities including Beijing and Tianjin. The return of the cities to China hinged on the Chinese government's agreement to modern reforms including the creation of sanitary administration. While the government initiated sanitary and public health administration under the pressure of foreign powers, private efforts in this regard had begun by local elite and literati since the late nineteenth century. Moreover, the 1910 plague epidemic triggered a widespread urban movement of sanitation to prevent plague, promoted mainly by local gentry and merchants as well as physicians of Western and Chinese medicines. Newspapers were influential in shaping public fear of the plague and actions of prevention. Chinese doctors of Western medicine collaborated with the YMCA and medical missionaries in carrying out major public health education campaigns in the 1910s to promote hygiene and disease prevention. The chapter examines the tensions of Chinese and foreign relations, traditional cultural norms and modern concepts, practice of sanitary and epidemic control, and the attempts of various groups to shape the future of China. These early efforts were influenced by Social Darwinian interpretations of personal health and national strength and the political implications of modern medicine and public health for the state and people.

Science lent the credibility and legitimacy of modern medicine and public health as essential elements of a modern nation. Chinese intellectuals, who started the New Culture and the May Fourth Movements in the 1910s–1920s, promoted science as the new cultural framework to re-invent China. Science also provided the cultural authority and identity of modernizers in the larger political and social movements to destroy the old world and create a new society of China. Modernization of medicine was not merely a medical matter but a political fight against reactionary forces in national revolutions. Chinese medicine, being integral to traditional culture, was considered an obstacle of holding China back from progress by radical intellectuals. In this context of cultural renaissance and ascendance of science entered the American medical enterprise of the Rockefeller Foundation, which exerted profound influence on the leaders of modern medicine in China. Chapter 2 studies these broad changes with attention to the Science Society of China and the intellectuals who shaped the new cultural orientation of scientism and vernacular (*baihua*) writing to popularize science among the masses, particularly the modern terminology of medical science and disease prevention during the outbreaks of epidemic diseases. Chinese intellectuals also started the Rural Reform and Mass Education Movement with pilot programs to integrate health modernization into the socio-economic development of rural reconstruction. The unique role of Peking Union Medical College in medical education and the training of public health leaders in China showed that the RF's medical enterprise focused on the production of health leaders, who eventually dominated the health bureaucracy and shaped the policies and development of the Nationalist health system.

Chapter 3 takes a close look at the construction of a modern national health system by the medical elite of the Nationalist government and the creative development of health programs by the CCP in their revolutionary regions. The LNHO and the RF provided significant assistance to the Nationalists in the institutional-building and professional-training of modern health. The Nationalist medical elite focused on building a modern health administrative system of institutions rather than the delivery of health service to people. They created beautiful designs of a national health system, even with a three-tiered rural health structure, but they were short on delivery, particularly in rural health construction. Extraordinary progress was made in establishing central medical research and training institutions but less successful in the development of local institutions during the politically tumultuous years of wars. The CCP, in contrast, built their revolutionary bases and worked with rural peasants on health programs from the bottom up. They relied on both Western and Chinese medicines in health service and encouraged the organization of health cooperatives and medical teams. With limited resources in medicine and professionals, they mobilized the masses to achieve health and social reforms. International aid was important to the CCP health development when medical assistance from different groups of the anti-fascist movement during World War II helped raise the standards of medical practice with new knowledge and technical equipment.

Chapter 4 examines the PRC's health development as an integral part of the socialist reconstruction of China. The alleged American germ-warfare during the Korean War had an unexpected impact on Chinese health policy and anti-disease movements. The Patriotic Health Movement combined national defense with disease prevention and provided the masses with the rally of political enthusiasm and national pride in carrying out activities of sanitation and anti-disease campaigns. Health movement became a patriotic political movement for national defense, economic production, and people's health in the overall transformation of social institutions and people's attitude and behavior. Through mobilization and the literacy movement, the masses learned the scientific knowledge of disease and health, and took an active role to fight disease and improve society and themselves. With the rapid development of diverse medical and health institutions, the health service was extended into rural villages with the training of millions of health workers in both Western and Chinese medicines, some of them part-time rural paramedics called barefoot doctors to serve fellow villagers. Free and low-cost healthcare was delivered to people through work-units and the rural commune system. What the Nationalist health planners had dreamed in their designs of a modern health system was now delivered by the health workers of the PRC in an actual health service. Thanks to the rural cooperative medical system, China was able to provide primary healthcare to 22 percent of the world population by using only 1 percent of health resources. China's low-cost healthcare system was hailed the model for developing countries that faced serious health challenges.

The economic reforms since the end of 1970s have fundamentally dismantled the socialist health system of free healthcare for the people. Instead, a health insurance system was introduced as part of the reform of the health sector. The result was a rapid increase of medical costs and inaccessibility of medical service in China, which gave rise to nation-wide complaints of the current health system and health service. The government has acknowledged the failure of health reforms in the 1990s and has issued a new reform plan of the health system in 2009. Chapter 5 discusses the marketization of economy and the collapse of the socialist healthcare system. It examines the operations and challenges of the New Rural Cooperative Medical System that was initiated in the beginning of the twenty-first century and the continuing efforts of the government to reform and re-build a health system with the provision of primary healthcare to people.

Notes

1 "On Hygiene," *Hankou ribao* [Hankow Daily], the 8th day of the Fifth month, reprinted in *Dongfang zazhi* [Eastern Miscellany], vol. 2, no. 8 (1905), 156–157.

2 British newspapers began to use the phrase "the sick man of the Orient" to describe China in 1896. Other newspapers followed suit. Several variations of the phrase, such as "the sick man of Huaxia," and "the sick man of East Asia," were in circulation at the beginning of the twentieth century according to Gao Cui (see his book, *From "The Sick Man of East Asia" to A Strong Country of Sports* [Cong "dong ya bing fu" dao ti yu qiang guo] (Sichuan renmin chubanshe, 2002), 9–12. In 1905, *The New York Times* (16 August 1905, 6) reported under the title "The Sick Man of the Far East": "China will henceforth be put in the same position in which Turkey has been for half a century. . . . She will become, by the ratification of the proposed treaty of peace, the Sick Man of the Far East." Western scholars usually use the phrase "the sick man of Asia."

3 Ruth Rogaski, *Hygienic Modernity: Meanings of Health and Disease in Treaty-Port China* (Berkeley CA: University of California Press, 2004).

4 Hu Cheng, "The Image of the 'Unsanitary' Chinese: Differing Narratives of Chinese and Foreigners – Observations of Public Hygiene in Shanghai, 1860–1911," *Bulletin of the Institute of Modern History Academia Sinica*, vol. 56 (2007),1–43.

5 Brett Bowden, *The Empire of Civilization: The Evolution of an Imperial Idea* (University of Chicago Press, 2009). See also, his *Civilization: Critical Concepts in Political Science*, 4 volumes (Routledge, 2009).

6 For the role of newspapers in shaping up public opinion and sentiment, see Joan Judge, *Print and Politics: "Shibao" and the Culture of Reform in Late Qing China* (CA: Stanford University Press, 1996); and Henrietta Harrison, "Newspapers and Nationalism in Rural China, 1890–1929," *Past & Present*, vol. 166 (2000), 181–204.

7 George Rosen, *A History of Public Health*, expanded edition (Baltimore: The Johns Hopkins University Press, 1993), 168–270; and Richard H. Shryock, *The Development of Modern Medicine* (Madison, WI: University of Wisconsin Press, 1980).

8 The three people's principles are people's nation (民族), people's rights (民权), and people's livelihood (民生).

9 Barry Buzan and George Lawson, *The Global Transformation: History, Modernity and the Making of International Relations* (Cambridge: Cambridge University Press, 2015).

10 Opium was always associated with the decline of China in the nineteenth century when China failed to stop the illegal drug traffic even by fighting the Opium War with Britain (1839–1942). In view of the wide-spread use of opium among Chinese people, physical well-being struck a painful cord in the national psyche but conveyed a unique meaning in the particular situation of China. The discourse of Chinese anti-opium movements concentrated on opium and the decline of China—the national shame and disaster. The Nationalist government launched anti-opium campaigns with anti-opium offices established in many counties; and the PRC government eradicated the opium epidemic in the 1950s via mass education and rehabilitation programs. Works on anti-opium movements include Alan Baumler, *The Chinese and Opium under the Republic: Worse than Floods and Wild Beasts* (Albany, New York: State University of New York Press, 2008);

and Kathleen Lodwick, *Crusaders against Opium: Protestant Missionaries in China, 1874–1917* (Lexington, KY: University Press of Kentucky, 2009). Tobacco smoking has developed into a social habit in China and the anti-smoking movement has recently gained momentum after its health hazards are aggressively publicized. Carol Benedict has written a history of tobacco smoking in China, *Golden-Silk Smoke: A History of Tobacco in China, 1550–2010* (Berkeley, CA: University of California Press, 2011). On anti-smoking movements in China, see Liu Wen Nan, *Jindai Zhongguo de bu xi zhiyan yundong yan jiu* [The Anti-Cigarette Campaigns in Modern China] (Beijing: Shehui kexue wenxian chubanshe, 2015).

11 Tan Chung, "Imperialism in Nineteenth-Century China (II)—The Unequal Treaty System: Infrastructure of Irresponsible Imperialism," *China Report*, vol. 17, no. 5 (1981), 3–33.

12 "Biographical File of W. W. Peter," Kautz Family YMCA Archives, University of Minnesota (hereafter YMCA Archives). The medal was awarded to people who had made significant beneficiary contributions to Chinese society.

13 The medal was displayed at a first-floor reading room at the Rockefeller Archives Center, North Tarrytown, New York.

14 Shirley S. Garrett, *Social Reformers in Urban China: The Chinese Y.M.C.A., 1895–1926* (Cambridge, MA: Harvard University Press, 1970); and Noel H. Pugach, "Standard Oil and Petroleum Development in Early Republican China," *The Business History Review*, vol. 45, no. 4 (Winter 1971), 452–473.

15 John Farley, *To Cast Out Disease: A History of the International Health Division of the Rockefeller Foundation, 1913–1951* (New York: Oxford University Press, 2004).

16 Mary E. Ferguson, *China Medical Board and Peking Union Medical College: A Chronicle of Fruitful Collaboration, 1914–1951* (New York: China Medical Board of New York, Inc., 1970), Appendix C, 245–253; and Mary Bullock, *An American Transplant* (Berkeley, CA: University of California Press, 1980), Appendix A, 233–237.

17 Margherita Zanasi, "Exporting Development: The League of Nations and Republican China," *Comparative Studies in Society and History*, vol. 49, no. 1 (2007),143–169.

18 Edmund S. K. Fung, *The Intellectual Foundations of Chinese Modernity: Cultural and Political Thought in the Republican Era* (Cambridge: Cambridge University Press, 2010).

19 Liping Bu, "Social Darwinism, Public Health and Modernization in China, 1895–1925" in *Uneasy Encounters: The Politics of Medicine and Health in China 1900–1937*, ed. Iris Borowy (Germany: Peter Lang, 2009), 93–124.

20 Sean Hsiang-Lin Lei, *Neither Donkey nor Horse: Medicine and the Struggle over China's Modernity* (Chicago: University of Chicago Press, 2014); and Bridie Andrews, *The Making of Modern Chinese Medicine, 1850–1960* (Vancouver: University of British Columbia Press, 2014).

21 Paul Starr, *The Social Transformation of American Medicine: The Rise of a Sovereign Profession and the Making of a Vast Industry* (New York: Basic Books, 1982).

22 Liping Bu, "Public Health and Modernisation: The First Campaigns in China, 1915–1916," *Social History of Medicine*, vol. 22, no. 2 (2009), 305–319.

23 Chow Tse-tung, *The May 4th Movement: Intellectual Revolution in Modern China* (Cambridge, MA: Harvard University Press, 1960).

24 On science as the cultural authority, see Gyan Prakash, *Another Reason: Science and the Imagination of Modern India* (Princeton University Press, 1999).

25 On the ideological identity of science, see Peter Buck, "Western Science in Republican China: Ideology and Institution Building," in *Science and Value: Patterns of Tradition and Change*, eds. Arnold Thackery and Evertt Menddelson (NY: Humanities Press, 1974), 159–184.

26 According to the Qing government's treaty agreements with foreign powers, Commissioner of the Maritime Customs Service of the Chinese government was

designated to a foreigner, whose authoritative power included, among other things, supervision of public health concerns such as quarantine during an epidemic. This treaty arrangement continued until the reorganization of Customs Services and the full tariff autonomy by the Nationalist government in 1928. Public health concerns including treaty ports' quarantine was under the supervision of the Customs Commissioner and the Customs Medical Officer. For instance, "the Quarantine Service in Shanghai was part of the Customs Service. Any quarantine action by the Port Health Officer must be acceptable to the Treaty Port Consuls, who often misused their extraterritoriality rights to protect the trade of their own nationalities at the expense of life during an epidemic." (See I. C. Yuan, "Doctor J. Heng Liu: Our Leader and Organizer of National Health Services," in *Dr. J. Heng Liu and Meidical and Health Development in China*, ed., Irene Ssu-chin Liu Hou, Taiwan Shangwu Yingshuguan, 1989), 181.

27 Health stations were sometimes called health demonstration units, centers, or areas. For the sake of convenience and less confusion, I use health station to describe them all.

28 Liping Bu, "Cultural Communication in Picturing Health: W. W. Peter and the Public Health Campaigns in China, 1912–1926," in *Imagining Illness: Public Health and Visual Culture*, ed., David Serlin (Minnesota: University of Minnesota Press, 2010), 24–39.

29 For a study of local propaganda work of the Nationalists, see Christopher A. Reed, "Propaganda by the Book," *Frontiers of History in China*, vol. 10, no. 1 (March 2015), 96–125.

30 Huang Wen, *Three People's Principles and Medicine* (Shaoguan, Guangdong: Shijie luntanshe, 1943).

31 *Propaganda Guide for the Health Movement* (Nanjing: Propaganda Department of the GMD Central Executive Committee, 1929).

1 Public health

A modern concept of national power

Introduction

The meaning of public health has evolved historically to indicate disease control, sanitation, disaster epidemic relief, and mental and physical health protection of the population as a whole.[1] At the turn of the twentieth century, the concept of public health carried a distinct significance of national power and social progress, as the advancement of nations was measured by national death rates and sanitary control. Administration of public health was the responsibility of local and central governments of modern nations. Ruth Rogaski used "hygienic modernity" to describe this modern phenomenon of national power, which she defined as a combination of state power, scientific progress, cleanliness, and the fitness of races.[2] Public health also became a contentious issue in the relations between Western imperialist powers and non-Western countries in regard to modern reforms and sovereignty. In 1901, administration of public health became a significant point in the negotiations between China and foreign powers for the return of Chinese cities after the suppression of the Boxer Uprising (义和团运动).[3] The Qing court had to agree to continue the sanitary work of foreign occupation before the powers would return Beijing and Tianjin to China. The matter of hygienic modernity came up again in 1910 when a pneumonic plague epidemic caused a full-blown public health crisis in northeast China. Foreign powers in the region expanded their control of city districts in the name of health protection, undermining China's sovereignty in controlling the epidemic and its territory. Known as the Manchurian plague in the West, this deadly epidemic took more than 60,000 human lives and caused financial losses of 100 million dollars.[4] The scale of mortality and socio-economic devastation was considered to have "rivaled or exceeded the Great Plague of London" in 1665–1666.[5] For the Qing dynasty, the Manchurian plague presented as much a public health crisis as a political challenge to keep China's sovereignty.

Northeast China had attracted active commercial and political activities of foreign powers during the scramble for China in the wake of the 1894–1895 Sino-Japanese war.[6] Russia and Japan each had penetrated the region with territorial concessions and railroad operations. Other powers, such as the United States,

Great Britain, Germany, and France, had established consulates in the region to represent their respective governments and their local businesses. After the outbreak of the plague, foreign powers, particularly the Russian and the Japanese, were eager to expand their territorial control with the pretext of plague prevention. Japan was preparing an invasion of the northeast, while Russia tried to enlist American support for the demand that "China should entrust to foreign physicians the care of deciding" the anti-plague measures.[7] Even Japanese and Russian medical scientists took an arrogant attitude towards Chinese medical scientists.[8] The plague crisis offered an unexpected opportunity for foreign powers to seek more territory gains, putting increasing pressure on the Qing government. Whether the Qing government could bring the plague epidemic under control was not only a matter of saving tens of thousands of lives but also a matter of proving China's ability to handle public health crisis as a sovereign country. It was apparent that successful management of the epidemic crisis was of immeasurable importance to China in maintaining its sovereignty.

China did not encounter the modern problems of urban squalor, pollution, and industrial diseases and poverty until the rapid growth of factories and trade in treaty-port cities after the 1860s. Cities like Shanghai, Tianjin, Hankou, and Guangzhou were major centers of foreign settlements, and by 1900, more than one hundred treaty ports were established under the unequal treaty system China had with foreign powers. The 1842 Treaty of Nanjing, which forced China to open up trade with and to cede Hong Kong to Britain after the Opium War, was a turning point in China's modern history in terms of its relations with foreign nations and its economic and social developments and political consequences.[9] The building of industrial factories in the treaty-port cities took away farmland, started environmental and health pollution, and initiated modern slums. Christian missionaries and foreign traders and soldiers introduced to China Western religion, medical science, capitalist enterprises, and modern killing and looting with gunboat diplomacy. The Qing government, which failed to fend off foreign assaults on the battlefields and at the negotiation tables, was slow and reluctant to reform in face of a fast changing world. It made frequent capitulations to foreign powers, which led to the decline of the Qing empire into a semi-colonial society, where traditional institutions of governance were weakened and new modern institutions such as those of hygiene and sanitation were barely created. The educated Chinese, particularly those influenced by Western thought and ideas and trained in the West, were anxious to explore what made the West powerful. One of their discoveries, as Yan Fu (严复, 1854–1921) first elaborated in 1895, was Western powers' emphasis on the physical fitness of the people. Ideas of Social Darwinism from the West and martial spirits of ancient China both contributed to the intellectual argument for a strong modern country of China via strong modern citizens.

This chapter investigates the changes of China after foreign powers introduced modern commerce and factories in the treaty ports with the rise of modern health hazards, and the shift of Western notion of China from "a splendor of the East" to "the sick man of Asia." It examines missionary medical activities in China and their impact on Chinese society in terms of relations between Western and Chinese medicines, and the contention on the validity of traditional Chinese culture and knowledge. It analyzes how Chinese modern intellectuals and health professionals promoted Western medicine at the expense of Chinese traditional culture and medicine, all in the name of science and national strength, and how the government created modern institutions of sanitation and hygiene during times of political and health crises, and the initiation of regulations on infectious diseases in the course of political transformation from a dynasty to a republic. Health education campaigns in the 1910s popularized the intellectual interpretation of individual health in relation to national strength. For the Chinese elite who shaped the social and political discourse of reform, public health was a political as well as a medical concept to promote national progress and modernization.

From salubrious cities to polluted treaty ports

Chinese cities were healthier than their counterparts in industrial Europe and America before they became treaty ports of foreign trade and industrial factories in the latter half of the nineteenth century. William Lockhart of the London Mission Society arrived in Shanghai in 1843 to find the city salubrious and the surrounding rural areas fertile, irrigated, and "well-drained and free from swamps." Local Chinese were "healthy and strong, as robust and well-fed a race as is usually seen in Chinese cities."[10] In contrast, many in industrial London and New York died of rampant outbreaks of infectious diseases such as cholera, typhoid, smallpox and yellow fever. Lockhart, who founded the first missionary hospital in Shanghai, was reminded of the difference in 1849 when Europe was struck by epidemics and China was spared.

> Shanghai is not to be regarded as an insalubrious city. Sickness, to an unusual extent, sometimes prevails in cities of the western world . . . , typhus and scarlet fever made fearful ravages in some places in Europe; and whilst cholera caused a great mortality in other parts of the world, China was mercifully preserved from its visitation.[11]

Lockhart was surprised that the water in the Huangpu River was "surcharged with decaying matter, and likely to cause sickness of a serious character, yet the people generally maintain a full average amount of health."[12] He observed that the Chinese had many habits conducive to health, such as drinking boiled water, wearing cotton-padded clothes in the winter, and having good ventilation of the house. "[D]uring certain periods, the Chinese suffer much from ague, diarrhea, and dysentery, but when their habits are remembered, the wonder is that they do not suffer more."[13] A decade later when Charles Alexander Gordon, the British colonial administrator who later served as Britain's surgeon-general, visited Shanghai in 1860, he was favorably impressed with Shanghai as well, in contrast to Calcutta:

> Villages appeared at intervals, and from their general looks seemed to indicate that their inhabitants were in the enjoyment of an average amount of personal comfort. Fields . . . extended to the horizon, small bulwarks being raised between them for the purpose of more ready irrigation and division according to the nature of the crops to be raised upon them.[14]

These accounts of personal comfort and farming activities indicated people's health and the prosperity of China in the mid-nineteenth century.

Chinese public bathhouses and teahouses attracted the attention of foreigners as well, about personal hygiene and health in China.[15] Lockhart highly praised tea-drinking in China in view of alcohol abuse in the West. He was impressed with the national habit of tea drinking and the sociopolitical role of teahouses in Chinese society.[16] He was fascinated with the tea sheds that Chinese gentry set up everywhere to provide free tea for the refreshment of weary and thirsty workers and travelers in the hot summer. All comers were invited to enjoy the tea, he wrote. The Chinese tea shed made an unexpected contribution to the modern West when the concept of tea shed was "worthily imitated in England by the establishment of drinking-fountains."[17]

In 1861 Lockhart came to Beijing and established the first missionary hospital, which eventually evolved into the Peking Union Medical College. As he did in other cities, Lockhart studied Beijing's "climate, its rainfall, the soil, the wells, the drainage of the city" and considered Beijing "really a healthy city."[18] John Dudgeon, who became a prominent missionary doctor in Beijing in the last three decades of the nineteenth century, was also impressed with Beijing's clean open space and sunny climate upon his arrival in 1864. He admiringly described the broad straight avenue of 120-feet wide stretching north and south through the city and the Hutong (胡同) lanes wide enough for two carriages to run abreast.[19] Like his fellow missionaries, Dudgeon examined Chinese diet, dress, housing and social customs, and their implications for health. He noticed that people in Beijing did not get sick even though there was miasma around them all the time.[20] Dudgeon was puzzled by this Chinese reality that contradicted the miasma theory of disease in the West. Before the germ theory was established in the 1880s, people in the West generally believed that diseases were caused by miasma.[21] The new germ theory of disease caused such a fundamental shift in Western medicine and health that William Sedgwick claimed: "Before 1880 we knew nothing; after 1890 we knew it all."[22] Dudgeon had written positively of Chinese lifestyle, urban conditions and hygiene. Scholars made different comments on Dudgeon's admiration of Chinese lifestyle and health. Gao Xi's biographical study reveals that Dudgeon did not judge China in Western terms but appreciated the healthy Chinese lifestyle on its own. Shang-jen Li argues that Dudgeon's "admiration of Chinese hygiene and his conception of the diseases of civilization were closely connected to his nostalgic vision of a paternalistic society."[23]

Lockhart and Dudgeon often expressed surprises when they considered the unsanitary conditions in parts of Chinese cities and the lack of widespread epidemics. Seeing no modern sewage system in Chinese cities, Lockhart criticized but was puzzled:

> Their cities being undrained, are always in a most filthy state; the canals into which the tide does not rise, are filled with putrid matter of every kind, and are seldom, if ever cleansed. The surprise is that the inhabitants can live at all among so much filth in the canals, streets, and in their own houses. . . . During the six years the port [Shanghai] had then been open, the mortality among the foreign residents had been small.[24]

Similarly, Dudgeon was not fond of the bad smell emitting from the carts of waste collectors and handlers in Beijing, and he was equally puzzled that people did not get sick. Collecting human and animal waste and rubbish was a traditional practice of the eco-recycle system in the agricultural society of China. Waste and rubbish were collected and made into fertilizers in a process that exposed them to sun-baking at confined sites in open air. Transportation of the waste by carts on the streets and the open-air processing let out far-reaching foul smell, to which foreigners were extremely sensitive.

In their studies of the health implications of all things Chinese, missionary doctors applied Western standards of their home countries to the Chinese situation and criticized the unsanitary conditions as the cause of disease, just as their colleagues did back at home in the sanitary movement and social reforms. They measured China against the health standards of Western countries, and took the lead on health concerns from the "medical and sanitary issues of the 1850s and 1860s" made visible by the sanitary reformists in London, New York, and Paris.[25] They also shared similar discourse in the description of city conditions, be it China, Europe, or the United States. In the late nineteenth century, the Hygiene Council of New York described the city streets "very filthy" with horse manure, dead cats and dogs and rats, and household and vegetable refuse.[26] The slums in London appeared little different from that of New York under Charles Dickens' pen.[27] The Chinese cities, which had now become treaty ports, were soon to gain the same characteristics of industrial cities of London and New York and the reputation of being filthy.

Europeans and Americans who came to China in the post-Opium War years made careful examination of the environment and all things pertaining to health for the very reason of their own survival in a foreign land. They chose the location of settlement best fitting for trade and for health. The British selected Lijiachang (李家场) as their settlement in Shanghai. The location had a river frontage and "is tolerably dry and free from any local circumstances that are supposed to generate malaria."[28] Residential houses and company buildings were constructed after 1845 when they obtained the land. The Americans came in 1848 and the area was incorporated into the International Settlement in 1863. They formed their own self-governing body called the Shanghai Municipal Council. When the French came, they acquired land south of the International Settlement, later known as the French concession. In accordance with the treaties their respective governments signed with the Qing, foreigners lived in their own settlements and enjoyed the privileges of extraterritoriality without being subject to Chinese laws. Epidemics were not a frequent threat in Shanghai as they were in European metropolis. In 1879,

> only three deaths from cholera [in the International Settlement where the population was about 3000], though apparently an epidemic was raging in Japan. The Chinese population seemed to be quite free of this disease, though for some years this disease seemed to have made its headquarters among the river population.[29]

The total death numbers, however, rose to 282 in 1888 in the International Settlement.

From the 1860s onwards, European and American businesses made their ways into Chinese treaty ports by building industrial companies and factories. In Shanghai alone, textile factories, chemical plants, hide and leather factories, ironworks companies, electricity companies, gas companies and works, lumber industries, power stations, water companies, banks, and insurance companies all emerged one after another, changing the idyllic farming landscape into an industrializing center in a short couple of decades. **(See Figure 1.1, Image of industrialization.)** Modern industries brought huge profits to the few wealthy foreigners, but devastated the environment and pauperized the masses of Chinese laborers. The double-edged sword of industrialization cut into Chinese land and society with profound impact. Hundreds of thousands Chinese migrated as cheap labor into the industrializing center of Shanghai from surrounding countryside and faraway rural villages. They looked for opportunities to work in the factories as farm land and traditional trades were swallowed up by the industrial companies. Almost all the companies and banks were owned by foreigners before the twentieth century.[30] Foreign population in the settlements increased rapidly. Statistics of the Shanghai Municipal Council showed 3600 foreigners in 1870 and more than 10,000 in 1905.[31] **(See Table 1.1, Population and death rates in the International Settlement.)** The working poor huddled in crowded and filthy makeshift huts with no sanitary water and toilets. One of the manifestations of the accumulation of poverty in Shanghai was the rise of shabby and squalid reed-huts on the banks of rivers adjacent to factories. The shabby reed-huts sheltered

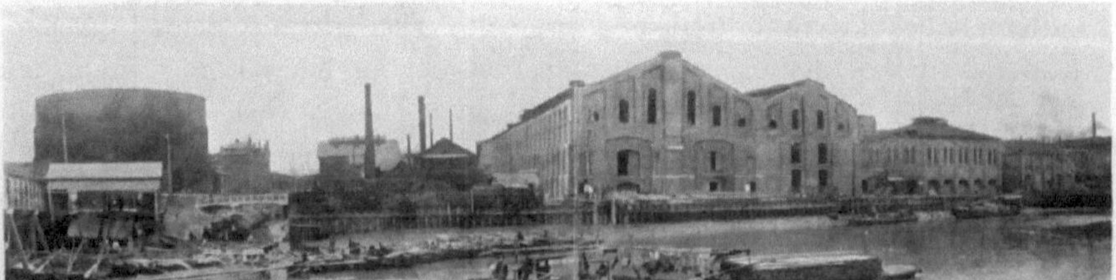

THE GAS WORKS.

Figure 1.1 Image of a gas company in Shanghai at the turn of the twentieth century

Source: Arnold Wright and H. A. Carwright, *Twentieth Century Impressions of Hongkong, Shanghai, and other Treaty Ports of China: Their History, People, Commerce, Industries, and Resources.* (London: Lloyd's Greater Britain Publishing Company, Ltd., 1908), 396.

Table 1.1 Population and death rates of Shanghai, 1887–1907

FOREIGNERS							*NATIVES*
Year	*Residents*					*Non-Residents*	*Death-rate of Chinese Population*
	Adults	*Children*	*Total Deaths*	*Population*	*Death-rate of Resident Population*	*Total Deaths*	
1887	64	20	84	3,731	22.5	46	...
1888	52	23	75	3,760	19.9	33	...
1889	39	28	67	3,789	17.7	25	...
1890	60	31	91	3,821	23.8	35	...
1891	61	38	98	3,980	24.6	45	...
1892	52	18	70	4,140	16.9	32	...
1893	45	21	66	4,310	15.3	31	...
1894	47	40	87	4,500	19.3	37	...
1895	45	35	80	4,684	17.1	44	...
1896	59	29	88	4,834	18.2	47	...
1897	42	27	69	4,909	14.5	32	...
1898	61	24	85	5,240	16.2	17	...
1899	75	29	104	5,510	18.9	28	...
1900	81	16	97	6,774	14.3	60	...
1901	91	37	128	7,000	18.3	91	...
1902	81	57	138	7,600	18.1	125	30.9
1903	86	46	132	8,300	15.9	82	21.2
1904	76	40	116	9,000	12.9	78	19.2
1905	96	33	129	11,497	11.2	112	14.2
1906	109	37	146	12,000	12.1	71	11.9
1907	153	92	245	13,700	17.9	83	20.0

Source: Arnold Wright and H. A. Cartwright, eds. *Twentieth Century Impressions of Hongkong, Shanghai, and other Treaty Ports of China: Their History, People, Commerce, Industries, and Resources* (London: Lloyd's Greater Britain Publishing Company, Ltd, 1908), 435.

the poor, migrant laborers and refugees. The slums continued to multiply as the city expanded in industrial commerce. Industries in treaty port cities, such as Shanghai, Tianjin and Hankou, caused disruption and breakdown of the traditional eco-recycle system of agricultural life. Industrial pollution, pauperization of Chinese laborers, and a lack of regular maintenance of public works in a semi-colonial Chinese society gave rise to fast growth of poverty, degradation of environment, and multiplication of diseases.

Hygiene and public health: a divide of foreigners and Chinese

Foreigners established hospitals and set up sanitary control services in their settlements. They conducted urban sanitation and disease prevention in China by using inspections and regulations, the usual methods that were practiced at their home countries. The Shanghai Municipal Council of the International Settlement had the power to administer taxation, police, education, public works, sanitation and public health. In 1861 the Council had a sanitary inspector in charge of street-cleaning and garbage collection. The next year it created a Unit of Waste and Rubbish (粪秽股) to oversee the removal of human and animal waste and rubbish. In 1863 the Office of Hygiene was created to take care of all sanitary and health-related affairs. The office was renamed the Public Health Department (卫生处) in 1898 with a medical doctor, Arthur Stanley, as the health officer.[32]

Modern sanitary facilities, such as the sewage system, indoor plumbing, and running water, were gradually installed in foreign settlements but not in the Chinese sections of the city. In contrast, Chinese sections became increasingly crowded with poor and migrant workers, and the general sanitation and public health deteriorated with lack of attention and resources for building and maintaining public works. The decline of the Qing government and the corruption of officials contributed to the worsening of conditions. Chinese reformist entrepreneur Zheng Guanying (郑观应，1842–1921) wrote in the 1890s:

> I saw wide and clean roads in the Settlement but filthy grounds in the Chinese districts . . . littered with smelling rubbish, and old and young would urinate and defecate anywhere. The diseased groaning here and there but no one paid them attention. I covered my nose and passed through. This demonstrated the failure of the government and no virtue of the wealthy. No wonder foreigners despise us.[33]

The unsanitary conditions and illnesses in Chinese treaty port cities became a key element in Western imagery of China as the "sick man of East Asia" at the turn of the twentieth century.

Epidemic diseases became a major concern of the Shanghai Municipal Council after Stanley served as the health officer. More than 30 kinds of diseases were listed as the causes of death; and smallpox, cholera, typhoid, scarlet fever, and tuberculosis headed the list of communicable diseases.[34] In a short time of three decades, Shanghai had changed from a salubrious city to a disease-ridden place. Arthur Stanley saw a different Shanghai from Lockhart, which he described as an unhealthy place. To prevent residents of the settlement from getting sick, the Public Health Department carried out vaccinations of smallpox. In 1904, "34,000 tubes of vaccines were sent out, an equivalent of 170,000 persons protected from smallpox."[35] Malaria was expected to be rife with the humidity and heat in the summer, but Stanley reported, with great pride, that all "the dreadful miasma . . . have, however, been dissipated by the lamp of science." He continued:

> During the past ten years much has been done by spreading sanitary knowledge, and by eliminating stagnant water to minimize the danger of malaria. It has been found that the parts of the Settlement most occupied by streets and well-built houses have been most free from malaria, while the outlying districts, where pools and slow-running and blocked creeks occur, have been most prone to malaria.[36]

Vital statistics gathered by the Health Department of the Municipal Council showed that death rates in the Settlement, though fluctuating in these years, were not much higher than that of London and New York in the same time period.[37] **(See Table 1.1 for death rates.)**

Death rates of Chinese, however, were higher as the data of Table 1.1 indicates, even though the statistical data were incomplete. High death rate, diseases and unsanitary conditions of China became the subjects of writings by missionary doctors who published in newspapers and popular and professional journals. Western media reports of China were increasingly dominated by the words "backward" and "weak."[38] Chinese elite from compradors to reformers and revolutionary intellectuals quickly picked up the discourse of "unsanitary" China to excoriate their government and to shame their countrymen into action of change. A 1905 editorial article in the *Hankou Daily* claimed that all problems of China had originated from the ignorance of hygiene:

> Our country and people do not know the importance of hygiene. Hence, roads are not repaired and gates are narrow and dim. When you travel, the road is full of dust; and when you enter a house, it is a world of darkness. . . . The foreigners' buildings are tall with big open windows to take in fresh air. It is a difference of heaven and hell when you compare foreigners' buildings with Chinese dwellings.[39]

The editorial of self-reproach used a simple image of contrast to depict the different result from attention to and ignorance of hygiene. There was no close examination of the underlying factors that created the divide of the world of healthy and wealthy foreigners and the world of un-hygienic and poor Chinese. The description of the living conditions indicated the huge economic gap and social divide between foreigners and Chinese. Similarly, Chen Duxiu (陈独秀, 1879–1942), the radical intellectual, thought that hygiene was the pivotal manifestation of civilization. He scolded his countrymen: "Westerners call these three nations unsanitary: India, Korea, and China. No matter where the Chinese go, they are humiliated not because of the decline of their country but because of their unclean habits."[40]

In the global colonial expansion of the West, diseases were racialized when the colonized non-whites were depicted as filthy and sickly creatures and the white colonizers the clean and healthy species. The dichotomy of the healthy civilized West vs. the unhealthy uncivilized non-West gave Westerners not only the medical justification to conquer non-Western societies but also the moral obligation of Christian missionaries to save the souls. Scholars have pointed out the crucial role of medicine in Western imperialist dominance of non-Western societies.[41] No one summarized it better than Louis-Hubert Lyautey, the French colonial administrator and marshal of France, about medicine and imperialism: "La seule excuse de la colonization, c'est la médicine."[42] Roy Porter pointed out that from Rudyard Kipling to Cecil Rhodes, tropical medicine and imperialist exploitation constituted rich sources of heroic stories of Western expansion into

Asia and Africa. The poverty and the myth of the diseased non-whites led to discrimination and injustice against them across national boundaries. Chinese in Honolulu and San Francisco, for example, were blamed for spreading diseases and suffered terrible mistreatment in America in the late nineteenth and early twentieth centuries.[43]

Missionaries and Western medicine

Christian missionaries brought Western medicine to China in the nineteenth century and used medical practice to open up Chinese society for evangelism. Pioneering missionaries to China, such as Peter Parker and Thomas R. Colledge, were medical missionaries whose practices led to more social interactions with local Chinese. Medical missionaries concentrated on surgery and treatment of the eye disease of trachoma, medical skills that Chinese physicians lacked, as their primary medical services.[44] Missionaries' medical practices proved so effective in opening up China that missionary societies adopted the strategy "to open a way through the body to the soul."[45] Missionaries built dispensaries and hospitals and schools in cities and rural towns as "a powerful evangelizing agency."[46]

Missionary groups exerted medical influence not only by establishing hospitals and medical schools but also by creating a missionary medical profession in China. They formed the Medical Missionary Society of China in 1838, which was re-organized as the China Medical Missionary Association (CMMA, 中华博医会) in 1886. Its official publication, *The China Medical Missionary Journal* (renamed as *The China Medical Journal* in 1907), was the first English-language medical professional journal in China, providing an authoritative voice of Western medicine and studies of diseases. Medical missionaries wrote extensively about diseases in China and published illustrations of abnormal illnesses in Western journals. Larissa Heinrich's study of the Lam Qua's medical portraits argued that missionaries were obsessed with the abnormal ailments of Chinese people and that their depictions of the abnormal sort contributed to a peculiar perception of the Chinese in Western imagination.[47] Missionaries' interpretation of ill health as external manifestation of moral degradation further justified their assumption of cultural superiority and leadership of reforms. In a more utilitarian sense, their depiction of encountering medical challenges in far-away lands helped mission societies solicit donations from their countrymen and countrywomen back at home to support the evangelical cause abroad.

Western medical textbooks and literature were introduced to China through translation as well. Chinese terms of Western medicine were created in the translation of modern medical knowledge from abroad. As the sciences of bacteriology and biology revolutionized Western medicine in the nineteenth century, medical missionaries increasingly used science to project themselves as representatives of a superior civilization and agents of advanced progress. They criticized China for lack of science and attacked Chinese medicine as superstition and quackery.[48] Western medicine became a force of contention in the endeavor to evangelize China by missionaries who dismissed the validity of Chinese medicine and its cultural traditions. Medical science and new "discoveries" of tropical diseases fed off the expansion of Western empires and their dominance in the global hierarchy of nations.[49]

It was ironic that when the West experienced the parallel of rise of science and decline of religion, science became an indispensable tool for Christian evangelism abroad. Since the late nineteenth century, criticism of China's lack of science became a common missionary discourse that claimed: "Millions were in soul and body sick unto death; but the science of healing was unknown [in China]."[50] To missionaries, "the health question in China is but one of the many sides to the problem of China's redemption."[51] The dual task of medical missionaries to practice Western medicine and to spread Christianity ushered in an era of fundamental transformation of Chinese culture and medical knowledge in the process of Western evangelization of China. Missionaries used their medical successes to demonstrate the power of God as well as the superior advancement of the West to impress native people. Their self-righteous impulse to "civilize" and to "save" others was propped up by their assumption of others as "backward" and "sickly" and themselves as superior and progressive. In the name of God and reforms, they imposed their religious beliefs and cultural values upon others and tried to transform traditional 'backward" societies into modern "progressive" nations.

However, Chinese language and culture as well as the lifestyles and social norms of Chinese patients posed challenges to medical missionaries who found communication with Chinese patients difficult. To better interact with Chinese, medical missionaries trained young Chinese to assist their work. The teaching language was the home language of the missionary societies, be it English, French, or German. The Japanese followed Western powers in this practice after Japan gained concessions in China. Foreign language requirement at missionary institutions reiterated the familiar pattern of Western colonization all over the world. Missionaries generally considered Chinese assistants very useful in the daily details of work because they had:

> excellent memory for facts and detail; faithfulness in carrying out methods once adopted; marked powers of observation; and the most extraordinary devotion to the principle of hard work . . . ; great delicacy in all operations . . . and particular fitness for, and adaptability to, the intricate and time-consuming problems of original investigation, and especially the use of the microscope.[52]

Missionaries sent selected young Chinese to study medicine in their own countries. Although most of those trained abroad were men, a few Chinese women were selected for the study of medicine as well. Missionaries' interest in training Chinese women may very well have been prompted by the frustrations they encountered in reaching out to Chinese women patients. By tradition and social norms, Chinese physicians and healers, who were male, did not physically examine female patients except feeling the pulses. In the case of missionary doctors, their practice relied on physical examination to determine the diagnoses.

Chinese women, however, for the sake of decency, refused to see male foreign doctors for cultural, if not other, reasons.[53] Mission societies addressed the cultural challenge by training Chinese young women as assistants and sending some abroad to study medicine, while recruiting increasingly more female missionaries to China. By 1900 China had 3000 Protestant and 886 Catholic missionaries; more than half of them were women.[54]

The most famous Chinese man who studied medicine abroad in the nineteenth century was Huang Kuan (Wong Foon, Wong Fun, 黄宽, 1828–1878), who obtained a medical degree at the University of Edinburgh in 1853. He was one of three Chinese young men—Yung Wing and Wong Shing being the other two—sent by missionaries in 1847 to study at Monson Academy in Massachusetts. They were expected to return to China upon completing a Christian education in America and to play a leading role in spreading the Gospel among their own people. Wong Shing became ill and returned to China shortly afterwards, while Yung Wing (Rong Hong, 容闳, 1828–1912) finished his education at Yale University in 1854 with honors and returned to China in 1859.[55] Huang Kuan enrolled at the University of Edinburgh in 1950 after Monson Academy. Upon completing medical studies, he returned to China under the auspices of the London Missionary Society. He practiced medicine in Guangzhou and devoted much of his time to the study of pathology and anatomy. Huang investigated the frequency of Asiatic cholera in Guangzhou and found the disease rare in the region. He wrote:

> the term *huo-luan* (霍乱), commonly used to signify cholera, seems to answer more to the English than to the Asiatic form of the disease. . . . Even to a Chinese physician the term *huo-luan* suggests none of the dreadful ideas usually associated with epidemic cholera in the mind of an European, which seems to show that *huo-luan* does not mean epidemic cholera.[56]

Missionaries sent several young Chinese women to America to study medicine in the late nineteenth century. They included Jin Yunmei (金韵梅, Yamei Kin, 金雅美, 1864–1934), Xu Jinhong (Hü King-eng, 许金訇, 1865–1929), Shi Meiyu (Mary Stone, 石美玉, 1873–1954), and Kang Cheng (康成, Ida Kahn, 康爱德, 1873–1930).[57] They were the pioneering women in modern Chinese medical profession who braved the academic demands of medical studies and survived the racial and cultural challenges in the United States.[58] Jin Yunmei, the first Chinese woman to complete an American medical education, graduated from the New York Infirmary for Women and Children in 1885 and spent three years' postgraduate work in New York hospitals.[59] She was invited by Yuan Shikai to lead the women's medical department in Tianjin in 1907. Xu Jinhong went to America to study medicine in 1884 when she was only 18 years old.[60] Xu received her medical degree at the Women's Medical College in Philadelphia with honors in 1894 and returned to China to work as a missionary doctor of the Methodist Episcopal Church in Fuzhou. From 1899 onwards, Xu ran the Woolston Memorial Hospital for women and children for 30 years, and trained women nurses.[61] When they were in the United States, American media treated Jin and Xu as celebrities for their extraordinary adventures in medical studies because very few American women were studying medicine at the time. Jin Yunmei even went on a lecture tour in 1904 before she returned to China. In Boston, she was portrayed as having "a charming personality" and was endeared for "her Bostonian accent of English."[62] Shi Meiyu and Kang Cheng studied medicine at the University of Michigan during 1892–1896. After they received their medical degrees, they returned to China and made fame for themselves in both missionary work and the medical profession. Shi Meiyu founded and led the Elizabeth Danforth Hospital in Jiujiang from 1900 to 1920; and Kang Cheng, at the invitation of local government officials, founded the Nanchang Women's and Children's Hospital. These returned women doctors set up a pattern of practice: they would subsidize the free service to the poor with the fees paid by the rich at their hospitals and dispensaries.

Missionary-trained Chinese doctors were accepted as members of the China Medical Missionary Association, but they rarely gained equal footing in the organization. Foreign missionaries continued their patronizing attitude toward their Chinese colleagues with the sense of racial and cultural superiority, even though some of them did not have as distinguished a medical training as their Chinese counterparts. When more Chinese were trained in Western medicine, sponsored either by missionaries or by their own means, tensions began to rise within the Western medical group. Some missionaries doubted, despite all the facts, the ability of Chinese to master medical science, as if that was the monopoly of the West. To other missionaries, "the native Chinese has many qualifications for making a worthy practitioner of scientific medicine . . . and may be depended upon to enhance the honour of our great profession by adding the strength of native talent to the sum total."[63] The divide eventually led to the formation of the National Medical Association of China (NMAC, 中华医学会) by Chinese professionals of Western medicine in 1915.

The training of Chinese accelerated the expansion of the army of medical missionaries. In 1905, a total of 3445 Western missionaries were working in China, including 94 female and 207 male missionary doctors working in 166 missionary hospitals and 241 dispensaries. Ten years later, the number of missionary doctors and nurses increased dramatically. The Protestant missions alone had 106 female and 277 male foreign physicians, 119 Chinese physicians, 509 Chinese medical assistants, and 142 foreign and 734 Chinese nurses. In contrast to the male dominance of medical profession in America and Europe, almost half of the medical missionaries (foreign and Chinese combined) were female in China. Moreover, 23 missionary medical schools and 36 nursing schools were operating in China, spreading the learning of Western medicine. Applicants had to be Christians in order to be admitted into missionary schools. By 1923, China had 53 percent of the Christian missionary hospital beds in the world and 48 percent of missionary doctors.[64] They provided medical services to about 1.5 million people—a small fraction of the 400 million Chinese, but their influence reached far beyond the patients. Through medical service, hospitals and schools, the missionaries penetrated Chinese society much deeper and broader than Western merchants who stayed in treaty ports. Relying on the power and support of their home governments, missionaries meddled with local affairs and village disputes to protect the Chinese converts against the non-converts, even though the numbers of Chinese converts were fewer than one million by 1900. Missionary activities were so extensive that China was thought to have more of an impact on the missionary movement than the movement on China.[65] Their involvements in local disputes, in addition to foreign powers' military aggression against China, gave rise to increasing resentments among Chinese against foreigners.

One hundred Chinese cities were made treaty ports under the unequal treaty system by 1900. Shanghai, Tianjin, Guangzhou, Hankou, and Dalian were major urban centers of foreign settlements and businesses. Foreigners enjoyed superior social status and accumulated wealth, while the Chinese population provided cheap labor and fell into inferior status with increasing poverty and diseases. In the Western-dominated sections of treaty-port cities, the electric streetlights, clean environment, tall buildings and rich companies symbolized the progress and power of the West. Newcomers of the colonializing powers would pick up the arrogant and uncouth attitude to look down upon China and Chinese with their chins up. Foreign control of Chinese industries and the comprador competition resulted in cruel exploitations of Chinese laborers and created the most shocking conditions for the working poor. In this semi-colonial world of China, a hostile relation developed between foreigners who lived like overlords and the Chinese who were distained and insulted in their own country. The foreign attitude of superiority towards the Chinese and the Chinese resentment of foreign presence in their country contributed to the growth of a grass-roots movement of Chinese nationalism that aimed at driving out foreigners at the very end of the nineteenth century, the Boxer Uprising.[66]

The Boxer Uprising, public health and modern reforms

The anti-foreign imperialist sentiment took a traditional movement of peasants uprising in 1900 to express the wishes to rid China of foreigners. This was the movement of the "Righteous Fists of Harmony," known in the West as the Boxer Uprising. The Boxers attacked missionaries and Chinese Christian converts before they moved to Beijing to lay siege of foreign legations. Western powers plus Japan formed an army of joint military forces, known as the Eight-Nation Military Forces (八国联军), to suppress the uprising and lift the siege. During the violent suppression of the Boxers, the cities of Beijing and Tianjin were looted, burned and destroyed. Hundreds of thousands Chinese were killed and their mangled bodies filled the streets along with debris and dead animals.[67] Beijing, Tianjin and other cities in north China were occupied by foreign forces during 1900–1902. The Qing government negotiated and signed the Boxer Protocol in September 1901 with the eight powers of military forces plus Belgium, Spain and the Netherlands. In the Protocol, China was dictated, as it had always been since the 1842 Treaty of Nanjing, by the victorious powers to pay 450 million taels of silver—twice the Qing government's annual tax revenue—as indemnity. This exorbitant amount led to future negotiations between China and the powers, and the eventual return of significant amount of the indemnities by first the United States and then the other powers.[68]

The foreign powers had to deal with the carnage of war and the enormous public health problems during their occupation of Beijing and Tianjin. The horrors of human suffering during the destruction of Beijing and Tianjin were widely reported and studied in the literature of Boxer Uprising, but the details of sanitation management and control of daily life by the occupying forces were less examined. Michael Hunt started the pioneering work with an investigation of how foreign forces regulated the life of Beijing through public health control.[69] Rogaski's study of Tianjin detailed the hegemony of hygienic modernity and the demolition of Chinese houses and city walls in the name of getting rid of germs under the foreign rule.[70] A provisional government of foreign forces occupied Tianjin for 25 months (much longer than they did Beijing) till August 1902, even after the Boxer Protocol was signed.[71] They would not return the city to China unless the Qing government showed willingness and ability to continue public health services and modern administration. The occupation government had set up sanitary institutions similar to those in the West and physically altered Tianjin to fit Western-style architecture. They conducted invasive control of people's daily life in the name of sanitation and public health. The military control of hygiene and sanitation, ironically, did not save Tianjin from a cholera outbreak in the summer of 1902. The foreign military government formed a sanitary police to deal with the epidemic by inspecting suspected cholera cases and homes. In the meantime, foreign powers used the epidemic as an excuse to extract more territory from the Qing and to expand their control over larger areas beyond their settlements.

Public health administration was a characteristic benchmark of advanced Western nations in the late nineteenth century when governments of England, France, Germany, and the United States began to take responsibility for public health under the pressure of social reform movements.[72] Industrial pollutions, unsanitary working and living conditions, filthy and crowded urban slums, and nutritional deficiencies contributed to the increasing outbreaks of epidemic diseases, such as smallpox, malaria, typhus, typhoid, cholera, and tuberculosis in Western industrial centers. Social movements across Europe were "concerned with the health of towns, the role of medicine as a political force, and with health as a right of citizenship and with the relationship between sickness, poverty and death."[73] Social reformers and sanitarians addressed the relation between poverty and disease that industrialization and urbanization had brought about. In England the Poor Law Commission was instructed to investigate the health of working classes throughout the United Kingdom. As a result, England passed the Public Health Act in 1848 and established the General Board of Health and local sanitary authorities "to coordinate the municipal responsibilities for environmental regulation which had previously been chaotically distributed between myriad local commissions."[74] In the United States, early public health efforts were locally oriented and concentrated in a few big industrial cities such as Boston, New York and Newark. Vital statistics showed that "one out of 44 people died in 1863 in

Boston and one of 44 that year in Philadelphia, New York's rate was one in 36."[75] Following the British example of setting up an administrative mechanism in public health control, individual states and municipalities in America began to create their own boards of health in the 1870s–1880s to tackle epidemics and sanitary problems that had risen with industrialization and the influx of large numbers of immigrants.[76] The public health movement was associated with many other social reform movements in the West, particularly the reforms of city-planning, school hygiene, women and children affairs, and municipal administration and responsibilities. In this Western context of sanitation and social reforms, the provisional government of foreign forces in Beijing and Tianjin carried the banners of hygiene and modern municipal administration of public health, and measured China against the standards of the West.

China's lack of modern sanitary administration and professional knowledge became its weakness in the negotiations with foreign powers. When Tianjin was finally returned to the Qing government, the task of meeting foreign demands of a modern administration fell to the shoulders of Yuan Shikai (袁世凯, 1859–1916), who had favorably impressed the foreign powers because of his role in suppressing the Boxer Uprising in Shandong. In 1902 the Qing court made Yuan Shikai Viceroy of Zhili (直隶总督) and Minister of Beiyang (北洋通商大臣). Zhili was a vast region surrounding Beijing the capital, consisting of today's Liaoning, Hebei and Shandong provinces with Tianjin as the center. The Viceroy was automatically made the Minister of Beiyang in charge of trade and foreign affairs. Yuan spearheaded the institutional modernization of Zhili by establishing modern police, sanitary service, transportation, city-planning, education, military and government organization.[77] Details of reforms and modernization in Zhili were recorded in the *Beiyang gongdu leizhuan* (北洋公牍类纂).[78] In regard to hygiene and public health, a sanitary department was created in the modern police system of Tianjin, to take care of street-cleaning, inspection and prevention of diseases, medical care, relief for the poor, and welfare services that used to be offered by Chinese merchant-gentry and government offices. Tianjin, like other Chinese cities, traditionally had various Chinese charitable organizations, such as Yuli Tang (育黎堂, originally created in 1687 for homeless people and changed names several times to become Jiuji Yuan 救济院 in 1912) and Guangren Tang (广仁堂, established in 1878 for disaster-affected women and children).[79] Furthermore, the Beiyang Sanitary Service (北洋防疫处) was created in 1902 in charge of sanitation and inspection of contagious diseases at ports and railway stations in Zhili. Yuan Shikai re-organized the medical school that was established by his mentor Li Hongzhang (李鸿章, 1823–1901) in 1881 into the Imperial Army Medical College. For women and children, the Tianjin Women's Hospital (天津公立女医局) was established in 1902 and the Beiyang Women's Medical School (北洋女医学堂), the first government-run women's medical school in China, was created in 1907.[80] Yuan Shikai invited Jin Yunmei, after learning about her as a distinguished woman physician, to head the women's medical department in Tianjin. The women's hospital and medical school were merged in 1909 as the Beiyang Women's Medical School and Hospital (北洋女医学堂和女医院) with Jin Yunmei as the supervisor.

The hospital had 22 beds, offering medical services to women and children as well as training women nurses. In 1915 Jin Yunmei went back to the United States with a plan to visit hospitals on the east coast and to update herself with the latest medical practices.[81]

In the modernization endeavor, Yuan Shikai relied heavily on Japan as the model, and used Japanese expertise to train Chinese technical personnel for the modern programs. Japan had successfully modernized itself by learning from the West and used primarily Germany as the model for Meiji reforms. Yuan invited Japanese instructors to train Chinese police with sanitary inspection, and employed Japanese doctors and professors at the Imperial Army Medical College. The police training manual included a wide range of sanitary responsibilities. They included (1) sanitary inspection of street-cleaning and maintenance of wells, rivers, and public toilets; (2) public health matters such as the examination and qualification of doctors and midwives, inspection of pharmacies and drug control, inspection of food hygiene and safety, inspection of slaughterhouses, barbershops and bathhouses, and health examination of prostitutes; and (3) prevention and inspection of eight epidemic diseases of cholera, dysentery, typhoid, typhus fever, smallpox, diphtheria, scarlet fever, and plague.[82] The job description of Chinese sanitary police was almost a direct translation of the Japanese sanitary police handbook. How effectively did the Chinese sanitary police implement these duties remains a subject of further studies, for there is little information available. Wu Liande once criticized that the Beiyang Sanitary Service "usually meant cleaning of the streets and removal of garbage."[83] Nonetheless, the modern initiatives of sanitation and disease prevention in Tianjin helped shape the construction of a modest modern infrastructure of sanitary police that proved handy later in the fight against the Manchurian plague in 1910.[84]

The Beiyang Sanitary Service marked the beginning of modern Chinese public health administration. Subsequently, sanitary bureaus were set up in major cities of different provinces. The modernization initiatives in Zhili strengthened Yuan's influence in the Qing court and the reforms under the "New Policy." The Qing court issued edicts of sweeping reforms to modernize China in the wake of the Boxer suppression. Yuan Shikai's experiment with a variety of modernization projects, such as police, education, and the military, gave the Qing court confidence to go ahead with national reforms. Yuan was instrumental in the creation of a Ministry of Education (学部) and a Ministry of Police (巡警部) of the Qing government. In 1905, acting on Yuan's advice, Empress Dowager Cixi issued a decree to end the traditional Confucian examination system in 1906 and to create, instead, a new school system, in which subjects of science were emphasized for study. Moreover, the Ministry of Police was established with a Sanitary Department in 1905, following the example of Meiji Japan. The central sanitary department was in charge of public health administration through local branches with the responsibility of disease prevention, vaccination, drug traffic inspection, water safety, and quarantine. The Ministry of Police was later changed to the Ministry of Civil Affairs (民政部). In 1906, several government hospitals were opened in major cities under the sanitary department of the Ministry of Civil Affairs.[85]

The Qing court took several steps to modernize medical education by introducing the learning of Western medicine. As early as 1865, John Dudgeon, the Scottish medical missionary, was hired by the Qing court to teach Western medicine in the Department of Science of *Tongwen Guan* (同文馆, the Academy of Foreign Languages). That was the beginning of modern medical education in China according to Chen Bangxian, the Chinese historian of medicine.[86] Work on modern medicine was slow and limited, however. In 1903, the Qing court added a medical laboratory to the Imperial University of Beijing, which became the Medical Academy in 1905 and taught both Western and Chinese medicines. To facilitate the training of Chinese in Western medicine, the Qing Ministry of Education made an agreement with the Japanese Ministry of Education about admission of Chinese students at Japanese medical colleges.[87] The Qing government also proposed a curriculum for Chinese medical colleges in 1905, which generated a heated debate among Chinese reformers. The curriculum, which included more than 30 required courses of science subjects, was similar to that of Japanese medical colleges except that anatomy and histology were not included. The explanation was that Chinese cultural ethics and customs were different from foreign countries and that things should not be forced upon the Chinese. The proposal recommended that instead of cadavers, models be used for the purpose of studying dissection. These recommendations signified the continuation of the Chinese traditional method of using models, not real human corpses, to study the composition of the human body. The proposal also recommended that since Chinese diet and customs were different from foreigners, internal medicine, surgery, women's and children's medicine should all consult and refer to the best of Chinese medical books while the rest should use the translation of the best foreign medical books.[88]

Critics of the proposed curriculum disputed the real reasons of the omissions of anatomy and histology. They pointed out three fundamental problems of the proposal. First, since anatomy and histology were of foundation medical studies, medical education without them was like a building without foundation. Second, the proposed curriculum conflicted with the third category of subjects in the reformed higher education curriculum, i.e. the pre-medical curriculum. As the basic courses on animals and plants and on German language were part of the pre-medical curriculum, students were expected to conduct scientific experiment and research in the tradition of German schools. Why should medical students not continue the basic medical science at college with anatomy and histology? Third, the proposal veered off the reform principle, because it tried to restrict medical studies by excluding anatomy and histology with the pretext of different culture and customs.[89] The debate of the curriculum clearly demonstrated the tension between the pro-tradition conservatives and the pro-reform modernizers. The exclusion of anatomy and histology indeed reflected the thinking of cultural conservatism, but the citing of cultural and dietary differences was not without ground in the argument for particular medical attentions. Medicine, as it directly interferes with individual bodies and the health of people, is increasingly understood in the context of local environments and individual lifestyles, particularly the ecology of disease.

The Chinese educated elite, particularly those who were influenced by modern medical education, were anxious to urge the government to accept Western medicine and emulate the West so that China would be modernized to join the "civilized world." Central to their concern was the potential of modern medicine to strengthen the Chinese nation in the struggle against foreign powers and their scramble to carve up China. They focused their attention on the relation between medicine and the society, and how medical modernization would be an essential step to revive the Chinese nation. To Chinese reformist intellectuals, scientific medicine and public health would not only make the Chinese people healthy but also advance China as a strong nation in the modern world. Little wonder a marked increase of publications on hygiene and public health appeared in Chinese newspapers and magazines at the beginning of the twentieth century.

Social Darwinism and national strength

Major newspapers, such as *Dagongbao* (*Ta Kung Pao*, 大公报) and *Shenbao* (申报), frequently reported and commented on medicine and public health, having a broad influence on public consumption of medical and health knowledge and the prevention of epidemics. Both newspapers published weekly medical supplements (医学周刊) to disseminate Western and Chinese medical knowledge as well as hygiene. The widely circulated magazine, *Dongfang zazhi* (东方杂志, *Eastern Miscellany*), regularly published articles and editorials on hygiene and medicine as well, where the discussion often centered on the relation between medicine, social progress, and national strength. In analyzing the importance of medical progress to the power of nation, one author criticized China's neglect of medical learning, praised the medical progress and power of the West, and commented on Japan's learning of Western medicine and modern success.[90] Chinese intellectuals increasingly interpreted modern medicine and hygiene as a measure and manifestation of national power and advance. Another writer simply stated that civilized nations with superior people all had detailed laws and regulations on hygiene, whereas nations that did not have hygiene laws were weak and had inferior people.[91] These writings all pointed to the connection of hygiene and modern Western medicine to national progress and power.

To many Chinese, the question of hygiene and public health was directly tied to China's struggle to survive foreign dominance. From the late nineteenth to the early twentieth centuries, educated Chinese were increasingly influenced by the social and political theories of the West, such as Social Darwinism and the racial argument of white superiority. Social Darwinian theories were first introduced to China by Yan Fu (严复， 1854–1921), who translated works of Thomas Huxley, John Mill, Adam Smith, and Herbert Spencer.[92] Yan Fu was sent by the Chinese government in 1877 to study technology at the naval schools of Portsmouth and Greenwich in England, but he spent time exploring Western political and legal theories and practices. After returning to China, he made recommendations on reforms but his ideas were not adopted by the Qing court. In contrast, his Japanese counterparts contributed significantly to their country's reforms of modernization.

Yan was disappointed with Qing's reluctance to reform. After the 1895 Sino-Japanese War, Yan Fu started a prolific career of translating Western works of Social Darwinism, partly spurred by China's defeat in the war and partly by his frustration with the Qing government. His translations formed the bulk of Social Darwinist readings in China that influenced reformists and revolutionaries alike in the nationalist movement to build a strong China. The translation of Western literature by Lin Shu (林纾, 1852–1924) further popularized Social Darwinian ideas in China.[93] The concepts of "natural selection" and "survival of the fittest" shaped Chinese intellectuals' interpretation of national survival in the age of global imperialist aggression. They conceptualized national strength in terms of people's physical fitness, moral virtues and knowledge of science. Popular magazines, professional journals, and newspapers all talked about competition (竞争) and evolution (进化), shaping a new intellectual orientation and discourse. Even school textbooks used Social Darwinian discourse to teach the "evolution" of the five thousand years of Chinese civilization.

The meaning of "competition" and "evolution" was understood on both personal and national levels. British philosopher Herbert Spencer's interpretation of individuals as cells of a social organism brought home to Chinese modernizers the vital importance of individuals to the well-being of the nation. They learned that Western nations all promoted public health and emphasized the physical education of people. Yan Fu believed that he had discovered the source of Western power when he noticed the different emphases between Western and Chinese education. In his observation of Europe, England in particular, Yan Fu noticed that Western education stressed the physical fitness of people, whereas Chinese education focused on learning and despised physical prowess. Yan Fu thought that physical strength was an important element of national strength, and he conveyed the idea to his countrymen by advocating physical fitness of the masses as one of the fundamentals to China's national revival. In his 1895 article titled "On Strength" (原强), Yan Fu articulated his ideas of training Chinese people to be strong in intelligence, physical fitness, and moral virtues (民智, 民力, 民德), as the three vital elements to achieve national greatness.[94] He advocated education of the masses, not a small number of elite, as the fundamental means to re-build China into a strong country. At the Global Chinese Students Association, Yan Fu criticized the many failures of the Qing's educational reforms and specified the criteria for each level of education. The importance was to educate the masses to raise national literacy, he emphasized.[95] Modern education was to make people strong, mentally and physically, in a world of competing nations. In light of the high illiteracy rate (almost 90 percent) in China, Yan Fu's articulation on mass education could not have been more urgent.

Other reformists also talked about the importance of education and physical fitness of the people as vital means to regain national strength. Liang Qichao (梁启超，1873–1929) asked why Western powers did not invade each other but scrambled for China. The reason, he argued, was not external but internal factors, for each of those Western nations was strong and China was weak. He believed that the only hope to gain national strength was to develop nationalism through creating new citizens of strong moral virtues, intelligence and physical fitness. Liang Qichao realized that the national crisis could not be handled by a statesman or a few heroes. Instead, if the 400 million Chinese people were made strong and be able to defend their country, then foreign powers would no longer be a danger to China.[96]

The Social Darwinian interpretation of national survival developed when China faced the danger of being carved up like a melon by foreign powers and the Chinese nation being wiped out as a result. The powers had intensified their scramble for China in the wake of the 1895 Sino-Japanese war. By the turn of the twentieth century, China was divided up into "spheres of influence" by Britain, France, Japan, Russia, and Germany; all of them had territory concessions in China. The profound national crisis led some frustrated Chinese reformists to seek the desperate strategy of encouraging provinces to go de facto independent from the central Qing government so that China might be saved in part for future national revival and unification.[97] Fear of the dismemberment of their country, coupled with the knowledge of Japan's success and the tragic fate of such distinctive civilizations as India, Egypt, and the Ottoman Empire, precipitated the literati's urgent calls for fundamental reforms of the traditional polity of the Qing system. Japan's military victory over China in 1895, ironically, made many Chinese realize that an Asian nation could become modern and strong through fundamental reforms. Japan's triumph over Russia in 1905 once again illustrated the successful results of its reforms. This time, Japan's victory discredited the racial argument of white supremacy and posed a serious challenge to the absolute Western dominance of Asia. An American YMCA secretary witnessed China ablaze with patriotism, for Japan's victory was "not only a release, but a revelation—a revelation that after all the European, even in arms, was not superior to the Asiatic."[98] The realization that race had nothing to do with a nation's status increased Chinese confidence in national rejuvenation with a nationwide patriotic movement. A similar impact was seen in India, where nationalist sentiment against the British rule surged. The rise of a new national spirit of patriotism marked the birth of modern Chinese nationalism that aimed at shaking off the yoke of foreign powers and making their country sovereign, modern and strong. Thousands of Chinese students went to Japan to study, hoping to find out the secrets of its success in order to save China.[99]

Japan was a compelling illustration of a formerly weak country that edged into the ranks of international powers by emphasizing literacy and physical fitness of its people through universal education and public health programs.[100] China tried to follow Japan in the reforms of modernization. The modern school system established after the abolition of the traditional examination system in 1905 emphasized science and Western learning.[101] The principal goals were to cultivate intelligence, physical fitness, and morality in training a new population of citizens in China.[102] Physical education (体育) was now being indigenized to serve the goals of building a strong country. The Spencerian concept of cells to a social organism informed the Chinese understanding of the relation of individuals to the nation. Contrary to Andrew Morris' claim that "the supremacy of the individual body" was accepted, the physical fitness of individuals was emphasized only to strengthen the county.[103] Chinese modernizers did not extol the personal achievement of physical prowess but the collective strength of the people for the sake of the nation. To reformers and revolutionaries alike, nothing but the strength and wholeness of the Chinese nation was supreme.

The Spencerian interpretation further shaped a changing image of China as a national body (国体). A new discourse emerged in public speeches about the "national body," which appeared in school textbooks, political tracts, literary pieces, newspapers, and magazines at the turn of the twentieth century. China was referred to as an ailing body that needed serious surgical operation and treatment. The discourse of national body intensified the relation of the individual to the nation in the sense that the country's fate was simultaneously the individual's fate. The infusion of the national and the personal existence was vividly expressed in anti-imperialist campaigns. When a student described the urgent situation of China's national crisis to people on the street, the very presence of his own existence began to embody the nation:

> . . . China, today, is like me—one body—whilst the eighteen provinces are like my head, arms and legs. The Japanese have occupied my head; the Germans have occupied my left shoulder; the French have occupied my right shoulder; the Russians have occupied my back, and the English my abdomen; then there is Italy which is riding my left leg and the United States is astride my right leg. Alas! Alas! As you can see, my body has been divided up and occupied by all these people! Tell me, how can I continue to exist?[104]

Chinese leading intellectuals considered mental and physical fitness the essential foundation of a strong modern nation. They believed that in a world of competing nations, the strong and superior (优) would survive and the weak and inferior (劣) would be weeded out. Modern medicine and public health appealed to Chinese officials and scholars in a new perspective of building national strength. Kang Youwei (康有为, 1858–1927) made a careful comparison between Japan's rapid adoption of Western medicine and public health measures and China's slow move in this direction.[105] Chinese medicine, meanwhile, faced increasing criticisms that it had low standards with widespread quackery. Although the Qing government had laws that required "any person practicing medicine without permission from the proper authorities" to be subject to a fine, enforcement of the law was lax when the empire declined.[106] The stress of the importance of medicine in national progress prompted more attention to rigorous supervision. In an attempt to show publicly that the government upheld high standards of Chinese medicine, Duanfang (端方, 1861–1911), the Viceroy of Liangjiang (Jiangsu and Zhejiang provinces), held an examination for 900 Chinese medical doctors in Nanjing in 1908. Those achieving three highest grades received government license; others were forbidden to practice. The Chinese medical scholar Ding Fubao (丁福保, 1874–1952) established a "Chinese and Western Medical Research Council" in Shanghai with a regular publication of *Journal of Chinese and Western Medicine* (中西医学报).[107] The purpose was to connect and combine the two medicines and to use modern scientific concepts to explain and theorize Chinese medicine.[108] Liang Qichao commented: "Today the practice of medicine is the noblest profession in the world."[109] Shanghai local gentry such as Li Shutong (李叔同) and Mu Shuzhai (穆恕斋) organized the "Society of Shanghai Studies" (沪学会) in 1904 to promote the change of habits to improve sanitary conditions and to strengthen the nation. Shanghai saw the publication of a vernacular newspaper on hygiene in May 1908.[110] Chinese modernizers urged the emulation of Western-style health system to create a clean and healthy Chinese nation.

The Manchurian plague and national sovereignty

The concept of public health was barely germinating in the public consciousness when a major epidemic of plague broke out in the northeast of China, a region referred to as Manchuria by foreigners, hence known as the Manchurian plague in the West. The great scholar on central Asia and Mongolia, Owen Lattimore, once pointed out that the name Manchuria:

> is of foreign origin and has no proper Chinese translation. It derives from the fact that foreign political rivalry for the control of China in the later nineteenth century first made Manchuria a region to be dealt with as a whole.[111]

The Chinese name for the region was simply the three northeastern provinces (东三省). I will use northeast rather than Manchuria in this discussion.

From October 1910 to March 1911, the northeast of China suffered the deadliest epidemic of pneumonic plague in modern Chinese history, costing more than 60,000 human lives and 100 million dollars financial losses.[112] The first signs of the plague appeared in Manzhouli (满洲里), a train station town on the Chinese border with Russia.[113] In six months, the disease invaded a "huge distance of 1700 miles" along railway lines and roads, infecting cities, towns, and villages in its path. It surged southwards, threatening the cities of Beijing and Tianjin and the provinces of Hebei and Shandong before it was brought under control.[114] The ferocious plague was suppressed only after extensive application of modern methods of quarantine, isolation, disinfection, and cremation. In bringing the plague under control, the Chinese government proved to international powers that China had the ability to deal with epidemic crisis and provide protection for the public. In the high time of foreign competition to scramble for China, the success to control the plague epidemic was of immeasurable importance to the Chinese government to maintain sovereignty over the northeast and the entire country.

The competition of foreign powers to expand their territory in the region revealed the intrigue of international politics during the plague crisis.[115] Japan and Russia, which had concessions in the region, were eager to expand their interest with the pretense of plague prevention. The international complication of plague management made the epidemic as much a public health crisis as a political struggle for China to keep itself intact. In the efforts to prevent the spread of the disease, Chinese authorities restricted railway travel, set up inspection points at railway stations, and distributed leaflets on methods of prevention. But the Russian government developed a scheme to bring "a joint pressure of the Powers" on the Chinese government. The Russian ambassador in Washington sent the State Department a memorandum on January 19, 1911, in which he criticized the Chinese anti-plague measures as "neither rational nor efficacious," and demanded that "China should entrust to foreign physicians the care of deciding upon such measures."[116] Japan, meanwhile, prepared for an invasion of the northeast of China, by moving its troops in Korea to the Chinese border and setting up barracks of thousands of soldiers in each of the twenty points along the railway. Moreover, Japan dispatched the 11th Division of the Japanese Army as re-enforcement and a high military advisor to inspect the installations. The Japanese repeatedly pressured Xi Liang (锡良, 1853–1917), Viceroy of the three northeastern provinces of Fengtian (奉天, Liaoning province today), Jilin (吉林) and Heilongjia (黑龙江), to let Japanese police handle the plague prevention. Adamantly upholding Chinese authorities in the region, Xi Liang made clear that "Japanese police activity outside Japanese sphere of jurisdiction was most unwelcome."[117]

The Russian and the Japanese reaction to the plague epidemic was nothing out of the ordinary in terms of their colonial ambitions in China. Before the outbreak of the plague, Japan and Russia had already decided on carving up China's northeast in their secret protocols of 1907 and 1910. The plague crisis only provided a convenient opportunity for the two to take advantage of the weakened China. They maintained that China did not have the scientific medical ability to prevent and control the plague. Even Japanese and Russian medical scientists adopted an arrogant attitude towards the Chinese medical scientists.[118] Under the predatory watch of foreign powers, China's fight against the plague epidemic became a fight to keep its sovereignty and a contest to prove its ability to control the plague epidemic.

High officials, such as Xi Liang and Alfred Sao-ke Sze (施肇基, 1877–1958) the special envoy of the Qing court, rose to the occasion and showed their political craftsmanship and administrative skills during the crisis. They managed to convince the Qing leaders to use modern medical methods to fight the plague and to keep Russia and Japan at bay. Their effective weapon to fend off the Russian and Japanese aggression was a young medical scientist by the name of Wu Liande (Wu Lien-teh, 伍连德, 1879–1960), who was a graduate of Cambridge University. Wu was serving as deputy director of the Imperial Army Medical College of the Chinese government in Tianjin. They asked him to head the anti-plague operation in the northeast. Wu came with an assistant to the hard-hit city of Harbin in December 1910 and immediately introduced modern methods of preventive medicine with full force of practice.[119] The success of bringing the plague under control within four months of his arrival was hailed as both a medical achievement and a political and diplomatic triumph for China. China hosted an International Plague Conference in April 1911, where the creation of North Manchurian Plague Prevention Service was recommended. The establishment of this new institution of public health with Wu Liande at its helm firmly consolidated the legitimacy of Chinese public health authority as well as Chinese political sovereignty in the northeast.[120] More importantly, the battle against the plague gave birth to a new system of public health management in China, staffed with medical scientists.

Modern prevention measures and traditional social customs

Wu Liande, in his prolific writing, had always described the Manchurian plague fight as the beginning of the Chinese modern public health system, despite the fact that Yuan Shikai initiated sanitary service in Zhili in 1902 and the Qing created a sanitary police in 1905. Scholars seemed to agree that the institutionalization of public health management and epidemic prevention with medical science started with the North Manchurian Plague Prevention Service.[121] Indeed, the Chinese government for the first time relied on Western-trained medical scientists to suppress the epidemic in 1910. As neither Chinese medicine nor Western medicine had a cure for plague at the time, the main efforts focused on prevention and containment. In the early stage of the anti-plague operation, the Chinese government isolated the sick and gave families money to bury their dead with coffins provided. When these measures of traditional administrative handling did not help to control the plague, the government, urged on by Wu Liande, abandoned them and began the modern methods of vigorous quarantine, isolation, disinfection, and cremation of the dead. In each city district, a man of some medical knowledge was put in charge if fully qualified doctors were not available, and under him were assistants, sanitary police, and disinfecting workers and bearers.[122]

The huge demand of house inspection, disinfection and isolation work led to the fast expansion of police in Fengtian. A small police was originally established in 1902, but by 1911 a total of 19,197 policemen at 218 police departments carried out the duty of inspecting major cities and towns in Fengtian province alone.[123] Military troops were also sent to assist the enforcement of anti-plague measures, as cremation and modern methods of plague prevention were not popular with the public. The deployment of tens of thousands of troops and policemen to fight the plague was unprecedented in Chinese history. To prevent the plague from reaching south of the Great Wall, traffic was stopped between the northeast and the rest of China. In the northeast, train passengers were inspected, and those suspected of infection were quarantined. The healthy ones were released after five or seven days of quarantine; those infected were sent to the plague hospitals, where few came out alive. Household inspection, disinfection, quarantine, and isolation were widely applied to residencies in the cities.[124] Despite these efforts, the plague continued to scourge cities and rural towns in big strides. When the Chinese New Year drew closer, laborers and migrant workers took to the roads to go home for the festival and to flee the plague. They tried to avoid official checkpoints of anti-plague authorities, thereby unwittingly helped spread the disease.

The Chinese government sought the cooperation and assistance of foreign health specialists such as missionary doctors and foreign medical scientists to fight the plague. When these men of medical profession plunged into the anti-plague operations, they risked their lives, too. The plague made no preference of race and profession. Medical professionals of Chinese and Western origin became infected when treating plague patients and died on duty. Even doctors who had received prophylactic vaccine, such as Xu Shiming (徐世明), Gérald Mesny, and Arthur Jackson, were struck down by the plague when working with patients. Arthur Jackson was a young athletic missionary of 26 years old with an education in arts and medicine from Cambridge University. He came to join the Scottish Presbyterian Mission in Shengyang in November 1910, and was asked to take charge of the anti-plague inspection in January 1911 on the Shengyang-to-Shanhaiguan line of the Imperial North China Railways. After eight days of inspecting hundreds of poor laborers in the third-class trains and housing them in small inns for quarantine, he fell ill with the plague and died within two days. Viceroy Xi Liang and the Chinese government set up a memorial fund for him at the Fengtian Medical College as token of appreciation of his service.[125] All the anti-plague workers—medical staff, police, ambulance men, cooks, house inspectors and anti-plague soldiers—risked their lives when fighting the disease. At an isolation station in Changchun (长春), the entire medical staff of 19 was infected and 18 of them died.[126] Altogether, a total of 297 out of 2943 anti-plague workers died.[127] The Chinese government established a compensation system for those who sacrificed their lives in the plague fight. A doctor would receive 10,000 taels of silver, while a student would receive 5000 taels.[128] The battle against the plague was won, but the fight cost the Qing government an enormous amount of monetary and human resources and further weakened the financial and social stability of the Qing system.

Of all the plague victims, the poor coolies and the illiterate villagers suffered the most because they had neither the economic means to seek better sanitation nor the health knowledge to protect themselves. Mark Gamsa described:

> Hovels with no sanitary facilities, where windows were kept shut throughout the long Manchurian winter, and the coal-heated *kang* (a raised brick and mud bed) was shared at night by men who had spent their days in hard physical labor, became the natural breeding grounds of infection.[129]

In a hamlet called Red Rock in the Daling District of Yushu County (榆树县), the plague spread to every household after Guo Laoshi (Guo the number 10), an inn keeper in the county town, came home for the Chinese New Year. Before his return, two merchants from Harbin had died in his inn, followed by the death of an inn clerk. Guo died on the eve of Chinese New Year. His family kept his corpse for five days according to local customs; that led to the deaths of 32 of his family of 53. The plague then spread to the whole hamlet, taking away another hundred lives.[130] The internalized value of cultural traditions and customs of daily life were hard to discard even in time of crisis. On the contrary, they became the only recourse available for people to turn to for solace and guidance. Traditions such as a proper burial in the hometown of the dead offered the living a sort of psychological comfort of obligation to the dead.

Eventually, dead bodies were piling up and lying around with no family members left to take care of them by late January 1911. "The son mourned the death of his father in the morning, but by evening the son himself died of the same disease," reported *Dagongbao*.[131] The terror of plague struck the heart of everyone, and the ghost of death, omnipresent, danced among the poor and the distressed. In Harbin, the many unburied dead lying on the frozen grounds became a public menace and getting worse. Facing this new crisis, Wu Liande made an unusual request to the Qing government, asking for permission to cremate the dead. Cremation of the dead was a taboo to the Chinese custom of keeping the body intact for burial. Granting the permission would be extremely unpopular, but the Qing government gave Wu the green light anyway. The decision may have been prompted by necessity rather than progressive thinking on the part of the Qing court; it nonetheless gestured the government's shift from traditional conservatism to modern methods of handling health crisis. Wu led more than 200 workers to collect the dead bodies in fierce cold winter. They divided the corpses into 22 piles with 100 each, and then poured gasoline to set them on fire. The open cremation stretched over one *li* (里, half a kilometer).[132] Other cities followed suit by building cremation sites. Not only the dead bodies but the belongings of the plague victims and their vacant houses were burned down in areas of the cities.

Local people were terrified that the dead and their belongings were treated in this disrespectful manner. To the common folks, the invasive and disruptive methods of plague prevention were unnecessarily harsh and insensitive to their way of life. They brought man-made disaster upon the nature-made plague to the people. Modern measures of isolating the sick from home and cremating the dead clashed with Chinese traditional values of filial piety and respect for the dead. Moreover, destruction of the infected houses and belongings added economic loss to the grief of the suffering family. "When a shop was forcibly closed and disinfected, and twenty-nine persons removed from it to an isolation station because of the death of a thirtieth, the merchants were highly incensed. . . . When the house-to-house visitation began it caused much fear."[133] In the beginning, the majority of the people did not understand the scientific rational behind the tough handling of the infected people and places. The isolated patients in the deadly quarantine stations became desperate when they were completely cut off from families and the outside world. Some tried to escape from the stations, which were guarded by armed soldiers. One anti-plague doctor reported that "isolation camps were at first a source of great dread."[134] Government regulations specified heavy punishment for anyone who attempted to escape. A public notice at Fengtian isolation hospitals read that if anyone dared to escape, he would be shot, in order to prevent the spread of the plague, for public good.[135]

Some merchants resisted the government's strict and sometimes excessive anti-plague measures by running their own anti-plague operation and keeping their shops open. In Shenyang, a merchant house set up isolation quarters for the sick on one side of the compound and treated plague cases with Chinese medicine with little precaution. As a result, the plague spread and took the lives of the doctors and the isolated patients. In consternation, the merchants allowed the police to disinfect and shut down the place. But it was too late, the plague had spread and 251 people died after their 12 days of experiment of self-operation.[136] Only through tragic events like that did people learn the terrible consequences of not cooperating with the anti-plague authorities. Sometimes, pure innocence and ignorance led people into plague traps. When a family died of the plague, neighbors "buried the bodies and helped themselves to the contents of the house—clothing, beddings, etc., even the matting on which the stricken had lain."[137] A few days later, people began to die until the whole village was lost. Individuals and families did not cooperate with the health authorities in the early stage of the plague because of fear of isolation and other measures of prevention more than the plague itself. Tragic experiences eventually made people realize the deadly transmission of the disease and the necessity of following the instructions of anti-plague officials.

Educational efforts were made by the Chinese anti-plague authorities. Large quantities of anti-plague placards and pamphlets were printed and distributed to instruct people how to prevent the entrance of plague into their communities and villages. But high illiteracy of the people hindered the educational effect.[138] In rural areas, it was common that the whole hamlet was illiterate. Communication of anti-plague notices and regulations to the common folks could only be achieved through public reading of government announcements and instruction, which had historically been a practice in Chinese society. In the adjacent villages of Shenyang, the provincial capital that housed the central anti-plague bureau, thousands of placards and leaflets were distributed to "be read in every village and homestead."[139] Some villages with effective leaders were able to conduct self-isolation by turning away out-of-town guests and returnees. Official reports attributed the self-defense to the educational effect of anti-plague leaflets sent by the government.[140]

Before the true culprit of the plague epidemic was scientifically identified, everybody assumed that rats caused the plague. People in the northeast and in big cities across China were encouraged with monetary rewards to catch mice to prevent plague. In the northeast, government regulations specified that every mouse caught alive would be rewarded with seven copper coins by the police. All the captured mice were destroyed at the mice burning sites. Fengtian province alone handled more than 80,972 mice.[141] In Hankou, the reward was two copper coins for a mouse brought to the police; and in Tianjin it was one copper coin for a mouse.[142] Newspapers like *Shengjin Shibao* (盛京时报), *Shengbao*, and *Dagongbao* widely reported the activities of mice catching to prevent plague. The newspapers even created a special section on plague prevention, disseminating preventive medical knowledge and encouraging people to adopt modern hygiene and sanitation. Rats and plague were therefore inseparably linked in people's minds. Only later did medical scientists find that the Siberian marmots—whose fur was so highly desired, not rats, were the transmitter of the devastating pneumonic plague.[143]

The plague fight extensively mobilized the Chinese bureaucratic system as well. The Ministry of Civil Affairs followed the example of Western nations by setting up a Health Board (*weisheng hui*,卫生会) to work with other government agencies and persons of Western medicine in making health rules and regulations.[144] In every *xian* (县, county), the lowest level of Chinese bureaucracy, anti-plague agencies were established. County officials mobilized village heads and elders to make sure government anti-plague notices were conveyed to the common folks and anti-plague measures carried out. However, local officials generally knew little of modern methods of prevention. In cities and urban centers where modern police force was put to action, plague prevention was more effective as inspection and disinfection were carried out.

In contrast to the violence and social disorder recorded in many societies at times of rampant epidemics, few violent social riots were reported during the 1910 plague epidemic, probably because of the deployment of military soldiers in the anti-plague operations.[145] Chinese resistance to modern prevention took the form of escaping the quarantine and hiding the sick and the dead. There was also suspicion among the Chinese that Japanese agents poisoned the wells in order to destroy the Chinese people and take Chinese land.[146] Studies of epidemics in different societies indicate that blaming the enemy was quite a common phenomenon. When China's northeast suffered the plague, southern Italy witnessed a cholera epidemic in 1910, where rumor of poisoning was widespread as well.[147] In the treaty ports of China, however, plague scare triggered widespread fear of epidemics and excessive regulations of health matters in foreign settlements. The British-controlled Shanghai Municipal Council drafted a health notification that required that no one in the International Settlement who was known suffering from plague, "smallpox, cholera, typhoid fever, typhus fever, diphtheria, scarlet fever, tuberculosis, anthrax, glanders, leprosy, hydrophobia, beriberi, and other infectious disease of which the Health Officer may from time to time require notice" was allowed to "milk any animal or wash any clothes or engage in any trade business or occupation."[148] The penalty for violation was "one hundred dollars or two months' imprisonment with or without hard labor."[149] There were 13,000 foreigners (4465 of them were British) and 410,000 Chinese living in the International Settlement in 1910.[150] Many of the Chinese residents were in service occupations, and they would lose their livelihood under this sweeping health regulation. When the Municipal Council sent health inspectors to homes of Chinese residents, tensions heightened. A few Chinese were taken away for isolation simply because they looked sick, and their homes disinfected. Some families faced the danger of being evicted or having their houses demolished. Resentment of wanton inspections and fear of mistreatment at the hands of foreigners led Chinese to health protests and riots. The Council deployed the physically mighty Sikh policemen to round up the Chinese and sent them to court. The arrested Chinese were put on public trial without being granted proper legal rights or protection. Despite their statement in court that they supported the health measures, the Chinese were punished with prison terms and hard labor.[151]

To protect the interests of Chinese residents, the Shanghai Chinese Chamber of Commerce made a request to the Council that the health measures be restricted to plague only and "not include other infectious diseases," because the enforcement of "such severe measure against ordinary infectious diseases would result in great inconvenience to the majority of Chinese residents who . . . do not have the services of foreign physicians but accustomed to treat these diseases in the manner prescribed by Chinese doctors."[152] They argued that the health measures should respect Chinese culture and social customs. Among the Chinese residents in the Settlement were wealthy merchants, financiers, and professionals of doctors and lawyers who had gained significant influence in the Shanghai business and political world. The Municipal Council had to negotiate with the Chinese elite and Shanghai magistrate because the daily life of the International Settlement depended upon Chinese services, not to mention the importance of keeping normal relations with Chinese businesses. Subsequently, the Council revised the health measures and specified only plague as the epidemic to be inspected in the public health notification. The Chinese elite's success in negotiation with the Municipal Council over health regulations indicated their ability to broker a compromise to alleviate the tension between foreign dominance and Chinese resistance and to win the right to take control of health matters by the Chinese themselves during the plague epidemic.

Newspaper reports and government health notifications contributed to public awareness of plague and the modern preventive methods. Both the central government and local authorities issued anti-plague regulations over bath-houses, inns and guest-houses and used inspection, isolation, disinfection and quarantine. Cities and towns also formed anti-plague organizations and emphasized the methods of isolation and quarantine to prevent the transmission of plague. They printed and distributed anti-plague pamphlets in colloquial Chinese for ordinary people. Media, particularly newspapers, played an extraordinary role in reporting the plague fight and disseminating scientific health information. They urged the establishment of anti-plague institutions across the country and encouraged people to change their unsanitary ways of life that were prone to spreading plague. Although plague vaccines were available to those in foreign settlements, they were too rare and expensive for ordinary Chinese. The Chinese medical scholar and doctor Ding Fubao appealed to the public that the most effective methods of preventing plague were to disinfect the house and pay attention to hygiene.[153] He even emphasized that public health should be an important work of local administration.[154] Wu Liande and his associates who worked at the forefront of the plague fight were acutely aware of the importance of public health education in the prevention of disease. They thought that the people were ignorant (*yumei*, 愚昧) and superstitious (*mixin*, 迷信), who had to be enlightened in the scientific knowledge of medicine. Medical scientists were determined to awaken the populace as well as the officialdom in the scientific knowledge of medicine, by which they meant Western medicine. Chinese medical scientists regarded the promotion of public health and modern medicine part of national modernization. Small in number, they nonetheless were ambitious to transform Chinese society through medical science. The reality was, however, that Chinese people relied on Chinese medicine as they had been for thousands of years and that they knew little about Western medicine, not to mention to use and trust it. The promotion of public health, in fact, served to spread the knowledge of Western medicine and create a science-based medical system to transform China.

Public health and Western medicine

In the first decade of the twentieth century, increasing numbers of Chinese students returned home after completing their education in Europe, America and Japan. Those who studied medicine were influenced by the latest development of bacteriology and biology, and the germ theory, which led to the preventive medicine to protect people from transmittable diseases. Hygiene and sanitary campaigns became a popular propaganda movement to disseminate information of preventive medicine in the West.[155] In China, the 1910 plague fight motivated more intellectuals and medical scientists to advocate public health and broader social reforms. They blamed the popular resistance to modern methods of disinfection and isolation on people's ignorance (愚昧) and superstition (迷信), the two most frequently used terms by Chinese intellectuals to describe the ordinary people in the first half of the twentieth century. They felt the urgency to enlighten Chinese people on the scientific knowledge of Western medicine and disease prevention. Germ theory, which explained the precise causation of diseases and prevention thereof, significantly popularized Western medicine as the scientific medicine of true knowledge and put pressure on Chinese medicine.[156] Medical scientists increasingly talked about public health and Western medicine in the same context, further promoting the intrinsic link between the two. They presented papers on public health at conferences of the China Medical Missionary Association, where both Chinese and foreign doctors turned their attention to the topic after the 1910 plague. Wu Liande called to awaken the sanitary conscience of China, and Diao Xinde (Tiao Hsin-teh, Edward Sintak Tyau, 刁信德, 1878–1958), who had just returned from America and took up a leading medical position in Shanghai, made a plea for a campaign of public health education in China. Arthur Stanley, the health officer of Shanghai Municipal Council, discussed the sanitary organization of China and how to initiate public health work in Chinese cities. Elliot I. Osgood, a medical missionary of the Christian Missionary Society, advocated a sanitary propaganda for China.[157] Every one of them advocated Western medicine in their call for sanitation and public health.

Western-trained Chinese doctors, who had been attending the CMMA conferences, contemplated forming a professional association of their own. Although Wu Liande had attempted to organize an association in 1910, he failed to secure sufficient interest and support. In 1914, Wu Liande and his associates made a survey of all qualified Chinese practitioners of Western medicine, and began organizational preparation. At the annual conference of the China Medical Missionary Association on February 5, 1915 in Shanghai, a group of 21 Chinese doctors gathered at dinner and voted to form a National Medical Association of China (NMAC, 中华医学会). They elected Yan Fuqing (F. C. Yen, 颜福庆, 1882–1970), a graduate of Yale University and Dean of Xiangya Medical College (湘雅医学院, Yale-Hunan Medical College) in Changsha (长沙) as president.[158] Yu Fengbin (C. V. Yui, 俞凤宾, 1884–1930) was elected the business manager, Diao Xinde the treasurer, and Wu Liande the secretary and editor of the association's journal, *National Medical Journal of China* (中华医学杂志). All of them were dedicated champions of public health. Yu and Diao had trainings in tropical disease and public health at the University of Pennsylvania in addition to their medical degrees. Three Chinese women doctors— Kang Cheng, Cao Liyun (Li-Yuen Tsao, 曹丽芸, 1886–1922) and Huang Qiongxian (黄琼仙, Ah Mae Wong, 黄阿梅, 1873–1933) were elected members of the five-member committee, which, together with other elected officers, took charge to draft the association's Constitution and Bylaws. Cao Liyun received her medical degree from the Women's Medical College of Pennsylvania in 1911. She took a one-year internship at the Mary Thompson Hospital for Women and Children in Chicago upon graduation. In 1912, she returned to China to work at the Friends Mission Hospital in Nanjing, which was the only hospital for women and children in the city. Cao actively engaged in the promotion of Western medicine and public health, as was seen in the health education campaigns in the 1910s.[159] Huang Qiongxian graduated from the University of Toronto in 1902 and became a leading physician in Shanghai after returning to China. The female founding members of the NMAC showed that women doctors played an active role in Chinese modern medical profession from the very beginning, but limited studies have been conducted about them. The NMAC was not exclusively Chinese in terms of membership. Leading public health advocates of Western origins were elected as honorary members, including Arthur Stanley; Edward H. Hume, Director of Hunan-Yale Hospital; H. S. Houghton, Dean of Harvard Medical School of Shanghai;[160] and G. E. Morrison, advisor to the Chinese government. By October 1915, the NMAC had 232 members.[161]

The National Medical Association of China distinguished the Chinese physicians of Western medicine as a group different from the medical missionaries, in their professional readiness to advocate medical science and public health in the broader social reforms of China. Yan Fuqing proudly announced that Chinese doctors would play an important role in China's health education and national modernization. There was professional competition and racial tension between the medical missionaries and the Chinese physicians of Western medicine. Missionaries' deeply entrenched racist views and their sense of superiority led to the treatment of their Chinese colleagues with less professional respect and trust, which the Chinese physicians resented. Wu Liande regularly called for tolerance and cooperation between the two groups in his addresses at conferences and publications. The two associations, however, professionally cooperated in promoting Western medicine and held joint conferences until 1932 when they merged into the Chinese Medical Association (中华医学会).

The NMAC gave the Chinese physicians of Western medicine a professionally unified platform to work with the Chinese government. Its constitution clearly defined the aim of the association as promoting the professional unity of Chinese physicians of Western medicine and serving the national effort to modernize and strengthen China through promoting "modern medical science in China" and arousing "interest in Public Health and preventive medicine among the people."[162] One of the first resolutions of the NMAC was to urge the Chinese government to establish a proper Public Health Service. In this sense, the NMAC stood out as a vanguard of the modern medicine to transform China from a traditional society to a modern nation. Intellectual modernizers perceived Chinese medicine as the symbol of traditional society and Western medicine the symbol of science and modernity. The NMAC provided the professional forum to make recommendations to the Chinese government regarding medicine and modernization. Many of the NMAC members had intimate personal connections with Chinese officialdom and the elite class who favored modern and Western orientation.

The official publication of the MNAC, *The National Medical Journal of China*, was published in both English and Chinese languages, a clear indication of attention to Chinese readership. The Chinese language section carried "not only matters of interest for doctors trained in Chinese but also helpful suggestions regarding health matters for the general public."[163] The contents in the Chinese section were not always identical with those in the English section of the journal, with the goal to disseminate modern medical knowledge to a broader Chinese audience. In this endeavor, the NMAC ran into a serious problem, that is, there was no unification and standardization of Chinese translation of Western medical terms. Chinese terminology of Western medicine had been translated by medical missionaries and the Chinese without a central agency to provide guidance. To tackle the problem, the NMAC formed a Terminology Committee with representatives from the China Medical Missionary Association, the Central Ministry of Education, the Jiangsu Educational Association (a nationally influential organization at the time), and the China Medical Pharmaceutical Society to undertake the task of standardization.[164] Funding from the Rockefeller Foundation facilitated the committee's work and the commercial publication of standardized Chinese terms of Western medicine.[165] The *National Medical Journal of China* regularly published Chinese terms of Western medicine with explanations to help Chinese understand them. The journal also published public health statistics about America, Japan, and European countries and compared them with other countries to emphasize the correlation between national health and national strength. These efforts helped raise the public's awareness of the importance of public health to national progress.

Western sanitary campaigns and public health movement began to influence China when missionaries started school hygiene and distributed information on epidemic diseases to school children. In 1910, the China Medical Missionary Association appointed a Committee of Medical Propaganda, but little was done due to the death of two committee members and the outbreak of the 1911 revolution that overthrew the Qing dynasty.[166] The situation changed when a young American by the name of William Wesley Peter (known as W. W. Peter, 1882–1959) came to China to join the missionaries. With endless energy and showmanship, Peter organized the first public health education campaigns in

Chinese cities in the mid-1910s, reaching out to the urban Chinese.[167] Peter finished his medical education at Rush Medical College in Chicago in 1910, and served as an active secretary of the Young Men's Christian Association (YMCA) without medical practice in America. He was sent to China by the Mission Board of the Evangelical Association. He arrived in Shanghai in November 1911 with his wife, Eleanor Elizabeth Whipple, who was also trained as a doctor. Peter went to work at a missionary hospital in Wuchang (武昌) in central China, where the Chinese revolution had started.[168] Like the rest of medical missionaries, Peter's work was to heal the body and save the soul by converting the patients to Christian belief.

Peter had come to China with the ambition to become a great surgeon, but his work at Wuchang changed his life. He saw the limited hospital services having a pitiful impact on the health of the large Chinese population. He noticed that Chinese patients knew nothing about infectious diseases and always thought illnesses as "caused by devils, spirits and revengeful gods, and hastened by night, and especially cold, air."[169] He was surprised that China had no laws to protect itself from disease-laden ships from abroad, nor laws against epidemics of contagious diseases from within. Chinese officials did not have knowledge about diseases, either.[170] Peter wanted to change his job to work on public health education.

Of the missionary societies and organizations in China, the YMCA was most active in health education in its social reform and service programs. It had distributed anti-tuberculosis and anti-cholera pamphlets and delivered health lectures. The Lecture Department of the YMCA, established in 1904, gave talks on the latest technological and scientific development to "capture the attention and interest of the Chinese literati and win their respect."[171] Receptive to Peter's ideas of public health education, the YMCA created a new Health Division under the Lecture Department, of which Peter was put in charge in 1913.[172] Peter took his new job with great enthusiasm and wanted to "become . . . an expert on hygiene, a director of public health." He pondered:

> to help me to reach this goal is my wife who had had a better pre-medical and medical training than myself. When we are called back to America [on furlough], we hope for some time for study and visitation with just this object in view.[173]

In the preparation for a health education campaign, Peter realized that there were more than just health issues to pay attention to. To get the health education program moving forward, he had to make it appealing to the interests of at least three different groups: the missionary/YMCA evangelical cause; the American commercial interests for their support and donations, and the Chinese personal and national concerns. To justify the health education campaign for American commercial interests, Peter articulated:

> China, plague-ridden and cholera-infested, is a distrinct [sic] menace to the health of America. China, handicapped by existing bad health conditions and

> therefore bearing more than the usual economic load due to high death rate and incapacity of wage-earners on account of preventable diseases, is to that extent less able to buy from America.[174]

He concluded that "[a] sick nation is a backward nation commercially." These appeals were also intended for the Chinese audience as well. Peter popularized the economic argument that "Health Pays Dividends" by pointing out that good health was a financial gain for the individual. He explained that good health not only offered "self-protection" for your life but also brought in "dollars and cents," because when you were healthy you were productive to make money, and when you were sick you had to spend money to see doctors. To appeal to missionaries, Peter articulated how the Church would benefit from health education. He pointed out that missionaries faced the questions of "[h]ow to develop contacts with previously inaccessible people so that they may be influenced toward the Kingdom [of Christ]" and "[h]ow to enlist those not yet in the Kingdom in service for others." Peter argued:

> The solution of these problems lies in the direction of finding some enterprise in which all classes in a city are interested. There are many who are not interested in education or religion with whom missionary workers have longed to get in contact. But everybody is interested in the health question, and a Health Education Campaign is one way in which the above problems may be solved.[175]

He declared that "our objective is not only four hundred million bodies, but four hundred million souls" and that the public health program "is a mighty weapon for extending the Kingdom [of Christ] in China."[176]

It was about this time that the Rockefeller Foundation (RF) organized a China Medical Commission to investigate opportunities to bring medical science to China. Peter tried to enlist the financial support of the RF but he did not succeed. The Rockefeller philanthropy's interest in China, and in Asia generally, was shaped by Frederick T. Gates (1853–1929), John D. Rockefeller's trusted advisor, even before the Rockefeller Foundation was organized. Gates, albeit a Baptist clergyman, was displeased with the denominationalist influence of missionary medical work in China. He criticized the "bondage of tradition" and the "ignorance and misguided sentiment" of missionaries. He wanted to re-train the medical missionaries into competent medical doctors with the aim to reform the denominational evangelism with medical science.[177] In the study of Gates' vision and plan to re-orient the transformation of China from the hands of missionaries to the solution of scientific medicine, few mentioned the voice of the Chinese who may have played a role in the solidification of Gates' rather radical scheme of vision. In 1912, a group of Chinese elite of medical practitioners, educators, officials and merchants, many of whom were educated in the United States, wrote Frederick T. Gates a "Memorial for the Endowment of a Hospital in China." The memorial letter was appended to the report of Charles W. Eliot

(1834–1926), formerly president of Harvard University, who submitted to the trustees of the Carnegie Endowment for International Peace his observations of China and Japan in 1912.[178] Frederick T. Gates was a founding trustee of the Carnegie Endowment as well as the trusted advisor of John D. Rockefeller, Sr. The memorial was the earliest evidence of the Chinese desire for Americans to build:

> a well-equipped hospital, which will not only serve as a model for the rest of China, but will confer untold benefit upon thousands of sick Chinese and serve as a center where the medical students and local practitioners may witness the highest development of medical science.[179]

Among the undersigned of the memorial were Wu Liande, Zhang Bolin (Chang Poling, Principal of Nankai Middle School), and Jin Yunmei.

The Chinese memorial letter may have further inspired Frederick T. Gates, after the Oriental Education Commission urged the foundation to focus on medicine in China.[180] In January 1914, the Rockefeller Foundation voted to establish a Commission to study the conditions of public health and medicine in China. Even William J. Bryan, the Secretary of State, lent a helping hand by providing the Commission letters of introduction to the American Minster in China, Paul S. Reinsch, to facilitate the work of the Commission. Members of the Commission visited missionary schools and talked with missionary doctors as well as YMCA leaders about possible collaborations.[181] At the suggestion of Roger S. Greene (a member of the Commission, formerly U.S. Consul-General at Hankou), the YMCA National Committee submitted in September 1914 a "Three-Year Plan and Budget" (1915–1917) to the Rockefeller Foundation, seeking financial support to cover the costs of office facilities, laboratory and fieldwork equipment, headquarters operation and salaries of five staff members of the YMCA Health Division.[182] The Foundation decided not to fund the proposed plan because the proposal appeared a scheme on paper with no operation programs, nor coordination with the China Medical Missionary Association, which was to initiate a similar public health program.[183]

The Foundation's comments on the proposal, nonetheless, led the YMCA Health Division to collaboration with the CMMA in developing a health education program that consisted of four inter-related components: lectures, exhibits, national exchange of lantern slides, and literature distribution. The YMCA recruited medical missionaries to write health articles for newspapers and pamphlets, showed lantern slides, and helped organize local health campaigns. Mission societies did not always cooperate, however, especially when the health education activities did not directly enhance their evangelical work. When Peter wanted to recruit C. H. Barlow, a missionary doctor with specialty on tuberculosis, of the Baptist Mission stationed in Shaoxing (绍兴) to develop a program of national exchange of health lantern slides for local shows and lectures, the mission society was reluctant to lend personnel and financial support.[184] Peter was, however, more successful in inviting medical leaders of different organizations to sit on the Advisory Committee of the YMCA's Health Division.

Henry S. Houghton served as chairman, and Wu Liande, Yan Fuqing, and C. H. Barlow were members of the Committee.[185]

In 1914, the China Medical Missionary Association asked Peter to help create a public health exhibit. Inspired by the traveling health exhibits in the United States, Peter purchased exhibition materials from American illustrated catalogues and then adapted them to Chinese audience.[186] The health exhibit was put on display at the national conference of the China Medical Missionary Association in Shanghai in February 1915. In an area of more than two thousand square feet, people saw maps, charts, diagrams, cartoons, paintings, pictures, placards, tracts and epigrams, as well as lantern slides and large mechanical and electrical devices that Peter and his staff created to illustrate deaths from tuberculosis and smallpox.[187] The conference also saw another display, created by Wu Liande and his associates, titled "Exhibit on the Manchurian Plague."[188] Wu's exhibit represented the public health education effort of the Chinese government, whereas Peter's the missionaries' program. These two exhibits, which were intended to publicize health knowledge among the general audience as well as the professionals, were so popular that requests came from different groups across the provinces to use the exhibits to launch health campaigns.

The public's interest in health exhibits inspired missionaries to use public health to spearhead evangelizing campaigns. The YMCA and the China Medical Missionary Association collaborated in coordinating public health campaigns to further penetrate Chinese society. Often, the sites of the health campaigns were chosen with the strategic consideration that evangelical campaigns would immediately follow the health exhibits to capitalize on the enthusiasm of the people at the gatherings.[189] Peter believed that the collaboration served as a step "to unite the C.M.M.A. and local Y.M.C.A. on a common program of work."[190] As a result, the CMMA formed a Council on Public Health in 1915 and allocated half of its budget (about $600) for the Council's work. Members of the Council included Henry S. Houghton, W. W. Peter, Yan Fuqing, Kang Cheng, F. C. Tooker of the Presbyterian Hospital in Xiangtan of Hunan province, and H. J. Smyly of Peking Union Medical School.[191]

The common interest in promoting public health knowledge led to the cooperation and collaboration of the missionaries and the Chinese modern physicians. The two groups, however, were motivated by fundamentally different goals. The Chinese physicians advocated scientific knowledge of medicine to strengthen China into a modern sovereign nation, whereas missionary societies utilized health campaigns to stage evangelical meetings to spread Christianity. The NMAC attempted to influence the modernization of China with the power of medical science, whereas the CMMA and the YMCA tried to shape the future of China with evangelical vision. The NMAC had limited resources to carry out a nationwide public health education, but the YMCA in collaboration with the CMMA had a stronger financial commitment and a wider network of mission societies. Despite their differences and tensions of relations, the NMAC, the YMCA and the CMMA decided to pool their professional expertise and resources to strengthen the movement of public health education. In March 1916, the National Committee of the

YMCA took the initiative to call upon the NMAC and CMMA to streamline their public health education efforts under one organization. The National Medical Association of China therefore joined the Council on Public Health to form the Joint Council on Public Health Education. The three groups utilized their wide social and political networks to generate support for public health education from the government and educational and commercial organizations. The Joint Council was headquartered in the Shanghai YMCA building, with Peter in charge of daily operation. It was made clear that the internal organization and policies of the three associations were not to be affected by the Joint Council.[192] With the participation of the NMAC, the evangelical agenda in public health campaigns receded, though the Christian message continued because of the leadership of the YMCA.

Health education campaigns: public health and national strength

Major health campaigns were launched in 1915 and 1916 in more than a dozen cities, such as Shanghai, Changsha, Xiangtan, Nanjing, Kaifeng, Hangzhou, Xiamen, Shantou, Fuzhou, Beijing and Tianjin. Local government officials, businessmen, educators and students, local branches of YMCAs and missionary groups were mobilized to work with the Joint Council's health team in organizing and running the lectures and exhibits of the campaigns. The aim of the health campaigns was to popularize scientific knowledge of medicine, raise people's awareness of sanitation and hygiene, and prevent disease. Science and public health were advocated as measures to gauge a nation's progress, modernity and strength. Local officials, merchants, and civic organizations wanted to bring the health exhibits and campaigns to their city because it would make their city look progressive and modern. Posters and bulletins were distributed in advance to the city where the campaign was to be held to publicize it. Like the health education tours in the United States and Europe, health campaigns in China emphasized graphic illustrations and demonstrative activities to attract attention and convey information to the visitors.[193] The visual materials and illustrative devices were particular useful and beneficial in transmitting health information and preventive medicine to those who could not read.

The health campaign in Changsha was one of the first launched by the Joint Council and sponsored by Hunan provincial government. It was conducted in the week of May 10–15, 1915, with the support of the governor and the police commissioner of the province. Changsha was the capital of Hunan, where the Hunan-Yale Hospital and Medical School was located.[194] Students were recruited to work as health instructors at the 35 sessions of lectures of the week-long campaign. Dozens of boxes of health exhibit items and devices were transported from Shanghai to Changsha. The display of the exhibition was so large that the Government Education Hall, the most spacious building in town, had to be used. At the center of the exhibition was a fifteen-foot tall model of a sanatorium designed by the Hunan-Yale Hospital and Medical School. More than 30,000 people attended the lectures, the exhibit, and the lantern slide shows. In addition to disseminating public health information, the campaign also raised $20,000 for a tuberculosis sanatorium, which was built near the Hunan-Yale Hospital two years later.[195] It was one of the first tuberculosis hospitals under the management of the Chinese Red Cross Society. A Public Health Society was also formed at the closing of the campaign, with the police commissioner elected as president and eleven influential men of Changsha as charter members of the society.

The health campaign lasted for a week with three major components—exhibitions, lectures, and slide and film shows. The exhibit materials and illustration devices grew into such a large collection that Peter had to hire several Chinese laborers to carry the materials on wheelbarrows when the Council's health team was on the road. Sometimes, urban residents were recruited to help stage public health parades on the streets to raise public awareness of how flies and mosquitoes carried germs to spread disease and kill people. The health campaign was a novel modern propaganda event in Chinese cities. It introduced modern knowledge of diseases to different social classes. It was challenging to make health topics appealing to the diverse audience of scholars, officials, businessmen, students, soldiers, ordinary urban residents and women. In order to attract people of every walk of life, the campaign had to find a common theme. Peter thought that self-protection and financial gain of public health would be persuasive to the Chinese people. Therefore, a big banner of "Health Pays Dividends" (卫生能生利) in both Chinese and English was hung high above the center stage of the lecture platform.[196] (**See Figure 1.2, Picture of lecture stage**) To his surprise, visitors to the health exhibits and lectures were not enthusiastic, though they were curious and eager to find out health information.

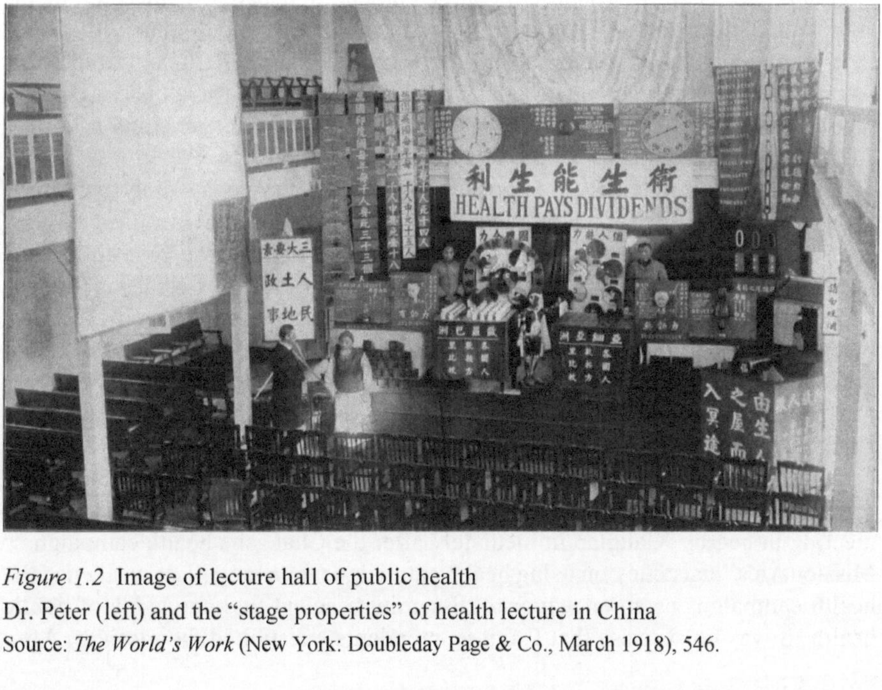

Figure 1.2 Image of lecture hall of public health
Dr. Peter (left) and the "stage properties" of health lecture in China
Source: *The World's Work* (New York: Doubleday Page & Co., March 1918), 546.

To Chinese laborers, merchants, literati, students, army officers, and government officials, the first and foremost concern was information about the fate of their country in the face of foreign scramble. They anguished over the imperialist powers' aggression and feared the nation's inability to survive. Just as the health campaign was being launched, China faced the new aggression of Japan. In January 1915, Japan made the infamous twenty-one demands, dividing the Chinese territory of Shandong province and attempting to gain control of Chinese political and economic affairs.[197] Japan's imperialist ambition alarmed Chinese people and heightened their nationalist sentiment. Patriotic feelings and the discourse of seeking national strength through modernization surged among the educated elite and the illiterate commoners alike. Discussions of progress and national strength filled the pages of newspapers and the conversations in tea-houses.[198] Social Darwinian ideas provided an intellectual interpretation of national survival of the fittest.

If the health campaigns were to catch the attention of Chinese people, it needed to address the major concern of every social class. Fully aware of that concern, Peter understood that the health subject had to be made relevant to China's struggle to build a strong modern nation. He shrewdly titled the theme of the health campaign lecture as "The Relation between National Health and National Strength." He elaborated on the relations between national health and national economic, educational, and moral strength.[199] He explained that the strength of a nation was demonstrated in the death rate of that nation. Strong nations like America and England had low death rates of 15 per thousand and 16 per thousand respectively; whereas weak nations like India and Mexico had high death rates of 33 per thousand and 35 per thousand.[200] Chinese audiences, apparently intrigued by his argument, wanted to know the death rate of Japan and compare that with China. Peter explained that although no statistics were available for China, "from information supplied by competent authorities . . . the number was not less than 40 [per thousand]."[201] Chinese health professionals in the 1920s generally acknowledged that the death rate of China was about 30 per thousand.[202]

The high death rate of China presented by Peter was devastating to Chinese visitors at the health campaign. They were not comfortable with the numbers, and some even questioned the information in disbelief. They became suspicious of the true intention of talking about China's high death rate and poor sanitation, particularly when it was done by a foreign missionary. At health lectures, when Peter explained that large numbers of Chinese were dying each year from preventable diseases, people in the audience would retort sarcastically that there were too many people in China anyway and deaths somehow kept people from being pushed into the sea.[203] The fact that missionary societies deliberately used health campaigns for evangelical activities undermined, to some extent, the credibility of the health lecture. The YMCA and the CMMA staged an evangelical meeting in nearby Xiangtan immediately after the Changsha health campaign.[204] Missionaries' insistency on using health campaigns for evangelism weakened the health campaigns as an endeavor to disseminate scientific knowledge of public health. It was no surprise that Chinese attendants questioned the motives. After the NMAC joined the YMCA and the CMMA to launch the health campaigns, no evangelical meetings were attached to the health campaigns. The focus on promoting health education and scientific knowledge about diseases, however, led to declining support of missionary societies to the health campaigns.

Chinese officials and merchants-gentry embraced public health campaigns to promote social progress and modernization. In provinces, local government conducted the campaign according to its own needs. In Nanjing, the week-long health campaign was organized and carried out by Jiangsu provincial government and the social elite in May 1915. Jiangsu Health Commissioner G. P. Wang oversaw the planning and daily operation of the campaign. Nanjing University supplied large assortments of specimens for the health exhibition and used medical students as health lecturers. The exhibition and lectures were held in the spacious Nanjing YMCA building and attracted more than 10,000 visitors. Nanjing University even cancelled a whole week of classes to encourage staff and students to participate in the campaign. A significant result of the campaign was the formation of the Jiangsu Public Health Association (JPHA) a year later, on 15 April 1916. The JPHA had five departments that emphasized prevention of epidemic diseases and home hygiene, study of hygiene and medicine, care of the sick, food and drug safety, and urban sanitary conditions. The prominent literati-merchant Zhang Jian (Chang Chien, 张謇, 1853–1926) served as president of the JPHA while Jiangsu provincial officials, key educators and leaders of local gentry filled other leading positions.[205]

Women attended the health events with great interest and curiosity. As was the social custom that men and women did not intermingle in public, they were kept separate at the health events. Campaign organizers set aside the last day of the campaign exclusively for women, called the Women's Day. Instead of lecturing on national health and national strength, the women were given a lecture on "The Care of Your Baby." It concentrated on baby care and home hygiene, with demonstrations on proper clothing for babies, methods of dressing and undressing, giving baths, preparing manufactured baby food, and making a good-sleeping baby bed. Women of prestigious positions were invited to speak on Women's Day to give importance and privilege to the campaign. During the Nanjing campaign, Mrs. Feng Guozhang (冯国璋), the governor's wife, addressed the Women's Day, with the call for more attention to health matters.[206] Women of different status—mothers and young girls—filled up the lecture hall. Some of the mothers even brought their babies to the lecture. Dr. Cao Liyun, the well-known female doctor in the city after her return from America, delivered the health lecture with a real baby in her arms to show the right way to bathe, clothe and feed an infant. Mothers in the audience were stunned that the baby was bathed on the stage and feared that he might not survive. A few days later, a local newspaper reported that the baby was doing just fine. Chinese mothers usually chewed rice before feeding it to their babies, and they also slept with their babies. These traditional methods were considered unsanitary and unsafe in modern hygiene. The lecture recommended mothers using manufactured baby food and demonstrated how to prepare it. Efforts to persuade Chinese women to adopt Western-style child-rearing, which was presented as the enlightened way of modern societies, stimulated active discussions. Women in the audience often interrupted the lecture with inquisitive questions of this and that.[207]

The health campaigns were great social events for local people. A witness recalled the unforgettable moment of instant excitement: "Goodness, parades, meetings, I don't know what all."[208] Between health shows and lectures, people went to teahouses to enjoy a cup of tea and continued their conversation about hygiene and diseases. The fanfare and curiosity of urban residents made the campaign as much a learning opportunity as a social event for local people. Merchants also exploited the opportunities for commercial purposes. At the Changsha campaign, people received free copies of a booklet called "Hygiene and Sanitation Indispensible [sic]," which was not distributed by the campaign organizers. The pamphlet contained good health information but ended by saying: "Now the way to secure all the advantages of hygiene and sanitation mentioned in this book is to buy Dr. Williams Pink Pills for Pale People <u>in large quantities</u>."[209]

The campaign made tours in provinces of Hunan, Henan, Jiangsu and Zhejiang, and it had yet to come to Beijing, the capital of China, to win the central government's recognition and to stimulate its interest in public health. Interior Minister, Zhu Qiqian (Chu Chi-chien, 朱启钤, 1872–1964), who was an advocate for public health, decided that the Ministry of Interior would sponsor the health campaign in Beijing during the week of May 22–29, 1916. The Ministry formed a Public Health Campaign Committee and raised more than $2000 from other government agencies and local business and educational groups. Normally, it would cost $300 to conduct a health campaign; with that large sum, the Committee wanted to make the Beijing campaign a model with national and international publicity. A grand opening reception was held on May 20 in the Central Park next to the Forbidden City, where the Interior Minister gave a formal speech to a large audience that included prominent government officials, educational and business dignitaries, and foreign guests such as the British ambassador Sir John Jordan and the American ambassador Paul S. Reinsch. More than 18,000 people attended the lectures and exhibits of the Beijing campaign, including police and soldiers as well as students and teachers, and women. A glimpse of the program schedule detailed the different groups attending the health exhibits and lectures.[210]

> Monday: 10:30 a.m. for police; 4 p.m. for male students; 6 p.m. for foreigners
> Tuesday: 10:30 a.m. for soldiers; 4 p.m. for male students
> Wednesday: 10:30 a.m. for merchants and gentry; 4 p.m. for male students
> Thursday: 10:30 a.m. for general, men; 4 p.m. for male students
> Friday: 10:30 a.m. for general, women; 4 p.m. for women students
> Saturday: 10:30 a.m. for general, women; 4 p.m. for women students

Different from the campaigns in other cities, two days of public health lectures were delivered to women in Beijing, which discussed the need of public health reforms in general, and baby care. The large numbers of women attending the lectures indicated that women enjoyed more access to public life in Beijing, even though their space of public life was kept separate from men.

The center stage of the Beijing health campaign was set up in the Central Park, with a large hall for the presentation of health lectures and the display of health exhibits. Public health films and lantern slides were shown in the evening, free to the public. The health lectures concentrated on the discussion of hygiene and sanitation, and solutions to national public health. Several factors were singled out as a hindrance to the progress of preventive medicine in China, namely, the lack of scientific knowledge and vital statistics, the lack of investigators and interest in national health, and the insufficient number of medical schools and hospitals and doctors. The lectures predicted that China would be able to improve health conditions "if she proceeded with the work in the same scientific manner" as the West did, and that progress in public health depended upon the support of public opinion, education, legislation and finance in this matter.[211] While the Joint Council used the American model for China' public health modernization, Chinese leaders were concerned about the immediate actions. They urged every group of visitors to practice what they learned at the health lectures and exhibits. They called on the general public to make a clean and sanitary city of Beijing by launching a crusade against flies and mosquitoes to remove the causes of diseases.[212] Several high officials of the Yuan Shikai government gathered to discuss the relationship between national health and national strength at the farewell dinner. Peter recalled: "It was most gratifying to note their willingness to spend several hours at a most critical time in the affairs of the country to discuss the question [of public health]."[213] Indeed, it was a critical moment in Chinese history, for Yuan Shikai died seven days after, on June 6, 1916, and China fell into the disintegration of warlordism. The health campaign did not stop. It moved on to Tianjin and attracted 15,057 people there.[214]

The rapid turnover of officials in the government during the political turmoil of warlordism made the accomplishment of health campaigns difficult to sustain. A disappointed Peter wrote: "Most of the men holding office at the time health campaigns were held in their cities are now political bench-warmers. Until the ins become outs less frequently little progress can be made."[215] The Joint Council attempted to turn the uncertainty into a unique opportunity to inject new ideas and influence. In the following years, the Joint Council continued to emphasize that China should follow the example of other great nations in establishing national, provincial, and city boards of health, and that China should collect vital statistics and arouse public opinion so as to bring about modern health-conserving work.[216] These suggestions sounded lofty but unrealistic when China had no stable government and few public health specialists.

A major challenge to the health campaigns was to find enough medical students to work as health instructors for the health exhibition sessions and lectures. Professional training of public health specialists did not start until 1925 when John B. Grant created a Public Health Department at Peking Union Medical College. In Beijing, students from local medical colleges were recruited to help with health lectures and explanation of the health exhibits. In places where few modern medical students were available, the task fell to the Joint Council's health team to train a "health faculty" out of a variety of recruits—students, teachers, businessmen and YMCA secretaries. The method was to train a few key recruits, and then designate them as teachers to train other recruits. The "health faculty" size varied from a few dozens to a few hundred, depending on the local arrangements and the number of anticipated visitors. In Tianjin, the Joint Council trained 450 men as "health faculty," and each health session had a different group of health instructors. In Changsha, the Council trained 75 men as health instructors to work on all sessions of health lectures and exhibits.[217] As they were better-equipped with public health subjects, the trained "health faculty" were expected to work with local public health societies to continue the work of health education after the campaign was over. However, that was a weak point of the health campaigns, as few follow-ups were conducted by the Joint Council.

In 1917–1920, Hu Xuanming (S. M. Woo, 胡宣明, 1887–1965) was put in charge of the Joint Council's health program when Peter was on furlough in the United States and then served in France during World War I. Hu received his medical education at the Johns Hopkins Medical School and the Harvard-MIT School of Public Health after his graduation from the St. Johns University in Shanghai. He worked on the translation of dozens of English health bulletins into Chinese. As he had little training in Chinese literature, Hu enlisted W. E. Macklin, a medical missionary in Nanjing, to help him with the translation. Macklin was well versed in Chinese language and literary style after decades of work and study in China. They wrote and translated 21 topics, including "Sanitation of a Chinese City," "Mode of Infection and Prevention," "Tuberculosis," "Cholera," "Small-pox," "Sex Hygiene," "Kill the Fly," and "Prevention of Colds."[218] Hundreds of thousands of copies were printed and distributed to provinces across China. Hospitals as well as educational and commercial organizations purchased the pamphlets to distribute to their clients. Hu reported "a general desire among the Chinese" to get health education material and that students were eager to talk about health to urban residents and rural farmers as well.[219]

The Joint Council did not provide a professional guide to local health campaigns because it did not have a standardized manual of operation. Hu Xuanming thought that topics of health exhibits and lectures should be standardized to help local enthusiasts do health educational work themselves. He realized that the Joint Council should develop follow-up programs after the week-long campaigns to sustain the momentum of changing people's views of disease and health behavior.[220] These ideas of closer collaboration with local public health societies failed to materialize, due to limited financial and human resources of the YMCA during the war time. Peter later acknowledged that it was "relatively easy to effect a temporary local organization in times of emergency, but difficult to keep this organization alive when the crisis has passed."[221]

The most notable program by Hu Xuanming was the National Health Essay Contest that started in 1917. It received financial support from the China Medical Board of the Rockefeller Foundation, which considered it important to attract students to Western medicine. The first national essay contest in 1917 focused on students' awareness of public health and national strength. The theme was "Present Health Conditions in China and How They May Be Further Improved." Contestants defined their own essay titles. Fifty-one essays were submitted from students from primary school to college.[222] One of the first prize-winners was Wu Baoguang (吴葆光), a student from Peking Union Medical College, whose essay was "On China's Recent Health Conditions and Methods of Improvement."[223] Wu pointed out that public health was not an isolated issue and its success relied on the coordinated progress of other realms of the society. As methods to improve China's national health, he envisioned a comprehensive health system, which he presented in a chart that included three key components: health education, health administration, and moral and charitable health. (**See Figure 1.3, Chart of health system.**) Health education included specialized medical education—medical schools, midwifery training schools and nursing schools, general health education at schools, and family health education on the transmission and prevention of diseases. Health administration had two major branches: (1) government hospitals—general and infectious ones; and (2) a health bureau that had an investigation department supervising sanitary police and health standards, an information and propaganda department, and a research and experiment department. It is important to note that Wu put sanitary police under the health bureau, a significant shift away from the current practice of having it within the police system. The sanitary police would continue the duties of food hygiene, anti-drug operation, cleanliness, and vital statistics collection. Moral and charitable health included education about hygienic behavior in religious ceremonies and rituals that involved food and drinks, education about moral behaviors to prevent venereal diseases, establishing private hospitals, and hygiene and health in prisons and poorhouses. In discussing venues of health education, Wu mentioned that, besides schools, most cities had lecture institutes (*xuan jiang suo*, 宣讲所) that gave talks on current affairs in the evening. Health subjects should be added to the lectures to inform the public about microbes and infectious diseases with pictures. He also recommended that talks over tea could be held once a week at the institutes where everyone was encouraged to freely share opinions with others. Family disease prevention should pay attention to hygiene in a wide range of things, such as carbon monoxide, wet nurses, baby care, vaccination, disease-carriers—mosquitoes, flies, fleas, bedbugs and lice, house animals, servants, the toilet, the house, the kitchen, water and rice use, alcohol, and the sick. Wu's discussion of such a broad range of health issues was truly impressive. It indicated the serious contemplation on national health construction among the young students, especially among the medical students.

In 1919, 61 essays were submitted in the national contest from eleven provinces, including 14 from female students. Jiangsu province took the lead with 25 essays and Zhili (Hebei) the second with 13 essays. The first prize of the college category went to John Wu of the Comparative Law School in Shanghai,

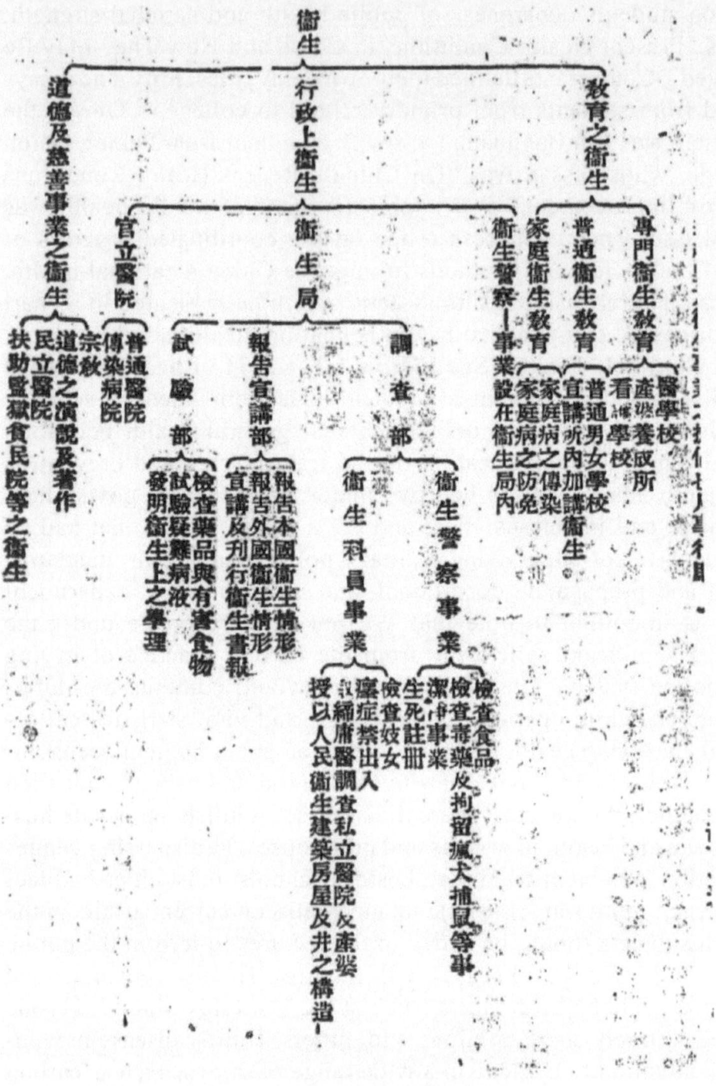

Figure 1.3 Wu Baoguang's chart of the health system

Source: Wu Baoguang (吴葆光), "On China's Recent Health Conditions and Methods of Improvement," *The New Youth* (*La Jeunesse*) vol. 3, no. 5 (July 1917), 1–2.

who wrote in English "The Relationship between National Health and National Wealth"; the first prize of the middle school category went to Ou-Yang Qing of Yeuh Yuen Middle School in Changsha, who wrote in Chinese "Personal Hygiene"; and first prize in the primary school category went to Miss Sheng Chen-xiang of Baldwin School for Girls in Nanchang, who wrote in Chinese

"What Makes One Sick?"[224] These essays clearly showed the influence of the Council's health campaigns in shaping people's views of disease and the relation between personal health and the society.

The health education program attracted support from other organizations, such as the YWCA, the Chinese Christian Education Association, and the Nurses' Association of China. With the addition of these organizations as sponsors, the Joint Council was re-organized into the Council on Health Education in 1920. Peter, after wartime service in France working with Chinese laborers, returned to China in January 1920 and became the director of the Council.[225] He stayed in the position till 1926 when he left China for good. He also served on the advisory board of the Shanghai Municipal Council during the campaign against epidemics and venereal diseases in 1920.[226] Moreover, he worked with the Chinese and Foreign Famine Relief Committee and the Huai Valley Conservancy Board.[227]

The staff of the Council increased from four to fourteen in 1920 with an annual budget of $26,000 from sponsoring organizations and individuals. The Council stayed in the same building of the China YMCA at Quinsan Gardens of Shanghai. Its major work included preparation and distribution of "health literature such as bulletins, leaflets, cartoons, posters, lecture charts, and books; lantern slides and film shows, and exhibit material," and participation in "local health programs such as health conferences, campaigns, better baby weeks, vision conservation and health examination in schools."[228] In 1920, the Council sold more than 132,000 copies of health bulletins across China and delivered hundreds of health shows of lectures, slide/film shows, and exhibits.[229] Health campaigns emphasized the preventive methods of disease, such as securing clean water and sanitation, keeping flies away from food, using anti-mosquito bed-nets, and killing rats. Health shows concentrated on infectious diseases like cholera, tuberculosis, plague, smallpox, venereal diseases, and malaria. Objectives of the health show in each city varied according to the city's particular needs. It could be promotion of a local public health society or vaccination of smallpox. Men of influence—government officials, army officers, businessmen and educators—were enlisted to support the health shows in the city. Local government was responsible for the organization of the health event and the expenses incurred.

In popularizing preventive medicine, the Council used simple devices such as the "Anti-Tuberculosis Story Calendar" and the "Brother Fat vs. Brother Lean" story to explain tuberculosis to the illiterate. Incidentally, "Brother Fat" stood for the healthy while "Brother Lean" for the sickly at that time. The Council would be called upon for help whenever an epidemic broke out. When Wuhu of Anhui province had an outbreak of smallpox in 1920, the Council sent a team to hold health meetings and conducted 5000 anti-smallpox vaccinations by working with local doctors and nurses.[230] The anti-cholera campaign in Fuzhou in June 1920 was one of the larger health campaigns. With the sponsorship of Fuzhou Health and Sanitation Committee, more than 2380 volunteers worked as assistants for the daily health parades, lectures, and a large outdoor health exhibit about cholera. The parades reportedly had covered 90 percent of Fuzhou streets with an audience of 220,000 people. The campaign seemed to have influenced the people because Fuzhou remained cholera free when it hit the region again.[231]

In 1923, the China Medical Board made a two-year grant of 27,000 Mexican dollars (one U.S. dollar was worth two Mexican dollars then) to support the Council's general work and another five-year grant of $22,500 (Mex.) to support a special campaign to promote Western medicine among students at middle schools and colleges.[232] The Board expected the Council to popularize Western medicine and to arouse students' interest in medical studies. Subsequently, the Council devoted activities to the promotion of Western medicine, with an annual national health essay contest, lectures for middle school and college students, presentations at education centers with exhibits, interviews and correspondence with students, arrangement of students' visits to local hospitals and medical schools, and scholarships of $100 (Mex.) each for eight medical schools to be awarded to the freshmen who won the first place in the competitive school entrance examination.[233] The theme of national essay contest shifted away from national strength to "Medicine as Life Work."[234] Ambitious to spread health education across China, Peter spent three months in Sichuan in 1924 organizing a Western Council on Health Education, much to the disappointment of the China Medical Board, whose interest was the promotion of scientific medicine among students.

The Council was dissolved in 1927. In its lifetime, the Council brought public health education campaigns to major cities of 13 provinces, making health knowledge available to urban Chinese of all social classes, many of whom would otherwise never have such opportunities. It helped raise Chinese people's awareness of sanitation, disease prevention, and the importance of public health in building a modern nation. The health shows and exhibitions left unforgettable impressions on the visitors, but often failed to sustain the momentum with follow-ups. John B. Grant criticized that the health campaigns left nothing permanent behind after they departed.[235] And yet, local public health societies were indeed formed in some cities, and health propaganda work continued with local government's support for annual week-long health campaigns in spring and summer. Curiosity about health campaigns drew large crowds, where people socialized and engaged in conversations about hygiene and sanitation, and national strength. They learned about China's high death rates, and that flies and mosquitoes spread diseases.

Government policy, modern medicine, and public health

For the politicians of the newly created Republic of China, promoting modern medicine and public health meant projecting a politically progressive image and winning support of a variety of modernizers—scholars, students, newspapermen, merchants, and urban residents. The Yuan Shikai government, albeit chaotic and ineffective, supported modern medicine and public health by issuing orders and regulations. It even tried to do away with Chinese medicine in a short episode of 1914. The term "modern medicine" was used interchangeably with Western medicine, but it also meant any modern medical practice and concept, such as anatomy and prevention of disease. The new Republican government promulgated a standard curriculum of modern medicine for medical schools in 1912. To further promote modern medical studies and practice, the government issued a Presidential Mandate in 1913 to legalize dissection of dead bodies, which the Interior Ministry provided specific regulations about.[236] For the purpose of teaching anatomy, medical schools requested prisons to provide dead bodies that no relatives or families had come to claim.

Yuan Shikai regarded sanitation as an important measure of progress and modernity. In 1913, Beijing Police Bureau issued regulations on a wide range of matters pertaining to public health and public safety under the name of *weisheng* (卫生). They included, but were not limited to, food hygiene, sanitation, midwifery, and carbon monoxide poisoning. The term "*weisheng*" has been translated to mean sanitation, cleanliness, hygiene, and health in China. In the early twentieth century, it seemed already a term for many things. For instance, "Regulation Regarding Midwifery License" included 12 specific rules about professional training requirement, practice, licensing, and operation fees. The regulation required that midwives must register and obtain a license after meeting professional criteria. Foreign women must present training documents of graduation.[237] The Yuan Shikai government also tried to license the practice of geomancers (阴阳生) in 1913. Of course, practitioners had to pay for the license and registration. There was little evidence that the regulations were regularly enforced. Beijing also had modern facilities like the gas heating system installed in some residents' homes; but accidents of carbon monoxide poisoning often occurred and law suits followed. The judicial and health units of Beijing Police Bureau collaborated in posting public notices and regulations to warn people of the danger and instruct them on how to prevent carbon monoxide poisoning. The police notice read: "Because ordinary people did not know about weisheng, deaths often happen due to carbon monoxide poisoning in winter. Please make sure to carry out the regulations to prevent harm and to save lives. It pertains to weisheng."[238] By using "weisheng" to refer to public safety, the police had broadened the meaning of *weisheng* beyond the conventional sense of public health.

In 1915, Yuan Shikai issued a Presidential Mandate on Sanitation to exhort local magistrates to report on the progress of sanitary work.[239] Newspapers and public notices published and circulated government regulations on public health and related matters so that people were made aware of them. For instance, the Beijing Police Bureau issued regulations on bone-meat workshops (骨头肉作坊) as a measure to protect neighborhood *weisheng* in 1913. Because bone-meat workshops produced terrible smells when they boiled butchered animals, the regulations banned the workshops from residential areas, and allowed them to operate only in outdoor space with few residents around. The regulations specified that only bones of pigs, sheep and cows were allowed for the shops to process, and no bones from diseased animals were allowed. The bones had to be processed immediately within two days to prevent meat from getting rotten. The regulations required that all shop equipment be cleaned, and the dates for shop operation were set from October to March only.[240] On September 20, 1914, *Jinghua ribao*

(京话日报, Peking Vernacular Daily) reported an incident of *weisheng* violation with the title "You ai weisheng" (有碍卫生, An Obstacle to Sanitation/Public Health). A neighborhood community complained that a terrible smell came from a newly opened sheep head meat processing shop (羊头肉锅房). It made people feel nauseated and they lost their appetite. Worse still, the shop threw sheep dung on the street, making the community filthy and unsanitary.[241] They accused the shop of violating health regulations and called the police to investigate the matter. The Metropolitan Police of Beijing had a regulation of 10 rules on sheep meat processing shops as early as March 1914, which required that all such shops be operated in an open space outside of the city where few people lived.[242] The residents complained that the shop's violation of the regulation caused harm to health. They were quick to use public health regulations to protect themselves and their community against unsanitary operations. The story indicated that the idea "*weisheng*" had become popular discourse of local people who were highly conscious of government health regulations in the mid-1910s.

Government favorable policy on Western medicine played a role in the increasing tension between Western medicine and Chinese medicine. Physicians of Chinese medicine worried about their own practice and existence. To seek protection, Chinese medicine doctors organized a committee in 1914 and sent representatives to meet with Yuan Shikai and the Minister of Education, Wang Daxie (汪大燮, 1859–1929), in the hope of getting their support for Chinese medicine.[243] To their astonishment, the Minister of Education responded by proposing to abolish Chinese medicine and Chinese herbal drugs. The entire Chinese medical and pharmaceutical world was incensed with vehement opposition to the government's threat. Chinese medical practitioners all over the country were mobilized to form a Delegation for the Salvation of Chinese Medicine (医药救亡请愿团). They successfully forced the government to withdraw the proposal, and Wang Daxie resigned as a result. This was the first attempt of the Chinese government to abolish Chinese medicine. The second happened in 1929 under the Nationalist government, which failed as well. Yuan Shikai, however, did not stop undermining Chinese medicine. Being a shrewd politician, Yuan knew that any support for the "old-style" Chinese medicine would appear politically unwise, because the "old style" medicine was criticized as unscientific and superstitious while modern medicine was promoted as scientific and progressive. Instead of working with Chinese medicine men, Yuan took further steps to restrict them. He issued a presidential mandate in September 1915 that required candidates for government positions in medicine, pharmacy and veterinary fields to have qualifications similar to the West and Japan, which literarily made training in Western medicine the standard for government employment. Physicians of Western medicine did not hide their joy over the failure of Chinese medical practitioners' political lobby. They felt that the presidential mandate had given the official recognition of Western Medicine and "the time when their [Chinese medicine men] influence prevailed had passed."[244]

The first modern "Regulations on the Prevention of Infectious Diseases" and the "Regulations on Medical and Pharmaceutical Examinations" were promulgated in 1916 as measures to protect people's lives and safeguard medical practice and standards.[245] As a testimony of commitment to disease prevention, the government made vaccination compulsory in Beijing. The regulations had two far-reaching implications: one was the modern understanding of infectious disease; and the other was the negative impact on Chinese medicine and the intensification of antagonism between practitioners of Chinese medicine and those of Western medicine. Regarding the concept of disease transmission (*chuanran*, 传染), Chinese medicine had different explanations for different infectious diseases such as smallpox, cholera, plague, and leprosy. It did not group these diseases under one category because they were interpreted as caused by different things according to Chinese medical theories.[246] In contrast, Western medicine grouped infectious diseases into one category according to germ theory and pinpointed germs as the single causation. In the 1916 regulations, the Chinese government defined eight diseases to be notified and regulated by the government, a significant step to demonstrate the modern state's responsibility to the health of people. The diseases were cholera, dysentery, typhoid fever, smallpox, typhus, scarlet fever, diphtheria, and plague. The list was similar to the one used by the Japanese government, but did not include many of the infectious diseases Chinese medicine had traditionally defined, such as leprosy, malaria, and tuberculosis. The list was also different from the one created by the Health Commission of Guangdong province, which had pioneered in establishing a government public health department in 1912. The Guangdong provincial government listed leprosy, puerperal septicemia and hydrophobia (rabies) in addition to plague, cholera, smallpox and diphtheria as the notifiable infectious diseases.[247] Following the modern methods, the Chinese government built several isolation hospitals in Beijing and other cities to house patients of infectious diseases in the 1910s.

Modern methods of prevention of infectious diseases and epidemics differed from traditional Chinese measures. Traditional Chinese measures encouraged avoidance and fleeing from epidemics (*biyi*, 避疫) whereas modern Western methods focused on quarantine, isolation and disinfection.[248] Chinese medicine encountered increasing attacks from modern medical doctors mainly because its diagnosis and explanation of diseases differed from Western medicine and the newly minted germ theory. The difference in medical theories made Chinese medicine unwelcome to those who were eager to jump on the bandwagon of modern science. Moreover, the fact that Chinese medicine rarely pinpointed one specific cause of a disease became the focal point of attack by groups of modern science and medicine. The elite of Western medicine emphasized the inability of Chinese medicine to specify the exact cause of disease, especially in the fight against infectious diseases, as evidence of the unscientific and superstitious nature of Chinese medicine.

The medical and public health fields became a contesting ground of the competing medical groups during national struggles for progress and modernity. Science in the early twentieth century held unique significance for Chinese intelligentsia in their search for a new national order and identity of China in the modern world. In advocating science to save China, Chinese physicians of

Western medicine, like medical missionaries, dismissed Chinese medicine as incapable of treating diseases and preventing epidemics because it could not produce the same kind of pathological explanation as Western medicine did. In the meantime, the vast Chinese population continued to rely on Chinese medicine, showing little interest in Western medicine. The gap between the modern medical elite and the common Chinese was deep and wide, but medical modernizers used health campaigns to promote Western medicine at the expense of Chinese medicine. Among the modernizers who saw modernization little different from Westernization were the Western-oriented medical elite and intellectuals who did not hesitate to reject Chinese culture and tradition in their embracing of the West. Deng Songnian (Tsung-nien Tang, 邓松年) was one of those medical modernizers. A graduate of Beiyang Army Medical College, he served as a medical officer of the North Manchuria Plague Prevention Service before studying at Harvard University in 1920. Deng was an advocate of modern public health and state responsibility for people's health. He was disappointed with the Chinese government in the realm of public health work, but fascinated with the power of the British Empire and its leading politicians' advocacy of public health. Invoking British Prime Minister Benjamin Disraeli's statement that public health was the first duty of statesmen, Deng urged Chinese officials that "the health of the people is the power of the nation." He wanted the Chinese government to promote scientific medicine and do "away with superstition and quackery." He admired the West but had little confidence in his own culture and people. He once mentioned that the ability of Chinese traditional physicians "to tell the true cause of disease is just as hopeless as to ask a native mason to build a huge bridge, such as the Manhattan Bridge of New York, at the mouth of the River Yangtze."[249] Deng's views reflected the mentality of a growing group of Chinese intellectuals who adored the modern West while having little positive to say about China. His indiscriminate acceptance of Western medicine as the scientific truth and his rejection of Chinese medicine represented the attitude of total Westernization among Chinese intellectuals in the 1910s–1920s.[250]

In juxtaposition to the total Westernization mentality, there was, among the Chinese general public, a strong suspicion of foreign enterprises in China. The Council on Health Education, which was led by an American YMCA secretary and sponsored predominantly by missionary organizations, was a foreign enterprise in the eyes of many Chinese. Urban residents, who attended the health campaigns and watched the health parades, felt that they already knew the sanitation and public health problems. The question was what to do about them. The Council, however, was not able to provide pragmatic solutions. Chinese public health activists looked for economically efficient and socially practical means to solve health problems. They were disappointed that the Council talked about the technical approaches and neglected the socio-economic conditions that caused unsanitary conditions and diseases. Moreover, tensions between missionary groups and Chinese medical professionals led to the erosion of their working relations in the movement of public health education. After Peter resumed the leadership of the Council in 1920, Hu Xuanming left to work for the Guangzhou municipal government and headed the Health Department of the city. In 1921–1925, Hu worked with Chinese leaders and medical professionals in organizing a Chinese National Health Association under purely Chinese leadership. The very idea of starting an indigenous movement of public health that the Chinese people would trust and support came from the realization that the Council on Health Education was seen as a foreign entity, to which Chinese people were slow to respond.[251] The Chinese National Health Association aimed to prepare public health education in schools and colleges, organized mobile units to fight epidemics, and established a health museum and a laboratory of research.[252] But the Association functioned only for a short time, and was ironically dependent on the Council's technical guidance and financial support.[253] It became defunct in the midst of the political instability and financial difficulty of 1925.

Conclusion

From the late Qing to the early Republic, the concept of public health as national power took hold of Chinese intellectuals and officials as a fundamental means to promote social progress and national modernity. The desire to transform the declining traditional society into a modern strong nation was expressed in the advocacy of scientific medicine and public health. Motivations of public health campaigns and the meanings of public health in China differed from those in the West. Public health movements in Europe and America began as a response to the social and health problems of rapid industrialization and urbanization, whereas in China, public health movements started as a response to the political and cultural needs to transform the country from a weakened traditional society to a strong modern nation. In the West, public health activists were deeply aware of the relation between the effects of disease, the efficacy of labor force and economic growth. Disease was measured in dollars and cents and health was examined in relation to commercial prosperity; hence, disease was considered a liability to commercial capital and economy.[254] In contrast, public health activists in China were elite modernizers who were concerned first and foremost with the political status of China in the modern world, i.e. China's unity and sovereignty. In their effort to modernize China, they took public health as a measure of national strength, social progress, and cultural modernity.

Fragmented efforts to disseminate knowledge of modern hygiene and Western medicine had been carried out in China since the nineteenth century. When modern hygiene was promoted in the West in terms of scientific medicine for the benefits of people's health and commercial economy, the self-governing bodies of foreign settlements in China's semi-colonial treaty-port cities also became concerned with the unsanitary conditions harmful to the health of residents and their commerce. The British-controlled Shanghai Municipal Council of the International Settlement set up an Office of Hygiene in 1863 to follow the practice back in England, as modern industrial factories increasingly polluted the environment and pauperized the labor in Shanghai. By 1898, the office had evolved into the Public Health Department with a medical officer in charge.

Sanitary services such as garbage collection and street-cleaning were available in foreign settlements only, leaving out the Chinese sections of treaty ports. When health regulations were issued by foreign settlement authorities, contentions developed between foreign authorities and Chinese residents because the regulations directly restricted the daily life and livelihood of Chinese. Negotiations over health regulations became grounds of political struggle between the dominance of foreign powers and the resistance of Chinese population in treaty ports.

Public health was an issue of national sovereignty during the Qing's negotiations with foreign powers over the Boxer settlement. For the first time, the Chinese government encountered the demand to continue modern sanitary administration and public health as a condition to get back the cities of Beijing and Tianjin from foreign powers. The Qing's decision to reform and modernize led to the creation of a modern sanitary administration—the Beiyang Sanitary Service, and a police system first in Zhili in 1902, and then the Central Police with a sanitary department in 1905. The sanitary police oversaw epidemic prevention and control, urban sanitation, hospital supervision, inspection of food hygiene and pharmaceuticals. All of these were administrative modernization under the "New Policy" of the Qing government. The broad responsibilities of the sanitary police were not effectively implemented for lack of professional expertise and low literacy of policemen. Nonetheless, the sanitary police system proved vitally important for Governor Xi Liang to rely on when he dealt with the emergency of a plague crisis in northeast China in 1910. In the face of the worsening plague epidemic and the pressure of foreign powers' demands, the Chinese government had to come up with the means to fend off Russian and Japanese schemes of territory expansion in the name of health protection. Public health matters of the Manchurian plague, as in the Boxer negotiations, became a focal point of international politics when foreign powers used them as convenient pretext to exercise colonial ambitions. In bringing the plague under control, the Chinese government proved to the international powers that China had the ability to deal with epidemic crisis and to provide safety for the public, therefore, defusing a possible sovereign crisis of China. These experiences added multidimensional meanings to "plague control" in China. The term was understood as control of disease, national suffering, and foreign erosion of Chinese land, society and culture.

The suppression of the pneumonic plague epidemic gave medical scientists an opportunity to claim the superiority of Western medicine over Chinese medicine, despite the fact that neither Western medicine nor Chinese medicine proved capable of curing or preventing the disease at the time.[255] In view of local resistance to modern methods of isolation, disinfection and cremation, medical scientists emphasized the urgent need to educate Chinese officials as well as the populace the knowledge of scientific medicine. They firmly believed that ignorance and superstition led Chinese people to resist modern methods of preventive medicine. The Chinese people, therefore, had to be enlightened with modern science.

The question of public health was directly tied to the image of China, which was depicted by Western media as "the sick man of East Asia" at the turn of the twentieth century. China's decline and struggle to remain sovereign in the encounter with foreign powers gave rise to profound self-doubt and self-reappraisal of the Confucian tradition of moral and sociopolitical order among the Chinese educated class. Chinese intellectuals anguished over the question of whether the Chinese race (人种) and country (国家) would be able to survive the constant assault of foreign powers. In this "orientational crisis," as Hao Chang called it, Chinese intellectuals sought a new order to make sense of the world they lived in. [256] An increasing number of them considered Chinese traditional culture and polity an archaic obstacle to national advance in the modern era of Western dominance. Some Chinese intellectuals turned completely to the West for remedies for China's woes, while others insisted on preserving China's national essence in the modernization reforms to strengthen the country.

Social Darwinian writings deeply influenced Chinese intellectuals in their search for new ideas and means to strengthen China. Since the late nineteenth century, ideas of "evolution" and "survival of the fittest" shaped Chinese intellectuals' interpretation of national survival in the age of global imperialist aggression. The generation of Yan Fu and Liang Qichao conceptualized national strength in terms of people's physical fitness, moral virtues, and knowledge of science. The concept of science, a key element of modernity that spread globally along with the rise of the West, came to dominate Chinese intellectual orientation in the early twentieth century. Science was taken not only as the absolute truth but also the yardstick to measure the truth of every theory and practice. Chinese intellectuals saw science as the source of Western power and advocated modernization through science to save China from foreign dominance.[257] As this chapter shows, modernity and science came in different forms and shapes to influence the change in China. In the promotion of public health and modern scientific medicine, different groups tried to realize very different goals according to their own values and visions of China's future.

Western argument of an international order of racial hierarchy based on skin colors, in which the Chinese were defined as an inferior "yellow race" to the superior "white" West, also influenced Chinese perceptions of international relations with some Chinese literally buying into the racist theory that the Asians were an inferior race doomed to be conquered and ruled by the advanced white race. Some Chinese went along with the argument of racial pre-determination and even developed their views of a hierarchical racial order, possibly seeking some comfort that the Chinese, as a yellow race, were not at the bottom of the racial structure projected by the white West.[258] The myth of racial hierarchy was fundamentally discredited when Japan staged a military triumph over Russia in 1905. It proved that race had nothing to do with the fate of a nation; instead, fundamental reforms were *the* key to rejuvenate the nation.[259] Nationalist confidence rose and China looked at Japan as a successful example of modern reforms. Patriotic Chinese young men and women went to Japan to seek modern knowledge and the secrets of success. Modern medicine became a favorite subject of Chinese students who wanted to save lives and improve their country, though many turned out to be more interested in revolution than a medical career.

The Yuan Shikai government promulgated a modern curriculum of medical education and legalized dissection of dead bodies for medical studies. A series of sanitation and public health regulations was issued by the new Republic. Infectious diseases were categorized according to international standards and regulated by the government for the first time. The initial step of modern administration of medical education and public health was further facilitated by the establishment of hospitals to treat and isolate infectious diseases. However, the government promoted modern medicine at the expense of Chinese medicine, and even required Western medical education as the qualification for government positions. These policies and requirements contributed to the increasing tensions between Western and Chinese medicines.

Public health education campaigns launched by the Council on Health Education popularized germ theory and Western medicine to a wide range of social classes in terms of hygiene, sanitation, and disease prevention in Chinese society. The campaigns aimed to accomplish the goals of spreading public health knowledge, arousing local interest, and making connections with government officials to develop favorable relations to work on public health matters. Leaders of the campaigns were not public health professionals but doctors of Western medicine who took a genuine interest in popular education about preventive medicine. They staged public health campaigns to popularize medical science in the hope of informing people of preventive knowledge. The campaigns also served to spread the ideas and concepts of Western medicine as fundamental ingredients of the modern transformation of Chinese society. In fact, doctors of Western medicine championed the importance of scientific knowledge of medicine in China's transformation from a traditional society to a modern nation. In educating Chinese urban residents about public health and preventive medicine, the Council relied primarily on the American model and transferred American methods and materials to China, which tended to alienate Chinese audience with a feeling of foreign imposition. As efforts to improve the health education effect, the Council created a variety of programs such as the national health essay contests for students, and distributed large quantities of posters and pamphlets to educational and commercial institutions across China.

Health education campaigns helped raise the public awareness of individual health and national strength. Moreover, they contributed to the development of a modern discourse of public health in Chinese society before the professional training of public health was established at medical schools. Popular understanding of the idea of *weisheng* went far beyond the conventional sense of hygiene and sanitation, as the urban community used it to protect itself from health hazard and the police used it to warn against carbon monoxide poisoning. With the introduction of modern ideas and practices of hygiene and public health, the ancient Chinese concept of *weisheng* gained new meanings along with the social and political transformations of China.[260]

Notes

1 George Rosen, *A History of Public Health*, expanded edition (Baltimore: The Johns Hopkins University Press, 1993), 1.
2 Rogaski, *Hygienic Modernity*, 1.
3 The eight powers were Britain, Germany, France, the United States, Russia, Italy, Austria-Hungary, and Japan.
4 Chi-min Wong and Wu Lien-teh, *History of Chinese Medicine* (Shanghai: National Quarantine Service 1936, reprinted by New York: Ams Press, 1973), 592.
5 William C. Summers, *The Great Manchurian Plague of 1910–1911: The Geopolitics of an Epidemic Disease* (New Haven: Yale University Press, 2012), 11.
6 Robert A. Bickers, *The Scramble for China: Foreign Devils in the Qing Empire, 1800–1914* (London: Allen Lane, 2011).
7 Imperial Russian Embassy, Washington, to Secretary of State Knox, January 19, 1911, NA [National Archives in Washington, D.C.], 158.931/64. Cited in Carl F. Nathan, *Plague Prevention and Politics in Manchuria, 1910–1931*(East Asian Research Center, Harvard University, 1967), 21–22, and footnote 86.
8 International power politics and the complication of plague control in northeast China was recorded by Wu Liande. See Wu Tien-teh, *Plague Fighter*: *The Autobiography of a Modern Chinese Physician* (Cambridge: W. Heffer and Sons, 1959), chapters I–III.
9 James L. Hevia, *English Lessons: The Pedagogy of Imperialism in Nineteenth Century China* (Durham, NC: Duke University Press, 2003).
10 William Lockhart, *The Medical Missionary in China: A Narrative of Twenty Years' Experience* (London: Hurst and Blackett, Publishers, 1861), 235.
11 Ibid., 244.
12 Ibid., 40.
13 Ibid., 244.
14 Charles A. Gordon, *China from a Medical Point of View in 1860 and1861; to which is added a chapter on Nagasaki as a Sanitaria* (London: Baillière & Co., 1863), 82–83.
15 The origins of Chinese public bathhouses developed with commerce in cities where merchants far away from home needed a place to clean themselves. A kettle was hung in front of the door to indicate a bathhouse. See Fan Xingzhun, *Zhonguo yüfang yixue sixiang shi* [An Intellectual History of Chinese Preventive Medicine] (Beijing: Renmin weisheng chubanshe, 1954), 58–68.
16 For the socio-political functions and public life of teahouses, see Di Wang, *The Teahouse: Small Business, Everyday Culture, and Public Politics in Chengdu, 1900–1950* (CA: Stanford University Press, 2008).
17 Lockhart, *Medical Missionary in China*, 37–48.
18 J. G. Cormack, "Early Days of Western Medicine in Peking," *China Medical Journal*, vol. XL, no. 6 (June 1926), 520.
19 John Dudgeon, *Medical Reports*, July–September, 1871, p. 76; cited in Gao Xi, *Dezhen zhuan: Yi ge Yingguo chuanjiaoshi yu wan Qing yixue jindai hua* [Dudgeon: An English Missionary and Medical Modernization in Late Qing] (Shanghai: Fudan University Press, 2009), 392.
20 John Dudgeon, *Medical Reports*, July–September 1872, p. 42; cited in Gao Xi, *Dezhen zhuan*, 393.
21 George Rosen, *History of Public Health*, 263–65.
22 E. O. Jordan, G. C. Whipple and C-E. A. Winslow, *A Pioneer of Public Health: William Thompson Sedgwick* (New Haven: Yale University Press, 1924), 57.
23 Shang-jen Li, "Discovering 'The Secrets of Long and Healthy Life': John Dudgeon on Chinese Hygiene," *Social History of Medicine*, vol. 23, no. 1 (2010), 21–37.
24 Lockhart, *Medical Missionary*, 244.
25 Kerrie L. MacPherson, *A Wilderness of Marshes: The Origins of Public Health in Shanghai, 1843–1893* (New York: Lexington Books, 2002), 39.

26 David Rosner, "Beyond Typhoid Mary: The Origins of Public Health at Columbia and in the City," in *Living Legacies at Columbia*, ed. William Theodore De Bary (New York: Columbia University Press, 2006), 272.
27 Charles Dickens exposed the dreadful conditions of disease and poverty in London slums in many of his novels, as his life paralleled the sanitary movement in England. See Socrates Litsios, "Charles Dickens and the Movement for Sanitary Reform," *Perspectives in Biology and Medicine*, vol. 46, no. 2 (Spring 2003), 183–199.
28 Lockhart, *Medical Missionary*, 235.
29 *Collection of Historical Documents of the Public Health Department of Shanghai Municipal Council*, vol. 2 (1865–1928), 285. Shanghai Municipal Archives, U1-16-4698 (2).
30 Arnold Wright and H. A. Cartwright, *Twentieth Century Impressions of Hongkong, Shanghai, and Other Treaty Ports of China: Their History, People, Commerce, Industries, and Resources* (London: Lloyd's Greater Britain Publishing Company, Ltd, 1908), 438–682.
31 Public Health Department of the Shanghai Municipal Council, 1928, p. 27, Shanghai Municipal Archives, U1-16-227. Also see Xiong Yuezhi and Ma Xueqiang, eds., *Shanghai de waiguo ren, 1842–1949* [Foreigners in Shanghai, 1842–1949] (Shanghai guji chubanshe, 2003).
32 J. H. Jordan, "Shanghai Municipal Council—Public Health Department," *Chinese Medical Journal*, vol. 49 (1935), 993; and "Public Health of Shanghai Municipal Council," Shanghai Municipal Archives.
33 Zheng Guanying, "Road Construction" in *Collections of Zheng Guanying*, ed. Xia Dongyuan (Shanghai renmin chubanshe, 1982), vol. 1, 663.
34 Wright and Cartwright, *Twentieth Century Impressions*, 434–445.
35 *Collection of Historical Documents of the Public Health Department*, vol. 2, 87–88. Shanghai Municipal Archives, U1-16-4697.
36 Wright and Cartwright, *Twentieth Century Impressions*, 434.
37 *Collection of Historical Documents of the Public Health Department of Shanghai Municipal Council*, vol. 2, 1865–1928, 374. Shanghai Municipal Archives, U1-16-4698 (2).
38 Ariane Knüsel, *Framing China: Media Images and Political Debates in Britain, the USA and Switzerland, 1900–1950* (England: Ashgate, 2012).
39 "Weisheng lun [On Hygiene]," reprinted in *Dongfang zazhi* [Eastern Miscellany], vol. 2, no. 8 (1905), 157.
40 Chen Duxiu, "My Patriotism," *The New Youth*, vol. 2, no. 2 (October 1, 1916), 1–6, 4.
41 David Arnold, ed., *Imperial Medicine and Indigenous Societies* (Manchester University Press, 1988); Roy MacLeod and Milton Lewis, eds., *Disease, Medicine and Empire: Perspectives on Western Medicine and Experience of European Expansion* (New York and London: Routledge, 1988). There was a long history of medical exchange between China and other nations before the arrival of modern European imperialism. See Ma Boying, Gao Xi, and Hong Zhongli, *Zhongwai yixue wenhua jiaoliu shi* [History of Cultural Exchanges of Medicine between China and Foreign Countries] (Shanghai: Wenhui chubanshi 1993).
42 Roy Porter, *The Greatest Benefit to Mankind: A Medical History of Humanity* (New York: W. W. Norton & Company, 1999), 463.
43 Robert Barde, "Plague in San Francisco: An Essay Review," *Journal of the History of Medicine and Allied Sciences*, vol. 59, no. 3 (2004), 463–470; Nayan Shah, *Contagious Divides: Epidemics and Race in San Francisco's Chinatown* (Berkeley, CA: University of California Press, 2001); and Charles McClain, *In Search of Equality: The Chinese Struggle against Discrimination in Nineteenth-Century America* (Berkeley, CA: University of California Press, 1994). Immigrants were often blamed for the outbreaks of diseases and other problems in America. See Howard Markel, *Quarantine! East European Jewish Immigrants and the New York City Epidemics of 1892* (Baltimore: Johns Hopkins University Press, 1999).

44 Shang-Jen Li, "Miraculous Surgery in a Heathen Land: Medical Missions to Nineteenth-Century China," www.ihp.sinica.edu.tw/~linfs/rh/active/miraculous.pdf, accessed May 16, 2010.

45 Walter R. Lambuth, *Medical Missions: The Twofold Task* (New York: Student Volunteer Movement for Foreign Missions, 1920), 107.

46 Ibid., 125.

47 Larissa N. Heinrich, "Handmaids to the Gospel: Lam Qua's Medical Portraiture," in *Tokens of Exchange*, ed., Lydia Liu (Duke University Press, 1999), 239–75. Some scholars pointed out that clinical photographs in the mid-nineteenth century frequently concentrated on "people suffering from extraordinary physical illness or disabilities." See Daniel M. Fox and Christopher Lawrence, *Photographing Medicine: Images and Power in Britain and America since 1840*, Greenwood Press, 1988, 25. In China, cameras were rare in the nineteenth century and missionary doctors used paintings to represent the deformity and illness of Chinese patients.

48 It was a myth that China did not have scientific investigations before the arrival of science from the West. The Chinese term "*gewu zhizhi*, 格物致知" shorterned as "*ge zhi*,格致" has the same meaning as "*ke xue*, 科学," science. Missionaries, when they went to evangelize other societies, knew little about those societies but assumed their backwardness and the need for sweeping changes in the image of the West.

49 David Arnold, ed., *Imperial Medicine and Indigenous Societies*; *Colonizing the Body: State, Medicine, and Epidemic Disease in Nineteenth-Century India* (University of California Press, 1993); Bridie Andrews and Chris Cunningham, eds. *Western Medicine as Contested Knowledge* (Manchester University Press, 1997); and Warwick Anderson, "Immunities of Empire: Race, Disease, and the New Tropical Medicine, 1900–1920," *Bulletin of the History of Medicine*, vol. 70, no. 1 (1996), 94–118.

50 Harold Balme, *China and Modern Medicine: A Study in Medical Missionary Development* (London: United Council for Missionary Education, 1921), 5–6.

51 Lambuth, *Medical Missions,* 72.

52 W. Hamilton Jefferys and James L. Maxwell, *The Diseases of China, Including Formosa and Korea* (London: John Bale, Sons & Danielsson, LTD, 1914), 12.

53 Wang Hsiu-yun, "Refusing Male Physicians: The Gender and Body Politics of Missionary Medicine in China, 1870s–1920s," *Bulletin of the Institute of Modern History Academia Sinica*, vol. 59 (2008), 29–66.

54 Patricia Ebrey and Anne Walthal, *Modern East Asia: From 1600* (Houghton, 2009), 316.

55 Yung Wing, *My Life in China and America* (New York: Henry Holt and Company, 1909). Yung Wing successfully persuaded the Qing Court to send young Chinese to study in the United States to gain modern knowledge of science and technology. In 1870, a total of 120 young Chinese boys were sent by the Chinese government to the United States for their entire education from grade school to college. See Thomas E. LaFargue, *China's First Hundred: Educational Mission Students in the United States, 1872–1881* (Pullman, WA: Washington State University Press, 1987).

56 *Customs Medical Report*, No. 6 (1873), 49; cited in Wu Lien-teh, J.W.H. Chun, R. Pollitzer and C.Y. Wu, *Cholera* (Shanghai: National Quarantine Service, 1934), 13.

57 Weili Ye "'Nü Liuxuesheng': The Story of American-Educated Chinese Women, 1880s–1920s," *Modern China*, vol. 20, no. 3 (July 1994), 315–346; Connie Anne Shemo, *The Chinese Medical Ministries of Kang Cheng and Shi Meiyu, 1872–1937* (PA: Lehigh University Press, 2011); and Kwok Pui-lan, *Chinese Women and Christianity, 1860–1927* (Atlanta, GA: Scholars Press, 1992).

58 More scholarly attention and studies should be directed at Chinese women physicians and their contribution to medicine and scientific culture in modern China.

59 "Chinese Women Doctors: Dr. Yamei Kin Tells of Training Schools at Tien-Tsin." *The New York Times*, July 21, 1915, 20. Weili Ye, *Seeking Modernity in China's Name* (Stanford University Press, 2001), 116.

60 "A Chinese Lady to Study Medicine." *The New York Times*, May 9, 1884, 5.

61 Ryan Dunch, *Fuzhou Protestants and the Making of a Modern China, 1857–1927* (New Haven: Yale University Press, 2001), 193–194. There was confusion about Xu Jinhong's Chinese name in English works. Kwok Pui-lan gave one version in *Chinese Women and Christianity*, and Weili Ye gave another in "Nü Liuxuesheng." Dunch set the record straight in his book.
62 "Dr. Yamei Jin." *Boston Evening Transcript*, April 23, 1904.
63 W. Hamilton Jefferys and James L. Maxwell, *Diseases of China*, 12.
64 Wong and Wu, *History of Chinese Medicine*, 844–849.
65 Xi Lian, *The Conversion of Missionaries: Liberalism in American Protestant Missions in China, 1907–1932* (State College, PA: Pennsylvania State University Press, 1997); and Henrietta Harrison, *The Missionary's Curse and Other Tales from a Chinese Catholic Village* (CA: University of California Press, 2013).
66 Chinese scholar Guo Moruo summarized that Chinese nationalism "was just two slogans, 'eradicate the traitors within, resist aggression from without.'" (Kuo Mo'jo, "A Poet with the Northern Expedition," trans. J. W. Bennett, *The Far Eastern Quarterly*, vol. 3, no. 2 (February 1944), 168. Chinese nationalism, like that of the decolonization movements in other countries, emphasized national sovereignty and "a conscious loyalty to a unified China, lest China be swallowed up by the colonial powers." John A. Harrison, *China since 1880* (New York: Harcourt, Brace & World, Inc., 1967), 131.
67 James Ricalton, *China through the Stereoscope: A Journey through the Dragon Empire at the Time of the Boxer Uprising* (New York: Underwood and Underwood, 1901).
68 Michael H. Hunt, "The American Remission of the Boxer Indemnity: A Reappraisal," *Journal of Asian Studies*, vol. 31, no. 3 (May 1972), 539–559; and See Heng Teow, *Japan's Cultural Policy toward China, 1918–1931: A Comparative Perspective* (Cambridge, MA: Harvard University Asia Center, 1999).
69 Michael Hunt, "The Forgotten Occupation: Peking, 1900–1901," *Pacific Historical Review*, vol. 48, no. 4 (1979), 501–529.
70 Rogaski, *Hygienic Modernity*, chapter 6.
71 Lewis Bernstein, "After the Fall: Tianjin under Foreign Occupation, 1900–1902," in *The Boxers, China, and the World*, eds. Robert Bickers and R. G. Tiedemann (Rowman & Littlefield Publishers, 2007), chapter 7.
72 George Rosen, *From Medical Police to Social Medicine* (New York: Science History Publications, 1974) and *A History of Public Health*; Richard H. Shryock, *The Development of Modern Medicine* (Madison, WI: University of Wisconsin Press, 1980); John Duffy, *The Sanitarians: A History of American Public Health* (University of Illinois Press, 1992); and Dorothy Porter and Roy Porter, "What Was Social Medicine? An Historiographical Essay," *The Journal of Historical Sociology*, vol. 1 (1988), 90–106.
73 Elizabeth Fee and Dorothy Porter, "Public Health, Preventive Medicine and Professionalization: England and America in the Nineteenth Century," in *Medicine in Society: Historical Essays*, ed. Andrew Wear (Cambridge University Press, 1992), 250.
74 Ibid., 253.
75 David Rosner, "Beyond Typhoid Mary: The Origins of Public Health at Columbia and in the City," *Living Legacies* (Spring 2004), 3. www.columbia.edu/cu/alumni/Magazine/Spring2004/publichealth.html. Accessed February 15, 2010.
76 John Blake, *Public Health in the Town of Boston, 1630–1822* (Cambridge, MA: Harvard University Press, 1959); Barbara Rosenkrantz, *Public Health and the State: Changing Views in Massachusetts, 1842–1936* (Cambridge, MA: Harvard University Press, 1972); John Duffy, *A History of Public Health in New York City, 1625–1866* (New York: 1968); Stuart Galishoff, *Safeguarding the Public Health: Newark, 1895–1918* (Westport, CT, 1975); Judith Walzer Leavitt, *The Healthiest City: Milwaukee and the Politics of Health Reform* (Princeton, NJ, 1982); Elizabeth Fee and Roy M. Acheson, eds., *A History of Education in Public Health: Health That Mocks the Doctors' Rules*

(Oxford University Press, 1991); and Nancy Tomes, *The Gospel of Germs: Men, Women, and the Microbe in American Life* (Harvard University Press, 1999).
77 Stephen R. MacKinnon, *Power and Politics in Late Imperial China: Yuan Shikai in Beijing and Tianjin, 1901–1908* (Berkeley and Los Angeles, CA: University of California Press, 1980).
78 Gan Houci, *Beiyang gongdu leizhuan zhengxubian* (Tianjin: Tianjin chuban chuanmei jituan and Tianjin guji chubanshe, 2013).
79 "Tianjin Jiuji Yuan" and "Tianjin Guangren Tang", Tianjin Municipal Archives.
80 Li Hong'e, Wang Yandong, Liu Jindiand Li Dongning, "Ji Zhongguo di yi suo gongli hushi xuexiao—beiyang nu yi xuetang [The First Nursing School of China—Beiyang Women's Medical School]," *Weisheng zhiye jiaoyu* [Health Vocational Education], vol. 28, no. 14 (2010), 35–37.
81 "Chinese Women Doctors: Dr. Yamei Kin Tells of Training Schools at Tien-tsin," *The New York Times*, July 21, 1915, 20. Jin Yunmei did not return to resume her position of the director of Beiyang Women's Hospital and School the next year possibly because Yuan Shikai died and the leaders of China changed. Kang Cheng (Ida Kahn) was chosen to serve as the director of the hospital and school in 1915–1918, during which she was reported spending her days in busy social life in Tianjin and leaving the management work to her staff. As a result, the hospital and school verged on bankruptcy, only to be saved by a new director called Cao Liyun, who served during 1918–1922.
82 Cui Lianyu, "Qingmo weisheng jingcha de chuangli ji lishi zuoyong" [The Creation of Sanitary Police in Late Qing and its Historical Function], *Zhonghua yishi zazhi* [Chinese Journal of Medical History], vol. 18, no. 2 (1988), 97–98.
83 Wu Lien-teh, "The Prevention of Infectious Diseases in China," *China Medical Journal*, vol. XLIII, no. 4 (April 1929), 343.
84 Carol Benedict, "Policing the Sick: Plague and the Origins of State Medicine in Late Imperial China," *Late Imperial China*, vol. 14, no. 2 (December 1993), 60–77.
85 Wong and Wu, *History of Chinese Medicine*, 567.
86 Chen Bangxian, *Zhonguo yixue shi* [Medical History of China] (Shanghai: Shangwu yinshuguan, 1937; reprint, 1998), 228–29.
87 Ibid., 230–31.
88 "Yike daxue zhangcheng shangque [Discussion on the Curriculum of Medical College]", *Dongfang zazhi*, vol. 2, no. 11 (1905), 259–260.
89 Ibid., 260–261.
90 Gu Yin, "On the Relation of China's Future and Medicine," *Dongfang zazhi*, vol. 2, no. 6 (1905), 107–114.
91 "On Hygiene," *Dongfang zazhi* (1905), 156–157.
92 His translation included Thomas Huxley's *Evolution and Ethics* (Tian Yan Lun), John Mill's *On Liberty* (Qunji Quanjie Lun), Adam Smith's *The Wealth of Nations* (Yuan Fu), and Herbert Spencer's *A Study of Sociology* (Qunxue Yilun). See Benjamin Schwartz, *In Search of Wealth and Power: Yen Fu and the West* (Cambridge, MA: The Belknap Press of Harvard University Press, 1964); and James Reeve Pusey, *China and Charles Darwin* (Harvard University Press, 1983).
93 Tsu Jing, *Failure, Nationalism, and Literature: The Making of Modern Chinese Identity, 1895–1937* (Stanford University Press, 2005). Magazines like *Science* (科学), *Eastern Miscellany* (东方杂志), *The New Youth* (新青年) and newspapers like *Dagongbao* (大公报), *Times* (时报) and *Shenbao* (申报) provided rich data on the popular obsession with Social Darwinian concepts in early twentieth-century China.
94 Liu Mengxu, ed., *Yan Fu juan* (Hebei Jiaoyu chubanshe, 1996, 550).
95 Yan Fu, "The Relation between Education and the Nation," *Eastern Miscellany*, vol. 3, no. 3 (1906), 29–34.
96 *Liang Qichao ping lun wen ji* [Collection of Liang Qichao's Essays] (Taiwan Xinsheng baoshe, 1990), 20–1; and Li Huaxing and Wu Jiaxun, eds., *Liang Qichao xuan ji* (Shanghai: Shanghai renmin chubanshe, 1984), 209–10.

97 Chiu-Sam Tsang, *Nationalism in School Education in China* (Hong Kong: Progressive Education Publishers, 1967).

98 Flectcher Brockman, General Secretary of the National Committee of the YMCA of China, "Report of Fletcher. S. Brockman," *Annual and Quarterly Reports of Field Secretaries of the YMCA*, 1905–1906, p. 47. University of Minnesota, YMCA Archives.

99 Wang Qisheng, *Liuxue yu jiuguo* [Studying Abroad and Saving the Nation] (Guangxi Normal University Press, 1995); and Saito Keishu, *Zhongguo ren liuxue riben shi* [History of Chinese Students in Japan], trans. Tan Ruqian and Lin Qiyan, (Hongkong: Chinese University Press, 1982.)

100 Susan L. Burns, "Constructing the National Body: Public Health and the Nation in the Nineteenth Century Japan," in *Nation Work: Asian Elites and National Identity*, ed. Timothy Brook and Andre Schmid (Ann Arbor: The University of Michigan Press, 2000).

101 Individual educators had in fact started their own educational reforms by establishing new schools in local communities without the central government's formal policy. See Marianne Bastid, *Education in Early Twenthieth-Century China*, trans. Paul J. Bailey (Ann Arbor, MI: Center for Chinese Studies, The University of Michigan, 1988); and Sally Borthwick, *Education and Social Change in China: The Beginnings of the Modern Era* (Stanford: Hoover Institution Press, 1983).

102 During the reform, some schools made a genuine effort to create an effective education with the purpose of strengthening the nation, but many only followed the trend with a name change of the school. Such superficiality inevitably led to the failure of many new schools. For contemporary accounts of educational reforms, see, for instance, Guo Moruo's *Childhood* (少年时代); Chiang Yee's *A Chinese Childhood*, and Li Boyuan's *Modern Times* (文明小史). Nevertheless, the three goals of "morality, intelligence, and physical fitness," very much influenced by the West, remained the principles of Chinese modern education throughout the twentieth century under the Nationalist and the Communist school systems despite different political ideologies. They are the three-good standards (三好标准) in modern education in China.

103 Andrew Morris, "To Make the Four Hundred Million Move," *Comparative Studies in Society and History*, vol. 42, no. 4 (2000), 879.

104 Li Boyuan, *Modern Times: A Brief History of Enlightenment,* trans. Douglas Lancashire (Hong Kong, Research Center for Translation, Chinese University of Hong Kong, 1996), 172.

105 Kang Youwei, *Riben shumu zhi* [Bibliography of Japanese Books] (Shanghai, 1898), 18.

106 Wong and Wu, *History of Chinese Medicine*, 406.

107 Ding Fubao was an influential figure in modern Chinese medical history. His prolific translation and writing and his active involvement in the research and debate on Western and Chinese medicine significantly contributed to medical modernization in China.

108 Ding Fubao, *Zhongxi yifang huitong* [Combining Chinese and Western Medical Prescriptions] (Shanghai, 1910).

109 Liang Qichao, "Yixue shanhui xu" [On the Medical Philanthropy Society], in *Yin-bing shi wenji* [Collection of the Ice-Drinking Studio], Shanghai, 1916. It is no surprise that Sun Yat-sen and Lu Xun who wanted to change China started with medical studies.

110 "Background of Shanghai Public Health," Shanghai Municipal Archives.

111 Owen Lattimore, *Inner Asian Frontiers of China* (Boston: Beacon, 1962), 105.

112 Wong and Wu, *History of Chinese Medicine*, 592; Jiao Runming, "The Plague in Northeast China from 1910 to 1911 and Measures Adopted by the Government and the Public," *Jindai shi yanjiu* [Modern Chinese History Studies], no. 3 (2006); and Cao Shuji and Li Yushang, "Origins of Plague Epidemic in Chinese History: A Discussion of the Concept of 'Unison of the Universe and Man' in Traditional Times," in *The Relation of the Universe and Man in Chinese Economic History* (Chinese Agriculture Publisher, 2002).

113 The plague originated in neighboring Russian towns in the spring–summer 1910. Many Chinese laborers were recruited to hunt for the fur of Siberian marmots, which was highly profitable in international markets. When the plague broke out, the Russian government took strict control and drove out the Chinese with possible infection. The men who first died of the plague in Manzhouli were returnees from Russia. For a full account of the plague epidemic, see Fengtian Central Bureau of Plague Prevention, *Report on the Plague in the Northeast Three Provinces* (Fengtian, 1912); and *Report of the International Plague Conference Held at Mukden, April, 1911* (Manila Bureau of Printing, 1912).

114 Wu Lien-teh, *Plague Fighter*, 32–33. At the centennial anniversary of the plague, Wu Liande and his contribution to modern public health are commemorated in Chinese literature and public ceremonies. See Wang Zhe, *Guoshi wushuang Wu Liande* [The Unique Countryman Wu Liande] (Fujian jiaoyu chubanche, 2007). The city of Harbin built a Wu Liande Memorial Hall, the first for a medical scientist in Heilongjiang province.

115 Carl F. Nathan, *Plague Prevention and Politics in Manchuria, 1910–1931* (East Asian Research Center, Harvard University, 1967).

116 "Imperial Russian Embassy, Washington, to Secretary of State Knox, January 19, 1911, NA [National Archives in Washington, D.C.], 158.931/64, cited in Carl F. Nathan, *Plague Prevention*, 21–22, and footnote 86.

117 Nathan, *Plague Prevention,* 32.

118 For the international complication of the plague control in northeast of China, see Wu, *Plague Fighter*, chapters I–III.

119 Preventive medicine was nothing new in China. It can be traced back more than two thousand years in the texts of *Huangdi neijing* [*Yellow Emperor's Classics of Internal Medicine*] and other Chinese classics such as *Shi jing* (诗经), *Shi ji* (史记), *Huai nanzi* (淮南子) and *Sanhai jing* (三海经). It emphasized personal and environmental hygiene, and attention to diet, clothing, and bodily care. While isolation and quarantine were known concepts in traditional China, family home was the base for patient care in China. Preventive care in Western-style hospital system came into practice only after missionaries introduced hospitals in the nineteenth century. See Fan Xingzhun, *Zhonguo yüfang yixue sixiang shi* (Beijing: Renmin weisheng chubanshe, 1954); and Lü Suying, *Zhongyi hulixue* [Nursing in Chinese Medicine] (Beijing: Renmin weisheng chubanshe, 1983).

120 By that time, the Qing dynasty had been overthrown and the newly created Republic was in deep financial difficulties. The Viceroy of the northeast, Zhao Erxun (赵尔巽), appropriated 140,000 taels of silver of government revenue to build hospitals and research facilities of the Plague Prevention Service, but funds to maintain the Service had to be negotiated with foreign powers that controlled China's Maritime Customs, the only source of steady income for China, but it was designated to pay indemnities to foreign powers. The powers at first vetoed the scheme, but were later persuaded to agree to the withdrawal of 60,000 taels annually from the Chinese Maritime Customs for the maintenance of the Service. Regulations were drawn by the Chinese diplomat Yan Huiqing (颜惠庆) to put the Plague Prevention Service under the aegis of the Ministry of Foreign Affairs of China. (Wong and Wu, *History of Chinese Medicine*, pp. 593–94.)

121 Carsten Flohr, "The Plague Fighter: Wu Lien-teh and the Beginning of the Chinese Public Health System," in *Annals of Science*, vol. 53, no. 4 (1996), 361–380.

122 Dugald Christie, *Thirty Years in the Manchu Capital* (New York: McBride, Nast & Company, 1914), 246.

123 Yu Yongmin, "Qingmo minguo shiqi Liaoning yiyao weisheng shilüe" [A Historical Review of Medical and Health Work in Liaoning Province, 1881–1949], *Zhonghua yishi zazhi* [Chinese Journal of Medical History], vol. 19, no. 4 (1989), 193–99; and Wang Jiajian, *Qingmo minchu wo guo jingcha zhidu xiandaihua de licheng (1901–1928)*

[*Modernization of the Chinese Police System in the Late Qing and Early Republican Era, 1901–1928*] (Taibei, Shangwu yinshu guan, 1984). Carol Benedict discussed the police role in the plague fight in China's northeast in her article, "Policing the Sick: Plague and the Origins of State Medicine in Late Imperial China," *Late Imperial China*, vol. 14, no. 2 (1993), 60–77.

124 Jiao Runming, "Plague in Northeast China," *Modern Chinese History Studies*, no. 3 (2006), 106–124.

125 Wu, *Plague Fighter*, 34–35; and Dugald Christie, *Thirty Years in the Manchu Capital*, 237–244.

126 "Isolation Station Closed due to the Infection of the Entire Staff," *Shengjing shibao*, eighth day of the second month, year 3 of Xuantong reign.

127 Wu, *Plague Fighter*, 37. Wu provided a chart of the specific professions of the anti-plague employees.

128 Jiao Runming, "The Plague in Northeast China," 116.

129 Mark Gamsa, "The Epidemic of Pneumonic Plague in Manchuria 1910–1911," *Past and Present*, vol. 190 (2006), 155.

130 Jiao Runming, "The Plague in Northeast China," 109.

131 Cui Xianyuan, "To Chinese Physicians of Western Medicine on Plague Prevention," *Dagongbao*, fifteenth day of the first month, year three of Xuantong reign, p. 3.

132 Jiao Runming, "The Plague in Northeast China," 114.

133 Dugald Christie, *Thirty Years in the Manchu Capital*, 248.

134 Ibid., 248.

135 Jiao Runming, "The Plague in Northeast China," 115.

136 Dugald Christie, *Thirty Years in the Manchu Capital*,250

137 Ibid., 252–53.

138 There were no reliable statistics of illiteracy rate in China at this time but it was estimated at above 85 percent.

139 Dugald Christie, *Thirty Years in the Manchu Capital*, 252–253.

140 *Report of the International Plague Conference*, 269.

141 *Report on the Plague in the Northeast Three Provinces* (Fengtian, 1912), part 2, chapter 6, 7–9.

142 Jiao Runming, "The Plague in Northeast China," 115.

143 The price of the marmot fur skyrocketed in international market before the outbreak of the plague. From 1907 to 1910, the price increased more than 6 times and the export of marmot fur from Manzhouli alone increased from 700,000 to 2,500,000. Human greed led to ferocious hunting for marmots. The plague could be understood as a response of nature to human greed. See Xia Mingfang and Kang Peizhu, eds., *Ershi shiji Zhongguo zaibian tushi* [Illustrations of Disasters in Twentieth-Century China] (Guangxi shifan daxue chubanshe, 2001).

144 Chen Bangxian, *Zhonguo yixue shi*, 284.

145 René Baehrel, "Class Hatred in Times of Epidemic," *Les Annales* 7 (1952); Nancy M. Frieden, *Russian Physicians in an Era of Reform and Revolution, 1856–1905* (Princeton University Press, 1981); and Terence Ranger and Paul Slack, eds., *Epidemics and Ideas: Essays on the Historical Perception of Pestilence* (Cambridge University Press, 1996).

146 Karl-Heinz Leven, "Poisoners and 'Plague-Smearers'," *Lancet*, 354 (December 1999), SIV53; and Dugald Christie, *Thirty Years in the Manchu Capital*, 247.

147 Frank M. Snowden, "Cholera in Barletta 1910," *Present and Past*, 132 (1991), 67–103.

148 "Municipal Notification, No. 2064: Plague, Public Health Byelaws," 1910. Public Health Department of Shanghai Municipal Council, U1-2-374, p.133, Shanghai Municipal Archives.

149 Ibid.

150 Robert Bickers, *Britain in China: Community, Culture and Colonialism, 1900–1949* (Manchester University Press, 1999), 125; and Zou Yiren, *Jiu Shanghai renkou bianjian*

de yanjiu [Study of the Population Change in Old Shanghai] (Shanghai renmin chubanshe, 1980), 90, 115.

151 Hu Cheng, "Quarantine, Race, and Policies in the International Settlement: Clashes between Chinese and Foreigners after the Outbreak of Plague in Shanghai," *Jindai shi yan jiu* [*Modern Chinese History Studies*] no. 4 (2007), 74–90.

152 "Letter to Chairman of the Municipal Council from Chinese Chamber of Commerce, Nov. 13, 1910," U1-2-374, p. 117, Shanghai Municipal Archives.

153 Ding Fubao, "Shuyi bingyin liaofa lun [On the Cause and Cure of Plague]," *Shengjing shibao*, eleventh and twelfth days of first month, year three of Xuantong reign, p. 3.

154 Ding Fubao, "Jing gao ge sheng defang zizhi yiyuan [To All the Provincial Council Members]," *Dagongbao*, thirteenth and fourteenth days of first month, year three of Xuantong reign, p. 1.

155 Rosen, *History of Public Health*; and C.-E. A Winslow, *The Evolution and Significance of the Modern Public Health Campaign* (New Haven: Yale University Press, 1923).

156 When Western medicine was increasingly promoted as the scientific medicine, scholars and practitioners of Chinese medicine, such as Ding Fubao and He Lianchen (何廉臣, 1861–1929) actively engaged in the intellectual debate of scientific medical theories. They formed the pioneering Chinese Medical Society (中国医学会) and published medical journals such as *Medical News* (医学报) to deal with the emerging challenges to traditional concepts of Chinese medicine.

157 Wong and Wu, *History of Chinese Medicine*, 606–610.

158 Yan Fuqing had deep connections with Chinese officialdom. His cousin, Yan Huiqing (颜惠庆, 1877–1950), held important Chinese government positions as Deputy Minister of Foreign Affairs in 1912, Foreign Minister in 1920, and Prime Minister in 1922. For his life and contribution to Chinese medical modernization, see Qian Yimin and Yan Zhiyuan, *Yan Fuqing Zhuan* (Shanghai: Fudan daxue chubanshe, 2007). The English translation is published with the book titled *Fuching Yen—A Pioneer of Chinese Modern Medicine* (Fudan University Press, 2011). For Yale in Hunan, see Nancy E. Chapman with Jessica C. Plumb, *The Yale-China Association: A Centennial History* (Hong Kong: The Chinese University Press, 2001).

159 Little was written about Cao Liyun except a biographical type of memorial book by Mary H. McLean, titled *Dr. Li Yuin Tsao: Called and Chosen and Faithful*, possibly self-published in 1925. The University of Chicago Library has a copy. See also Judy Tzu-Chun Wu, *Doctor Mom Chung of the Fair-Haired Bastards: The Life of a Wartime Celebrity* (Berkeley, CA: University of California Press, 2005), 57–58.

160 The Harvard Shanghai medical school ended soon after the Rockefeller Foundation decided to build a medical college in Beijing. Houghton served as director of Peking Union Medical College in 1921–1928.

161 Wong and Wu, *History of Chinese Medicine*, 602–605. Among Chinese physicians of Western medicine, tension existed between the Japan-Germany trained faction and the Anglo-American trained faction, which lasted throughout the Republican era.

162 Ibid., 605.

163 Ibid., 606.

164 *National Medical Journal of China*, vol. 5, no. 4 (1919), 225.

165 *The Rockefeller Foundation Annual Report* (New York, 1923), 263.

166 Wong and Wu, *History of Chinese Medicine*, 564–65.

167 Liping Bu, "Public Health and Modernization: The First Campaigns in China, 1915–1916," *Social History of Medicine*, vol. 22, no. 2 (2009), 305–319; and "Cultural Communication in Picturing Health: W. W. Peter and the Public Health Campaigns in China, 1912–1926," in *Imagining Illness: Public Health and Visual Culture*, ed. David Serlin (Minneapolis, MN: University of Minnesota Press, 2010), 24–39.

168 W. W. Peter, "Annual Report for the Year Ending September 30, 1916," 14, Kautz Family YMCA Archives, University of Minnesota (hereafter YMCA Archives).

169 Peter, "Annual Report for the Year Ending September 30, 1914," 3, YMCA Archives.

170 Ibid.

171 Dr. David Z. T. Yui, "A Report of the Lecture Department of the National Committee of the Young Men's Christian Associations of China," YMCA Archives. The YMCA's social reform programs in China have been studied by various scholars, notably, Shirley S. Garrett, *Social Reformers in Urban China: The Chinese Y.M.C.A., 1895–1926* (Cambridge: Harvard University Press, 1970); Jun Xing, *Baptized in the Fire of Revolution: The American Social Gospel and the YMCA in China: 1919–1937* (Bethlehem, PA: Lehigh University Press, 1996); Charles Keller, "Making Model Citizens: The Chinese YMCA Social Activism, and Internationalism in Republican China, 1919–1937" (Ph.D. diss., University of Kansas, 1996); and Kimberly Ann Risedorph, "Reformers, Athletics and Students: The YMCA in China, 1895–1935" (Ph.D. diss., University of Washington, St. Louis, Missouri, 1994).

172 Peter, "Annual Report for the Year Ending September 30, 1914," 2, YMCA Archives.

173 Ibid., 6. Eleanor Elizabeth Whipple received her education at the University of Chicago (B.S., 1907) and Rush Medical College (M.D., 1911). She did not hold any official missionary position but served on the YWCA's Physical Education Committee and taught at YWCA schools. See "Secretary's Wife's Record" in "Biographical File of W. W. Peter," YMCA Archives.

174 Peter, "Annual Report for the Year Ending September 30, 1914," 6.

175 Ibid., 7.

176 Ibid.

177 John S. Baick, "Cracks in the Foundation: Frederick T. Gates, the Rockefeller Foundation, and the China Medical Board," *Journal of the Gilded Age and Progressive Era*, vol. 3, no. 1 (2004), 59–89.

178 Carnegie Endowment for International Peace, *Some Roads towards Peace: A Report to the Trustees of the Endowment on Observations Made in China and Japan in 1912* (Washington, D.C.: Carnegie Endowment for International Peace, 1914), Appendix II, "Memorial for the Endowment of a Hospital in China," 70–72.

179 Carnegie Endowment for International Peace, *Some Roads towards Peace,* 70.

180 The Rockefeller philanthropy funded the Oriental Education Commission to China to investigate possible opportunities to create a nondenominational university in China. The Commission reported that it was not possible because the missionaries would oppose it for fear of undermining their proselytizing. The Commission recommended the focus on medicine. Wallace Buttrick, first director of the China Medical Board, claimed that the Commission's report was central to the creation of China Medical Board in November 1914 because it turned Gates' thoughts to medical work in China. See John Baick, "Cracks in the Foundation," 64.

181 China Medical Commission of the Rockefeller Foundation, *Medicine in China* (New York: the Rockefeller Foundation, 1914).

182 Letter and budget proposal from Fletcher Brockman to Harry P. Judson, chairman of China Medical Commission of the Rockefeller Foundation, September 2, 1914, YMCA Archives.

183 Peter, "Annual Report for the Year Ending September 30, 1915," 13.

184 Ibid., 9; and "Annual Report for the Year Ending September 30, 1916," 7.

185 Peter, "Annual Report for the Year Ending September 30, 1915," 2.

186 For the cultural gap and the adaptation in health education propaganda, see Liping Bu, "Cultural Communication in Picturing Health: W. W. Peter and Public Health Campaigns in China, 1912–1926," in *Imagining Illness.*

187 Peter, "The Public Health Exhibit," Appendix 2 to "Quarterly Report, January–March, 1915," 3; and letter, W. W. Peter to F. S. Brockman, July 29, 1914, appendix to Peter's 1914 annual report, 9, YMCA Archives.

188 Peter, "Annual Report for the Year Ending September 30, 1915," 11.

189 Peter, "Report for Quarter Ending June 30, 1915," 2.

190 Ibid., 2.

191 Peter, "Annual Report for the Year Ending September 30, 1915," 2–3.
192 Peter, "Annual Report for the Year Ending September 30, 1916," 2–3; and Wong and Wu, *History of Chinese Medicine*, 611.
193 For health campaigns in the West, see C.-E. A. Winslow, *The Evolution and Significance of the Modern Public Health Campaign* (New Haven: Yale University Press, 1923).
194 For Yale-in-China project, see Reuben Holden, *Yale-in-China: The Mainland, 1901–1951* (New Haven: The Yale-in-China Association, 1964); Edward H. Hume, *Doctors East Doctors West, An American Physician's Life in China* (New York: Norton, 1946); and Jonathan Spence, *To Change China* (Boston: Little, Brown and Company, 1969), chapter 6.
195 Roger S. Greene to Wallace Buttrick, 9 June 1917, folder 551, box 26, series 1, RG 4, RF, Rockefeller Archives Center (hereafter, RAC).
196 French Strother, "An American Physician-Diplomat in China," *The World's Work* (New York: Doubleday Page & Co., March 1918), 547.
197 For details of the twenty-one demands, see http://en.wikipedia.org/wiki/Twenty-One_Demands. Accessed February 7, 2015.
198 For social life of teahouses in China, see Di Wang, *The Teahouse: Small Business, Everyday Culture, and Public Politics in Chengdu, 1900–1950* (Stanford University Press, 2008); and Lao She, *Teahouse*, Chinese-English Bilingual edition (Hong Kong: The Chinese University Press, 2004).
199 Peter, "Outline of Demonstrated Lecture." Appendix 6 to Peter's 1915 annual report, YMCA Archives.
200 E. G. Routzahn, *The Health Show Comes to Town* (New York: Russell Sage Foundation, 1920), 16–17.
201 "National Health and National Strength," *Peking Gazette*, 24 May 1916.
202 Huang Zifang, "Zhongguo weisheng chuyi [On Public Health in China]," *National Medical Journal of China* 13 (1927), 338–354.
203 Routzahn, *Health Show*, 17.
204 Peter, "Report for Quarter Ending June 30, 1915," 2.
205 "Constitution of the Kiangsu Public Health Association, 1916," pp. 1–2, folder 91, box 8, series 1, RG 4, RF, RAC; and Wong and Wu, *History of Chinese Medicine*, 616–17.
206 Feng Guozhang, one of Yuan Shikai's generals and protégés, was military governor of Jiangsu in 1913–1917. After Yuan Shikai died, he served as acting president in 1917–1918. This was Feng Guozhang's second wife, who was governess to Yuan Shikai's daughters before her marriage to Feng Guozhang.
207 Peter, "Quarterly Report, June 1915," 3.
208 *The Reminiscences of Dr. John B. Grant*, Columbia University Oral History Project (Oral History Research Office, Columbia University, 1961), 131.
209 Peter, "Annual Repot for the Year Ending September 30, 1915," 6. Dr. Williams Pink Pills were widely advertised in Chinese newspapers and magazines in the 1910s–1920s.
210 "Public Health Campaign," *Peking Gazette*, Friday, May 19, 1916.
211 "Public Health Campaign," *Peking Gazette*, Friday, May 24, 1916.
212 Ibid.
213 Peter, "Annual Report for the Year Ending September 30, 1916," 7.
214 Ibid., 13.
215 W. W. Peter, letter to E. C. Jenkins, 25 November 1917 folder 65, box 6, series 1, RG 4, RF, RAC.
216 W. W. Peter, "The Work of the Council on Health Education," *National Medical Journal of China*, vol. 6, no. 4 (1920), 235.
217 Routzahn, *Health Show*, 24–27.
218 S. M. Woo, "Report of Joint Council on Public Health Education, 1917–1919," *The China Medical Journal*, vol. XXXIV, no. 2 (March 1920), 186–88.
219 S. M. Woo, "Aims of the Joint Council on Public Health Education in China," *The China Medical Journal*, vol. XXXIV, no. 1 (January 1920), 71–75.

220 Ibid., 72.
221 Peter, "The Field and Methods of Public health Work in the Missionary Enterprise" *The China Medical Journal*, vol. XL (March 1926), 227.
222 "National Health Essay Contest," *National Medical Journal of China,* vol. 3 (1917), 65.
223 He had his essay published in *The New Youth* (新青年) vol. 3, no. 5 (July 1917), 1–9.
224 "National Health Essay Contest," *National Medical Journal of China*, vol. 5, (1919), 136–37.
225 Peter was sent to France in November 1918 by the National War Work Council of the YMCA to deliver health lectures in Chinese language (he spoke with Nanjing accent) to members of the Chinese Labor Battalion. As public health officer to Chinese laborers, Peter promoted public health and sanitation among the 140,000 Chinese laborers sent by Chinese government to work for the Allies during the war. The plan was for Peter to carry health data back to China for future recruitment of Chinese laborers. The armistice in November 1919 ended his work in France and he was able to return to China to continue his work of public health education. Peter personally regarded his time in France as "wasted." During his furlough, Peter studied at the Harvard-MIT School of Public Health and received a Certificate of Public Health in 1918. He eventually earned his doctorate in public health from Yale University in 1927. (See "Biographical File of W. W. Peter," YMCA Archives.)
226 Shanghai Municipal Council Minutes, November 17, 1920, Shanghai Municipal Archives.
227 "Biographical File of W. W. Peter," YMCA Archives.
228 Peter, "The Work of the Council," 234.
229 Ibid.
230 Peter, "The Field and Methods," 226–30.
231 Peter, "The Work of the Council," 234–35.
232 *The Rockefeller Foundation Annual Report*, 1923, 262.
233 Peter, "The Field and Methods," 229–30.
234 *The China Medical Journal*, vol. XXXVIII, no. 5 (May 1924), 433.
235 *The Reminiscences of Dr. John B. Grant*, 131–32.
236 Zhang Daqing, "Zhongguo jindai jiepou xue shi lue [Brief History on Anatomy in Modern China]," *Zhongguo keji shi zazhi* [Chinese Journal for the History of Science and Technology], no. 4 (1994), 18–28. In 1928, the Nationalist government issued new regulations on dissection, and amended them in 1933 (J29-3-589, pp.28–30, Beijing Municipal Archives.).
237 Beijing Police Bureau Regulations Regarding Midwifery License, 1913, J181-18-222, Beijing Municipal Archives.
238 Beijing Police Bureau, November 1914, J181-18-3552, Beijing Municipal Archives.
239 *National Medical Journal of China*, 1915, no. 1, 37.
240 Beijing Police Bureau, "Regulations on Bone Meat Workshops, 1913," J181-18-224, pp. 6–7, Beijing Municipal Archives.
241 "Investigation of the Peking Vernacular Daily's report on sanitation obstacle," September 1914, Beijing Police Bureau, J181-18-3550, Beijing Municipal Archives.
242 "Beijing Police Bureau's Regulations on No-Inner City Sheep Meat Shops," March 1914, Beijing Police Bureau, J181-18-2778, pp. 10–12, Beijing Municipal Archives.
243 Tensions between Chinese medicine and Western medicine peaked in the era of the Nationalist government, where Western-trained Chinese medical leaders attempted to abolish Chinese medicine but practitioners of Chinese medicine used all political influences to fight for their own survival. See chapter 3 of this book; and Xu Xiaoqun, "'National Essence' vs. 'Science': Chinese Native Physicians' Fight for Legitimacy," *Modern Asian Studies* 31, no. 4 (October 1997), 847–877.
244 Wong and Wu, *History of Chinese Medicine*, 600.
245 Wong and Wu, *History of Chinese Medicine*, 849. For the regulations, see Zhang Zaitong and Xian Rijin, eds., *Minguo yiyao weisheng fagui xuanbian, 1912–1948*

[Selected Health Laws and Regulations of the Republic of China, 1912–1948] (Shandong: Shandong daxue chubanshe, 1990).

246 For the Chinese concept of infectious disease, see Angela Ki Che Leung, "The Evolution of the Idea of Chuanran Contagion in Imperial China," in *Health and Hygiene in Chinese East Asia*, edds., Angela Ki Che Leung and Charlotte Furth (Durham: Duke University Press, 2010), 25–50.

247 Wong and Wu, *History of Chinese Medicine,* 596–97. The Municipal Health Commission of Guangzhou carried out modern work of notification of infectious diseases, disinfection and cleaning of infected premises, examination of dead rats, plague and smallpox prevention, freeing the city from lepers, and registration of deaths.

248 On the different methods of prevention of infectious diseases, see the discussion by Sean Hsiang-lin Lei, "Sovereignty and the Microscope" in *Health and Hygiene in Chinese East Asia*, 88–97.

249 T. N. Tang, "Scientific Medicine and Public Health," *National Medical Journal of China*, vol. 6, no. 1 (1920), 236–40. He gave a speech on the same topic at the Chinese Students' Alliance Conference in Princeton, New Jersey on September 9, 1920. Benjamin Disraeli and William E. Gladstone, the two political rivals dominating nineteenth century Britain, debated a great deal about public health in their political campaigns. Chinese health professionals often credited the two for emphasizing the health of the people as the power of the nation. Jin Baoshan (P. Z. King, 金宝善) mentioned Gladstone in his article "Beijing zhi gonggong weisheng," *Zhonghua yixue zazhi*, vol. 20, no. 3 (1926), 253.

250 A glimpse of the leading journals and articles in China during the first two decades of the twentieth century conveys very well this kind of mentality and attitude.

251 S. M. Woo, "The Problems of the Future of the National Health Association," *The National Medical Journal of China*, vol. 9 (1923), 132–33.

252 *The Rockefeller Foundation Annual Report* (New York, 1921), 308.

253 Woo, "The Problems of the Future of the National Health Association," 132–39.

254 George Rosen, *History of Public Health*, 168–269.

255 This type of claim was particularly clear in the writings of Wu Liande and other Western-trained physicians. See Wu, *Plague Fighter*. Medical missionaries had made similar argument since the nineteenth century and continued the argument in their account of the plague epidemic. See Dugald Christie, *Thirty Years in the Manchu Capital*. Even today, the pneumonic plague is "still impossible to cure unless identified within the first twenty-four hours," according to Mark Gamsa. See his "The Epidemic of Pneumonic Plague in Manchuria 1910–1911," in *Past and Present* vol. 190 (2006), 147.

256 Hao Chang, *Chinese Intellectuals in Crisis* (Berkeley, CA: University of California Press, 1987), 5.

257 Wang Zuoyue, "Saving China through Science: the Science Society of China, Scientific Nationalism, and Civil Society in Republican China," *Osiris*, vol. 33 (2002), 291–321.

258 Historically, the Chinese had interpreted human differences in terms of culture and geo-ecology. "Race" as a concept to differentiate human societies based on physical differences and skin colors was originally conceived and advocated by the West. It began to influence the Chinese perception of human differences after Western race theories and Social Darwinian evolutionary theories were introduced to China in the late nineteenth century. On the issue of race, see Michael Banton, *The Racial Consciousness* (London and New York: Longman, 1988); Michael Banton and Jonathan Harwood, *The Race Concept* (New York: Praeger, 1975); and Thomas Gossett, *Race: The History of an Idea in America* (New York: Schocken, 1963). On Western influence and Chinese racial interpretation, see James Reeve Pusey, *China and Charles Darwin* (Harvard University Press, 1983); and Frank Dikötter, *The Discourse of Race in Modern China* (London: Hurst and Company, 1992). Dikötter's

book is a comprehensive study but it failed to analyze the very Western influence of race concept on the changing interpretation of human differences in modern China.

259 Ironically, Japan used the same racist argument to justify its superior position in Asia, and sought to join the West as an equal, based on the racist argument.

260 Rogaski, *Hygienic Modernity*; Lei Xianglin, "Why Weisheng Does Not Mean Protection of Life—The Other Health, Self and Disease during the Republican Era," *Taiwan Social Studies Quarterly* 54 (June 2004), 17–59; and Yu Xinzhong, *Fangyi, weisheng, shengti kongzhi: Wan Qing qingjie guannian he xingwei de yanbian* [Prevention, Hygiene, and Body Control: Transformation of the Concept and Practice of Cleanliness in Late Qing] (Beijing: Zhonghua shuju, 2009).

2 Science, public health and national renaissance

Introduction

Chinese intellectuals continued the argument about national health and national strength with the emphasis on science in the New Culture and the May Fourth Movements. The ascendance of science as the unquestionable truth and the touchstone of everything made scientism the ideology of Chinese intellectuals in their search for solutions to China's problems—social, political, economic, and medical.[1] Peter Buck argued that science was an "ideological entity" for Chinese in the Republican era with profound iconoclastic implications, for science was understood as capable of providing standards by which Chinese traditions could be judged and found wanting. Science was seen as a "substitute religion" or a new "ideology" with which to replace a discredited Confucianism.[2] Science even gained the "cultural authority" to replace China's cultural traditions, as traditions were considered the cause of Chinese problems and science the panacea. Gyan Prakash's analysis of science and modernity in India is equally applicable to China in the revolutionary transition from traditional culture to the national renaissance of science.[3] To "save China with science" (*kexue jiuguo*, 科学救国) was the slogan and driving force of patriotic Chinese intellectuals. The New Culture Movement encouraged the use of plain colloquial language—vernacular (*baihua*, 白话)—as the medium of writing so that the masses would understand the written just as they did the spoken. Vernacular writing aimed to make science and new cultural concepts accessible to the masses. Hu Shi (胡适, 1891–1962), a leading figure of the New Culture Movement, championed the movement of vernacular writing and dissemination of science.

Civic organizations such as educational and social institutes, which had multiplied in cities, became a popular venue for intellectuals to lecture on current affairs and social and scientific ideas. Modern scientific terms such as *xijun* (细菌, germ) and *weishengwu* (微生物, microbes) became popular discourse of ordinary people during the cultural transformation. Police and social organizations printed in vernacular language public notices to instruct people on the prevention of transmittable diseases. Modern medicine was promoted as the scientific medicine for students to study while the understanding of human body was taught in school biology classes with the latest interpretations from the West.

Confucianism was attacked as the obstacle of China's progress, and Chinese medicine, being integral of traditional China, was discredited as medically superstitious and politically archaic. The global reach of the Rockefeller Foundation in the attempt to bring social transformation and modernization via medical science influenced China through the medical institution of Peking Union Medical College (PUMC) and the medical elite it trained.

This chapter examines the intellectual development of a science culture in China and how different players shaped the growth of local public health programs and the vision of a national health system. It pays special attention to the Science Society of China and the rise of science in China's intellectual life in a global context of student migration and knowledge circulation. The Rockefeller Foundation set up a new standard of medical education in China via the training at Peking Union Medical College. The college produced a small but influential group of medical elite who eventually dominated the Nationalist health modernization enterprise. The multiple roles of John B. Grant in the creation of public health profession and the promotion of preventive medicine, social medicine and state medicine forever linked him with the development of urban and rural health stations and the national health system during the Nationalist era. Chinese intellectuals and medical modernizers, while working with international colleagues and organizations, became the driving force in popularizing ideas of preventive medicine and social reforms, and experimented with local rural reforms via mass education and health programs.

The Science Society of China and the new culture of science

China witnessed the rise of science as a central force to shape and guide Chinese intellectual thought after the 1910s. The phenomenon appeared concurrent with the unfolding of the New Culture Movement that was spearheaded by Western-educated intellectuals. Students going abroad since the late nineteenth century had produced significant numbers of Chinese intellectuals and scientists who were determined to break away from traditional thought and customs.[4] These intellectuals ranged from reformists to revolutionaries, such as Yan Fu, Liang Qichao, Hu Shi, and Chen Duxiu. Tens of thousands of Chinese went to study in Japan after it rose as a regional power, with the ambition to learn the success of Japan and use it to save China from foreign dominance. Many Chinese students became disillusioned with Japan, however, when it attempted to subjugate China with territory demand and indemnity, topped with the infamous 21 demands in 1915. Japan proved no different from Western powers in the attempt to dominate China. The disillusionment with Japan prompted more Chinese students to go and study in the United States while the number to Japan declined. Nonetheless, Chinese students in Japan played a prominent role in the 1911 revolutionary leadership and the development of social sciences.[5] Chinese students in America and Europe, in contrast, were often attributed for their leading role in advancing natural science and scientism to re-shape Chinese intellectual orientation. Students' focus on science subjects abroad were intertwined with national crises at home. For many Chinese students, they were motivated to go abroad to study with the urgency "to save China with science" (科学救国). As a matter of fact, "to study abroad to save China" (留学救国) and "to save China with science" were two inter-related popular slogans for Chinese students who sought to acquire advanced learnings in the West and to return home well equipped to build China.[6]

Students began an organized effort to disseminate science by forming science societies and publishing science journals. In 1907, Chinese students in Paris established a Chinese Chemistry Association in Europe, the earliest science society of and by Chinese. In 1909 a biology research society was formed in China, which was followed by the organization of a Chinese Science Society in 1912 and a Chinese Engineering Association in 1913.[7] None of these early science societies and associations lasted long enough to make a meaningful impact on Chinese society until the formation of the Science Society of China (中国科学社, the Society hereafter) in 1915 by a group of Chinese students in the United States. The Society moved to China in 1918 when the founding members returned upon their completion of studies. It lasted till 1959 and was the most influential science organization before the Nationalist government established the Academia Sinica in 1928 and the Communist government established the Chinese Academy of Sciences in 1949. Leaders of the Society played leading roles in both Academia Sinica and Chinese Academy of Sciences.

The Science Society of China started with a group of Chinese students at Cornell University in June 1914 when they met to discuss the publication of a Chinese science journal.[8] They noticed that in the West all science journals were published by science societies. Following that pattern, they decided to form their own science society to sponsor the publication of a science journal in Chinese language. They named the journal *Kexue* (科学, *Science*), and intended to publish it monthly to communicate scientific research and scholarship among members of the society and to popularize science in China. They received enthusiastic responses when the proposal was circulated among Chinese students in the United States, Europe, Japan and China. In 1915, the Society had 77 members with a broad mission to promote science learning and industry in China. In addition to publicizing science among the literary public and initiating research among Chinese scientists, the Society aimed at writing and translating scientific books, standardizing Chinese scientific terminology, holding lectures to spread scientific knowledge, and building libraries, museums and research institutes.

The Society functioned as a platform for Western-educated Chinese intellectuals to push China towards a science-oriented system of learning and thinking, and to break away from Chinese traditional learning, in the endeavor to develop industries for national advancement and to join "the civilized nations" of the West. Chinese students' learning in the West was deeply informed by the national needs at home—national rejuvenation and modernization. The editors of *Kexue* explained:

> All civilized countries have established scientific societies to promote learning. These societies in turn have sponsored periodicals to publish advances in scholarly research and inventions of new theories . . . It is science, and only science, that will revive the forest of learning in China and provide the salvation of the masses.[9]

Their advocacy of science as a means of national salvation centered on two things: one was the industrial/material development driven by scientific knowledge and technology, and the other was the change of people's world outlook and mentality from old traditions of superstition to belief in science.[10] Their practical purpose of promotion and application of science carried unique Chinese historical characteristics.

The journal *Kexue* was a milestone of modern science in China. It began publishing in 1915 and was the first academic journal on science in Chinese language. Modeled after the journal of the American Association for the Advancement of Science, *Kexue* disseminated scientific knowledge and shaped the thinking of China's cultural and social transformation. Members of the Society conducted scientific research in China just like their counterparts in the West. Previously, learning of sciences was made mainly in the form of translating science books and essays from abroad. The Jiangnan Arsenal Bureau of Translation of the Qing government published large numbers of translated books during the Self-Strengthening Movement. In the 1870s, John Fryer, who was director of the translation bureau, collaborated with his Chinese associates in translating science textbooks from England for Chinese students and titled them as *Primers for Science Studies*, which included chemistry, physics, astronomy, geography, botany, and physiology.[11] John Fryer also published a monthly called *Ke Ji Hui Bian* [Chinese Scientific Magazine] in 1876. It was a collection of translated essays on Western science, but the magazine continued only for a short period. In contrast, *Kexue* of the Science Society of China was published every month to feature members' latest research reports and essays of a wide range of science subjects. One observer mentioned that *Kexue* published over a thousand essays on natural sciences during 1915–1924, more than all the publications on science by the rest of major journals and magazines combined together.[12] The purpose was to promote professionalism of scientific studies in China, with Western standards as the criteria. Like many Chinese intellectuals educated in the West, members of the Society believed that science was a product created, developed, and standardized by the Europeans and that China must obtain science from the West. *Kexue* consistently advocated the adoption of a scientific worldview. Essays in the journal took on a "symptomatic" characteristic, as one scholar pointed out, when they called for "Scientific Spirit," "Scientific Method," "Science and Education," "Science and Morality," and "Scientific Philosophy of Life."[13]

When the Society moved to China in 1918, executive offices were set up in Shanghai and Nanjing. Leading members of the Society included prominent intellectual figures of twentieth-century China: Zhu Kezhen the geographer and meteorologist, Hu Shi the philosopher, Zhao Yuanren the linguist, etc. Their broad understanding of science made the Society an inclusive association, welcoming scholars from disciplines of natural sciences as well as social sciences and humanities. Returned students from America, Europe and Japan joined the Society as an elite group. Membership increased from 363 in 1918 to 1005 in 1930. Membership was categorized into physical sciences (mathematics, physics, astronomy, chemistry, geology, and meteorology), biological sciences (biology, medicine, and agriculture), engineering sciences (chemical engineering, electrical engineering, civil engineering, mechanical engineering, mining, dyeing and fabric manufacture), and social sciences (psychology, education, economics and commerce, political science and sociology, history and philosophy). Fifty-eight members were in the field of medicine in 1930. The Society formed a Terminology Committee in 1916 to examine and approve terms and phrases of science, which essentially standardized the professional terminology of science in China. In 1920, the Society established a library, whose collection, by 1930, included 37,012 scientific works and more than 140 types of science journals published in Britain, America, Germany, France, Japan and other countries. The Society subscribed to such medical journals as *American Journal of Anatomy*, *Anatomical Record*, *Journal of General Physiology*, *Journal of Comparative Neurology*, *Zeitschrift fuer Zellforschung und Mikroskopische Anatomie*, and so on.[14] Apparently, anatomy and neuro science, subjects of less attention in Chinese medicine, were the center of interest. The Biological Research Laboratory in Nanjing, established in 1922, made it possible for Chinese scientists to conduct modern science research. Scholars have noted the Society's role in building scientific research institutions and in transforming Chinese society.[15]

The diverse backgrounds of members in disciplines and schools made the Society an academic community full of dynamics and rivalry, but the leadership remained in the hands of American-trained intellectuals. Wang Qisheng made the following observations about American-educated Chinese in spreading science: first, they presented a complete picture, rather than bits and pieces, of Western science to China; second, they paid attention to science popularization and science enlightenment, making science accessible to the public while exerting significant influence in changing Chinese people's mentality and worldview from traditional to modern scientific orientation; third, they investigated the technological and scientific achievements in Chinese history, therefore making contributions to the integration of Western and Chinese cultural achievements; and fourth, they unified and finalized scientific terms that had been causing confusion in China because of the different versions of translation by missionaries, Japanese sources, and non-specialists.[16] Many members of the Society took up teaching positions at major universities in Beijing, Shanghai, Nanjing, Wuhan, and other big cities, exerting broad influence on younger generations while they engaged in intellectual debates and political actions about the transformation of Chinese society. They energized the New Culture and the May Fourth Movements with "Science" and "Democracy" as the engines of national advancement, and called for radical social reforms and the restoration of national sovereign rights.

Like their counterparts in the West, members of the Society conducted laboratory research and wrote Chinese science textbooks. To address the urgent need of science education in Chinese schools and colleges, the Society offered summer institutes to train science teachers from the mid-1920s onwards.[17] About 30 different science courses, including biology, zoology, chemistry, physics, and qualitative and quantitative analyses, were taught at summer institutes, with evening lectures given by prominent scientists. The Society also organized public lectures and displayed scientific knowledge at institutes of popular lectures (演讲所) in many cities, disseminating new ideas and information on science. It even began a new publication, *Science Pictorial* (科学画报), for the masses in 1933. *Science Pictorial* made science more accessible to the less educated reading public, contributing significantly to the popularization of science in China.[18] In the effort to popularize science at schools, the Society cooperated with many organizations such as the Chinese National Association for the Advancement of Education, the China Foundation, the China Medical Board of the Rockefeller Foundation, and universities of Southeastern, Nankai, Shandong Christian, and Qinghua. However, concerns over science education were not always the same among these different groups. Chinese scientists and educators were interested in training qualified science teachers for secondary schools and colleges, but the China Medical Board was more concerned with the scientific knowledge of pre-medical students. Their common interests in promoting laboratory sciences ultimately drew them together in sponsoring science education and research.

The "faith" in science was promoted by scientists and non-scientists alike in the New Culture and the May Fourth Movements. Chinese intellectuals waged a war on old cultural traditions of Confucianism in their struggle to create a new science culture for China. They rejected the old-style writing and advocated *baihua* (plain language, the vernacular) writing so that the masses could understand the written media about new learning and knowledge. In the revolutionary cultural practice of *baihua* writing, Hu Shi and his associates thought of themselves no less the pioneers of a Chinese Renaissance than those of European Renaissance and Enlightenment. In fact, they were inspired by the European Enlightenment in their advocacy for a new culture in China. Chinese intellectuals believed that the rise of the West since the Renaissance had proven that the advancement of science was the secret of Western power. Likewise, China should embrace science for national rejuvenation and advancement.

Much of the rhetoric of science promotion and the attack on non-science was fired up by intellectuals of little training in science who wrote and published radical ideas and views in magazines and newspapers to influence public opinion. In his examination of the relation between medicine and the cultural iconoclasm in the May Fourth Movement, Ralph Croizier cited Cheng Duxiu, Lu Xun, Ba Jin, and Lao She— none of them were scientists but intellectual giants of twentieth-century China—as representatives of the movement that attacked and rejected traditional Chinese medicine and heritage.[19] According to the critics, the social implications of traditional Chinese medicine stood out in two negative ways: its non-scientific nature, which they equaled to superstition, caused many unnecessary deaths, therefore weakening China physically; and its authority that directed people's views and behavior, which they considered ignorant and superstitious, hence weakening China mentally.

The contention between Chinese and Western medical knowledge systems symbolized the political fight between the old and the new, the conservative and the liberal, the traditional and the modern, and the backward and the progressive. Zhou Zuoren (周作人, 1885–1967), younger brother of Lu Xun, was an important intellectual in the New Culture Movement. His writings on the question of medicine characterized the trend of thinking among revolutionary intellectuals: "The struggle between a new and old medicine is, I believe, not merely a professional question, but is a part of the reactionaries' flood of reviving the old. Therefore it cannot be minimized."[20] In the 1920s, any attempt to promote Chinese medicine was identified with warlords' political militarism to return China to the past and to obstruct the revolutionary endeavor of Guomindang. It was in this context of cultural and political struggle that revolutionary intellectuals "sharpened the attacks on Chinese medicine and made many progressives unwilling to see any value in it," Croizier pointed out.[21]

Medical and social understanding of the human body

Colleges of Western medical education had been on the rise in China since the turn of the twentieth century, particularly in places of Western influence. Notable private medical colleges included Medical College of Shanghai Aurora University (established in 1903), Medical College of Cheeloo University of Shandong (1904), Union Medical College in Beijing (established in 1906 and became Peking Union Medical College after the Rockefeller takeover in 1915), Southwest Union Medical College in Chengdu (1910), South Manchurian Medical College in Shenyang (1911), and Xiangya Medical College in Changsha (1914). Major public medical colleges included Guangdong Medical College (1909), National Medical College in Beijing (1912), Jiangsu Medical College (1927), and National Shanghai Medical College (1927). They were the centers to promote Western medicine and train doctors of Western medicine. In the meantime, physicians of Chinese medicine were under constant attacks by modernizers whose most powerful argument was that Chinese medicine could not offer scientific explanation of the cause of disease.[22] By scientific explanation, the modernizers meant germ theory.

Concepts of germ theory were translated into Chinese at the beginning of the twentieth century. In encounters with the West, China and Japan faced similar challenges in interpreting and assimilating Western cultural concepts and medical knowledge in their own languages because there were no equivalent terms and words for many Western concepts and ideas. Chinese and Japanese translators often resorted to sound translation, which inadequately conveyed the real meanings of the original text. Japanese translators sometimes made efforts to create new terms out of Chinese characters (*kanji/hanzi*, 汉字) to correspond with Western concepts, as in the case of translating "germ" into *jun* (菌). In the first decade of the twentieth century, Chinese scholars translated many Western works from Japanese versions, which proved a short-cut to learn from the West and to assimilate Western concepts. Ding Fubao, a well-known scholar deeply versed in both Chinese and Western medicines, translated Japanese medical books into Chinese and used Japan's *kanji* (汉字) terminology of Western concepts of germ and bacteria such as *jun* (菌, germ) and *xijun* (细菌, bacteria) for Chinese readers. These terms thereafter became accepted Chinese terms to explain the cause of disease scientifically. The concept of *xijun* as the cause of disease was popularized to urban residents through health education campaigns and lectures. Newspapers and health circulars during major outbreaks of plague and cholera epidemics further drove home the idea of *xijun* and the concept of transmittable disease (*chuanranbing*, 传染病).

The promotion of science and scientific medicine created a pro-science intellectual environment and culture. Advocates of science and modern medicine worked with various groups and organizations to propagate scientific medicine among ordinary people, particularly the young students. The China Medical Board of the Rockefeller Foundation funded the propagation of a Western medicine program to attract students to study modern medicine. In 1926, students from Fujian Christian University, Fudan University, Chengdu Provincial Girls Normal School, and Xiangya Pharmacy Preparation School won the top prizes of the National Essay Contest on medicine by passionately praising Western medicine as scientific medicine and rejecting Chinese medicine for lack of science. The first prize winner, Chang Tsung-liang, was a 22-year-old student from Fujian Christian University, who vehemently attacked Chinese medicine in his essay titled "'Old Style' Versus 'Modern' Medicine in China: Which Can Do More for the Health and Progress of the Country, and Why?" His conviction in science was brilliantly expressed:

> The very rock of ages upon which they [traditionalists] are depending has proved itself nothing but a medical iceberg melting now under the brilliant sunshine of science. . . . Everybody knows that modern China needs science. Modern medicine is a branch of science, whereas 'old style' medicine is but a fool's philosophy.[23]

Similar views characterized the other prize-winning essays, although there was acknowledgement of some usefulness of Chinese herbal medicine. Historian Ralph Croizier commented on these young essayists: "They hailed the dawn of science and the scientific medicine with the passion of converts; they rejected Chinese medicine with the indignation of polemicists."[24] These remarks would fittingly apply to the Chinese intellectuals who advocated a new culture of science with a revolutionary spirit for change.

National health essay contests were effective platforms to promote modern medicine across the nation and to shape the debate over the medical and social values of the two systems of medicine, in relation to China's future, as medical debate was shrouded in the political discourse of cultural conservatism vs. national renaissance. The science-minded Rockefeller officers regarded the work of the Council of Health Education as of low scientific standards but saw the usefulness of the Council in doing popular medical propaganda to attract students. W. W. Peter, director of the Council, had the charm of a great salesman, but his expertise as a public health professional was not highly regarded by the RF officers, who saw him as a propagandist rather than a solid public health professional.[25] In early 1921, the PUMC turned him down as a possible visiting lecturer in public health because he was not considered "up to academic qualification."[26] Peter, in fact, had regularly given public health lectures at different medical schools, including the PUMC in the winter of 1916.[27] Peter and his associates had created a large collection of health exhibition materials at the Council, truly the first of its kind in China, which included medical illustrations, charts, lantern slides, picture films, mechanical devices and many more. Medical colleges including Peking Union Medical College and local health campaigners rented or borrowed the health items in their public health lectures and campaigns. The China Medical Board acknowledged that the popular health education of the Council "serves to stimulate interest in study for the medical profession and incidentally gives the people an idea of the aims of the medical schools."[28] Public health education helped spread the ideas of Western medicine and promoted it as an essential ingredient of science and modernity.

School biology classes taught biochemical explanation of the human body with visual aid of posters and drawings to help students understand. Pharmaceutical advertisements, newspapers and magazines also contributed to spreading modern medicine to inform the public of the scientific effect of Western drugs—the chemical pills and concoctions—in curing illnesses, preventing diseases, and vitalizing the human body.[29] The idea of a strong body had fascinated Chinese modernizers since the late nineteenth century in their search for solutions to China's plight. They saw an intrinsic link between the strong physique of individuals and national strength in Social Darwinian light. The intellectual fascination with physical strength of the body continued in the agitations of Republican revolutionaries. Sun Yat-sen and his associates promoted military physical education to train the body for revolutionary activities. To the reformist and revolutionary Chinese alike, a strong country came from the strong bodies of citizens.

Mao Zedong, the communist leader of China, claimed that he became an ardent physical culturalist in his youth. He told the American journalist, Edgar Snow:

> In the winter holidays we tramped through the fields, up and down mountains, along city walls, and across the streams and rivers. If it rained we took off our shirts and called it a rain bath. When the sun was hot we also doffed shirts and called it a sun bath. In the spring winds we shouted that this was a new sport called "wind bathing." We slept in the open when frost was already falling and even in November swam in the cold rivers. All this went on under the title of "body training."[30]

Mao Zedong spoke of the relation of physical strength between the people and the nation. He pointed out that if China was weak it was because the Chinese people were weak. He discussed the three aspects of education that Yan Fu had advocated since 1895—the intellectual, the moral, and the physical. Like many of his contemporaries, Mao accepted military heroism and military drills as an integral part of physical education. He not only continued the late Qing reformist argument that the three aspects of moral, intellectual and physical education "are equally important" but also went one step further to emphasize that physical education complemented the other two—virtues (the moral) and knowledge (the intellectual)—in a fundamental way. For "both virtues and knowledge reside in the body. Without the body there would be neither virtues nor knowledge." Mao further elaborated: "Physical education not only harmonizes the emotions, it also strengthens the will." In his view, people should dare to make a change from the tradition of "flowing garments, a slow gait, a grave and calm gaze" to a new mode of body-building where one was able "to leap on horseback and to shoot at the same time; to go from battle to battle, to shake the mountains by one's cries, and the colors of the sky by one's roars of anger."[31]

There was a new promotion of learning the scientific details of the physical composition of the body in the 1920s–30s, in addition to the social understanding of the importance of strong physique in saving the nation and carrying out revolutions. Medical education in the areas of anatomy and physiology promoted "scientific" understanding of the human body and disease. Modern interpretation of the scientific composition of human body—an inward looking at the compartmentalized and itemized body in small units of chemical elements appeared the opposite of the Chinese interpretation of the body as a microcosm. The historical difference between Chinese and Western interpretations of the structure and functions of the human body, as Shigehisa Kuriyama illuminates, is of a rich variety developed over several millennia. The Chinese focused on the tracts and points (经络与穴位), the unseen, whereas Westerners were preoccupied with the muscles (肌肉), the seen. Europeans failed to grasp the Chinese concepts of tracts and points of acupuncture when they studied Chinese medicine in the seventeenth to eighteenth centuries because they could not see these entities.[32]

In the 1930s, Chinese modernizers introduced to Chinese students the interpretation of the human body as an industrial palace by Fritz Kahn (1888–1968), but with Chinese cultural adaptation.[33] A series of Chinese educational posters were created to convey Kahn's mechanical interpretation of the functions of the human body.[34] Chinese students also learned, via colorful images, that the human body was scientifically analyzable and quantifiable in terms of chemical composition. A comparison of Kahn's original image of man machine (**Figure 2.1, Man as machine**) and the Chinese posters (**Figure 2.2, Human body a factory**) to re-present Kahn's ideas, however, demonstrate significant modifications of the original in the process of transferring Western ideas to China. In the Chinese images, a man of 168 pounds has 98 pounds of water and 52 pounds of carbon and 18 pounds of other elements. His head is the general management office, his eyes windows, his ears telephones, his lungs bellows, and his arms cranes and clutches, etc.[35] Chinese visual re-presentation of Kahn's mechanical body added Chinese cultural characteristics to make the alien concepts easy to comprehend.

The promotion of scientific medicine and modernity was also contributed by the commerce of biomedical drugs, which marketed modern medicine to Chinese consumers especially in large cities of Shanghai, Tianjin and Beijing. The poster of an aspirin advertisement represented a flourishing commercial market for biomedicine in China in the 1930s **(Figure 2.3, Aspirin advertisement)**. The image showed that the Chinese advertising companies had embraced the industry's marketing ideology that beauty sells. The Chinese beauty, quite a modern one, held up an aspirin pill from Bayer Company and told the viewers the magic power

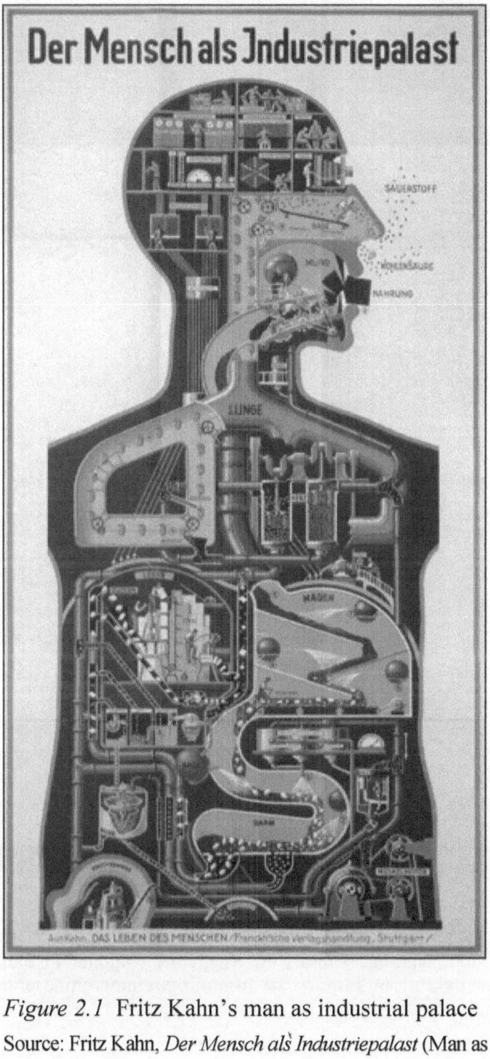

Figure 2.1 Fritz Kahn's man as industrial palace

Source: Fritz Kahn, *Der Mensch als Industriepalast* (Man as Industrial Palace) (Kosmos Verlag, 1926)

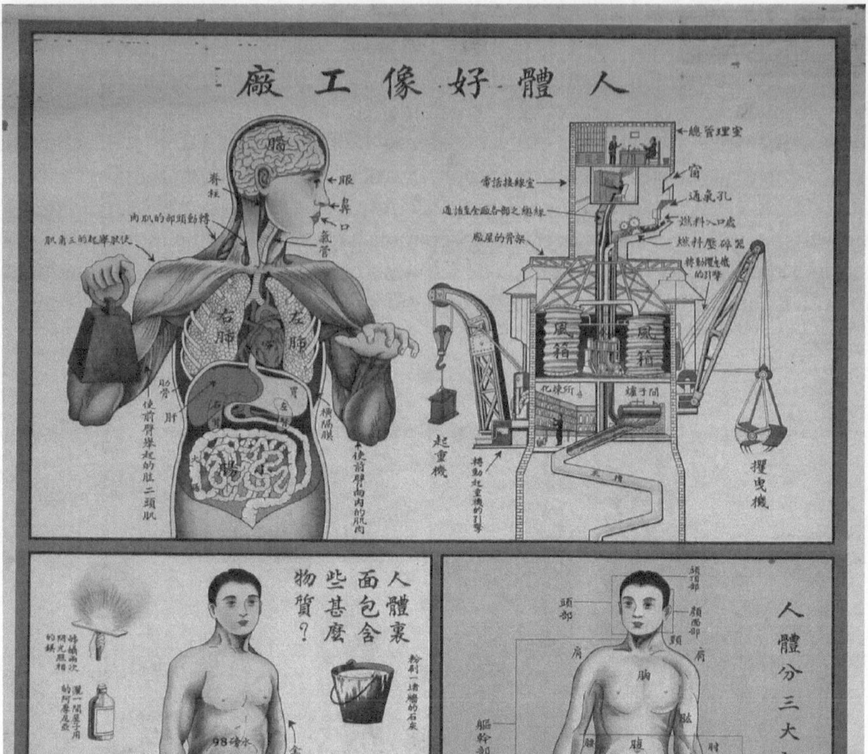

Figure 2.2 "Human body is like a factory." Chinese interpretation of Kahn's concept

Source: Chinese Public Health Collection, National Library of Medicine, National Institutes of Health, Bethesda, MD, USA. Online exhibit at http://www.nlm.nih.gov/hmd/chineseposters/understanding.html.

of the little pill against headache, feverish cold, and influenza.[36] The attraction was obvious. More importantly, Chinese merchants advertised modern hygiene and biomedicine in the name of national strength and social progress to tie individual health to national goals. Sherman Cochran argued that medical merchants played a significant role in spreading Western ideas and modern dreams in China in the first half of the twentieth century.[37] Medical commercials, in addition to educational health posters, popularized modern concepts of the human body and Western medicine to a broader public with the message of individual health, national strength and modern progress.

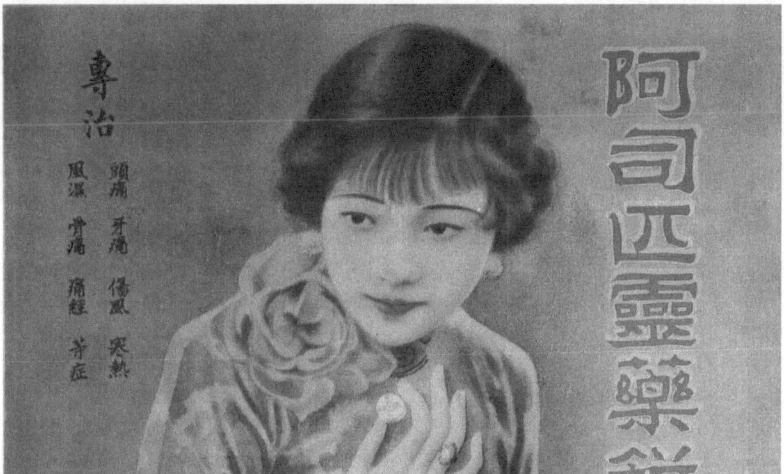

Figure 2.3 Chinese advertisement of aspirin pills

Source: Chinese Public Health Collection, National Library of Medicine, National Institutes of Health, Bethesda, MD, USA. Online exhibit at http://www.nlm.nih.gov/hmd/chineseposters/pharmaceutical.html.

Peking Union Medical College: an American outpost of medical science in China

The Rockefeller Foundation (RF) entered China with an ambitious enterprise of medical science in this pro-science intellectual climate. The RF took over the missionary Union Medical College in Beijing with US$200,000 on July 1, 1915 after careful surveys of the medical conditions in China.[38] The college was originally founded in 1906 by the London Missionary Society and then joined by five other British and American missions. It enjoyed the patronage and financial support of Empress Dowager Cixi (慈禧, 1835–1908) and many leading Chinese officials. Teaching was conducted in Chinese and the first class graduated in 1911. The graduates received a special diploma with the recognition of Chinese government.[39] By the time the RF purchased the school, it had 128 students, whom the China Medical Board (CMB) of the RF transferred to other schools to complete their medical education. The RF renamed the college Peking Union Medical College (PUMC) and rebuilt it after the model of the Johns Hopkins' School of Medicine, making it an American "outpost of modern medicine in the Far East."[40]

John D. Rockefeller, Sr. showed philanthropic interest in China when his Standard Oil Company made huge profits with monopoly of China's kerosene market.[41] In 1908 he sent a commission, composed of Drs. Ernest D. Burton and Thomas C. Chamberlain of the University of Chicago, to study the educational situation in China, Japan, and India. The commission submitted a report, recommending the establishment in Beijing of an educational institution for the teaching of natural sciences. After some consideration, medical science, rather than general science, was proposed as the educational focus. A second commission was sent to China in 1914 when the RF was organized, to investigate the needs and opportunities of medical work. In the summer of 1915, another commission went to China for further investigation, which was composed of key figures of the RF—William H. Welch, Simon Flexner, Wallace Buttrick, and Frederick L. Gates. They recommended the creation of two medical schools—one in Beijing and one in Shanghai.[42] Ultimately, the Shanghai school did not continue after the RF concentrated on Beijing. The RF created the China Medical Board (CMB) in 1914 to take charge of the foundation's interest in China, particularly the management of PUMC and "the gradual development of a system of scientific medicine in China."[43]

The re-organization and re-building of PUMC illuminated the RF's adept handling of cultural diplomacy in the transmission of medical science from America to China. The modern state-of-art medical facilities were housed in the new buildings constructed in traditional Chinese style, giving the appearance of perfect harmony with Chinese tradition. The Chinese architecture presented no disruption of the city's landscape but an appreciation of China's long civilization. (**Figure 2.4, PUMC building**). This was a good contrast to foreign powers' destruction of Tianjin traditional buildings to fit the modern sanitary demands during their occupation. American medical giants such as William H. Welch

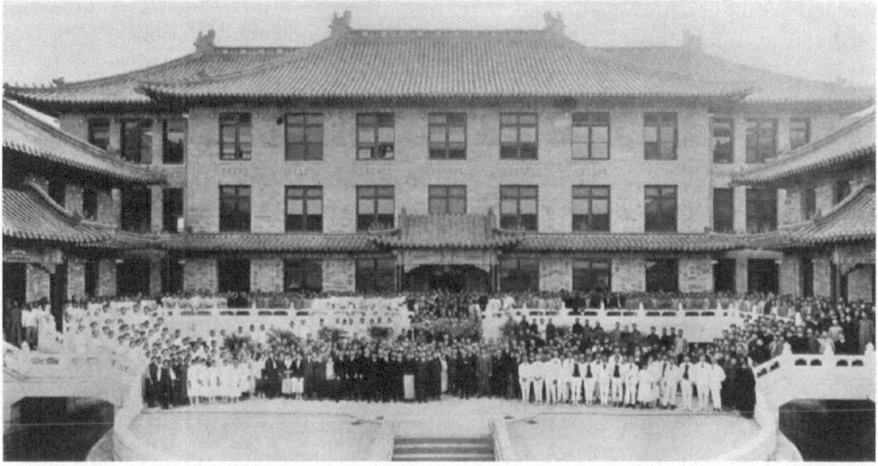

Figure 2.4 Staff and students of Peking Union Medical College, 1921

This picture was taken in the forecourt of the PUMC Hospital constructed by the Rockefeller Foundation. From left to right the groups are nurses, administrative staff, faculty and hospital interns; to the right on steps, students; in the background, laboratory assistants, hospital attendants, janitors, cleaners, cooks, laundrymen, gatekeepers, and other servants.

Source: Inside cover page, opposite the title page of the book, *Addresses & Papers, Dedication Ceremonies and Medical Conference: Peking Union Medical College, Sept. 15–22, 1921*, Peking, China (Rumford Press, Concord, New Hampshire, 1922).

and Simon Flexner, who sat on the China Medical Board, set the standards for the new PUMC in terms of faculty, students, and research facilities as well as the language of instruction. Selection of faculty was based on the qualifications of expertise in medical science. Medical curriculum and length of courses were all designed with the best of American medical schools, such as the Johns Hopkins Medical School, as the prototype and standards.[44] In order to guarantee the quality of students, PUMC created its own pre-medical school to strengthen the science courses of physics, chemistry and biology before medical college. Teaching was changed from Chinese to English language.[45] Applicants for PUMC must first pass the English proficiency test. The English test would limit the access of PUMC to students who had prior exposure to Western influence and education, such as those of missionary schools or the social elite. The CMB officials justified their decision on English language with the belief that "it is impossible to train students properly in modern medicine through the medium of this tongue [Chinese]."[46]

There were objections to the change of teaching language from Chinese to English. Medical missionaries generally favored teaching in Chinese, which was the language of instruction at the majority missionary medical schools, with the exception of the Hunan-Yale College of Medicine and a few others. The former faculty (missionary doctors) of the college objected to teaching in English and warned Welch: "Chinese students taught medicine in English are likely to be out of touch with the people and will not advance Chinese medicine."[47] But Welch insisted, and the RF reiterated once and again: "The aim should be to create as good a medical college as can be found anywhere in Europe or America."[48] They believed that English instruction was imperative for that purpose. John D. Rockefeller, Jr. encouraged: "Let us then go forward with one accord towards the attainment of this objective which will make permanent the establishment on Chinese soil of the best in scientific medicine that the world can offer."[49] The RF medical authorities were fully aware that such an education would produce students out of touch with the Chinese masses. Welch made it clear: "Our ultimate aim, though years ahead, was to train Chinese as teachers and leaders who would eventually take over the work."[50] Simon Flexner, who at first argued against English as the medium of instruction when Ernest Burton first recommended it, changed his mind and agreed with his colleagues after his visit to China in 1915. His reason for that was to keep rigorous standards of medical science. This mindset of the RF medical officers may have been shaped by the new enthusiasm for high medical education standards in America after the Flexner Report in 1910 revealed the woeful inadequacies of American medical schools.

Besides the tensions between the missionary community and the RF officers over the approach of medical education, there was little dialogue between the RF officers and Chinese leaders over medical education and China's modernization.[51] The RF's elitist view that excellence of science could only be obtained in English, reflected the similar mentality of European colonists who were convinced that science could be obtained only through the tongue of the colonizing country. Eric Andrew Stein mentioned, in his study of the Netherlands Indies (today's Indonesia), that Dutch colonists insisted on teaching medicine in Dutch. They held science and scientific medicine as a distinct European possession, believing that the Javanese did not have the capacity to comprehend the "truth" of science or keep the purity of science in their own language. They feared that the use of indigenous language would lead to a creolization of scientific thought.[52] The RF's insistence on teaching science in the English language indicated the Western assumption of monopoly over science and scientific "truth" and the arrogant attitude towards the intellectual modes of non-Western societies. The projection of the superiority of the West, on the basis of science, would undoubtedly foster an inferiority complex among the natives and, by the same token, their unquestioned acceptance of things from the West. The requirement of English defined the Western identity of PUMC in the eyes of Chinese. Some of the field officers of CMB and RF, however, had their reservations, and expressed their views years later. John B. Grant, chair of the Public Health Department of the PUMC, ventured to suggest that Chinese be the teaching language. Even Roger S. Greene, resident director of China Medical Board in Beijing and later director of PUMC, felt the need to enable "Chinese students to study without the mental strain involved in doing all their work in a foreign language."[53]

The Rockefeller approach of elitist science education contrasted sharply with the Chinese intellectuals who endeavored to popularize science by revolutionizing the writing from literary formality to plain vernacular. Chinese intellectuals purported to make science accessible to the masses, believing that it was a necessity in the modern transformation of China that the masses understood science. Paul Monroe of Columbia University was deeply involved in the US–China cultural and educational affairs. He served as chairman of PUMC Board of Trustees (1920–1926) and chairman of China Medical Board (1928–1934). He made the comments that a national educational system provided two essential functions: one was to select and train a small number of persons with superior ability upon whom the conduct of society must depend upon (in other words, the education of leaders), and the other was to educate the masses of people.[54] It was interesting to note that Chinese students who studied in America returned to advocate mass education, while the RF officials coming from a society that promoted democracy of education, focused on the education of elite leaders in China. The RF followed the pattern, in their effort to change China with medical science, that Americans were mentors of the Chinese in the modernization scheme.[55] They aimed to train a small group through the learning at PUMC to be different from the Chinese masses by mastering scientific knowledge in English and using it to change their country. The RF medical authorities were determined to depart from the missionary low quality of education "with their coolie constituency,"[56] and to initiate high standards of medical education with an elitist emphasis. Excellence in education and research was promoted in the training of a few able medical men to take up the leadership of China.

The PUMC began to admit students in the fall of 1919, and had only 13 students enrolled by 1921, the year the college was officially dedicated. Following the standards set up by Welch and Flexner, the college introduced rigorous science studies and research in the fields of anatomy, chemistry, biology, physiology, pathology, bacteriology, surgery, medicine, materia medica, ophthalmology, gynecology, and obstetrics.[57] As did the Rockefeller Institute for Medical Research in the United States, PUMC established a hospital for teaching and training purposes.

X-ray, this most advanced scientific instrument of diagnosis in the West at the time, was acquired by PUMC for research and medical practice. A Roentgenology unit was created with Paul C. Hodges in charge. Hodges, who had received his medical training at Washington University working with X-ray diagnosis, was a master of radiological instrumentation and made an "enduring contribution to the introduction of diagnostic radiology to China."[58] He trained his successor Dr. Chih-kuang Hsieh (Xie Zhiguang, 谢志光, 1899–1967), who became the first Chinese radiologist and headed the radiology department at PUMC from 1928 to 1948. Moreover, Hodges built X-ray machines that were able to operate on various electrical supplies and conditions. These machines were purchased and used by medical doctors, schools and hospitals in different parts of China, including Hunan-Yale Medical School in Changsha, St. James Hospital in Anqing, Dr. C. Lee in Wuxi, Dr. Thomas in Ningbo, Temple Hill Hospital in Yantai, Taylor Memorial Hospital in Baoding, and PUMC.[59]

The RF deferred direct engagement in hygiene and preventive medicine in China, presumably for the following reasons: (1) systematic protection of public health was a government factor; (2) confidence in scientific medicine was not sufficiently widespread to ensure Chinese people's cooperation for effective work; (3) the conditions in China to be dealt with, be it biological, social, or economic, were so different from those in the West that it was important to proceed with a careful study of local conditions and proper adaptations, and (4) no sufficient numbers of highly trained personnel necessary for public health program were available.[60] If these were the reasons for China, the RF certainly did not hesitate to conduct hygiene and preventive medicine programs in Sri Lanka and Java at that time, where local conditions were not any better than China. It is apparent the RF had a different strategy in China. Up till 1920 the China Medical Board made little effort in the popular education of preventive medicine and public health matters.

By 1921, however, the China Medical Board and the RF began to change their policy on hygiene and public health in China, due to internal and external pressures. Internally, there were pressing needs for someone to take care of the hygiene demands at the PUMC campus. Henry S. Houghton, director of the PUMC (1921–1928, 1937–1946), and Richard M. Pearce, director of the Division of Medical Education of the RF and acting director of the PUMC in 1920–1921, both made it clear to George Vincent, William H. Welch and Victor Heiser the needs of hygiene education in the RF's medical enterprise in China. Pearce wrote that not only the internal "matters of quarantine, student and staff health and control of sanitation" for the college employees put much burden on the professor of medicine but also the external demand to help with "famine relief, plague in Manchuria, and . . . preparing for a possible typhus epidemic" in Chinese society compelled the PUMC to take men from the department of medicine to participate in such work.[61] Pearce considered the engagement in public health services, though necessary, detrimental to the work of the department of medicine, because it prevented medical professors from doing their own work. As an advanced and best equipped medical institution in China, the PUMC could not:

> escape this responsibility in times of public calamity. . . . Every foreign institution is expected to do its share in order to help out the weak Chinese administration, and to decline to assist puts us in a bad light and weakens our prestige.[62]

Pearce continued that the PUMC was already losing "valuable opportunities to impress upon the community its usefulness in the field of public health" and losing contact with government authorities because the PUMC did not have a man to devote his entire time to hygiene work.[63] With reports like these, the RF began to re-position itself in the matter of public health.

The RF chose John B. Grant, out of several candidates, to go to China to take charge of hygiene and public health matters. Grant, who was born and grew up in China, had a MD from the University of Michigan and was a recent graduate of the Johns Hopkins' Public Health School. He had worked with the RF on the hookworm control program at Chinese coal mines in Hunan during 1917–1919. Grant sailed to China in August 1921, having been appointed as Associate Professor of Public Health of PUMC and representative of the International Health Board (later International Health Division, IHD) of the Rockefeller Foundation. He carried three major responsibilities: (1) to develop a curriculum of hygiene and preventive medicine for teaching purpose, (2) to establish an intramural "College Health Service" for the PUMC staff, which hopefully was to extend as a model to schools and colleges in China, and (3) most important of all, to "ascertain . . . the possibility of initiating public health activities in the country, which would be of a permanent and progressive character, aiding the quicker establishment of a national public health movement."[64] Wearing different hats, Grant had to define his identity on different occasions. When he was in Beijing, he was a PUMC professor; but when he traveled around China to survey public health situations, he was the IHD representative of the RF. His official titles and his fluency in Chinese language, not to mention his familiarity with and sensitivity to Chinese culture and social norms, opened up unusual venues to work with Chinese authorities and leaders of the medical profession. Grant would eventually exert a profound influence on China's public health profession and the creation of a modern national health administration system in China. Conducive to Grant's work, the Chinese government had already committed itself to scientifically preventing epidemics.

1917–1918 plague: epidemic prevention and popularization of science

The Republic of China encountered a major pneumonic plague epidemic in 1917–1918, which started in Suiyuan (绥远, today's Inner Mongolia area) and Shanxi (山西) in August 1917. The frightened locals, in an attempt to escape to safe regions, helped spread the disease towards the south and east, making the plague a national epidemic crisis.[65] The Beiyang government (北洋政府) did not receive reports on the epidemic until late in the year, but took immediate action by forming a Plague Prevention Commission (防疫委员会) and sending Wu Liande and other medical specialists to investigate and conduct containment. As in the 1910 plague fight, isolation and containment were the key methods in managing the epidemic, but different from 1910, plague had been defined as a notifiable infectious disease in the 1916 legislation on the Regulations on Infectious Diseases (传染病预防条例).[66] Hence, the government had the legal obligation to fight the epidemic. The Beiyang government issued a series of rules, in accordance with the 1916 regulations, on the responsibilities of local officials, doctors and patients, and the guidance of plague reporting and methods of prevention. Government's rules and regulations were published in major newspapers such as *Dagongbao* for public information. However, local officials, particularly those in Suiyuan and Shanxi, often ignored the regulations, as the central government was weak and ineffective in directing local government during the era of warlordism (1916–1926). Violence occurred when Wu Liande and other plague scientists were attacked during their investigation and examination of plague victims.[67] The violent incidents indicated an open resistance of the locals to the government's modern health management. The plague epidemic was brought to an end in May 1918, after ten months of devastation, fear and chaos, and the loss of 16,000 lives and hundreds of millions of dollars.

During the epidemic, active popular education on plague prevention appeared in many places, which was a significant progress from the 1910 plague fight. In addition to the government, local gentry and merchant classes (the traditional social groups called upon to help relief) and new social and educational institutions played important roles in disseminating knowledge of plague and prevention through media, public lectures, public bulletins and notices, and vernacular circulars. The public were made aware that the plague had no cure and that prevention was the key to fight it. Two areas were emphasized as ways to prevent plague—all for the purpose of preventing the transmission of the disease: (1) personal hygiene and sanitation of public places, and (2) food hygiene—banning all meat transportation from outside the city and regulating local butchery and meat shops and markets. It was feared that sick animals and rotten meat helped spread the disease.

The government and private institutions offered public lectures and distributed anti-plague notices to spread health information. In Beijing, the Model Institute of Popular Education (京师模范通俗教育演讲所) delivered vernacular anti-plague lectures and printed pamphlets to distribute in every district.[68] The Health Department of Beijing Police Bureau also distributed public notices and guides to officials as well as commoners. For instance, "Plague Prevention Guide for Officials" (官吏防疫须知) described the disease and the means of spread, and how local government should use various methods of prevention. "The Vernacular Bulletin of South-Gate Plague Prevention and Examination Station" (南口防疫检验所白话布告) and "The Vernacular Circular on Plague Prevention" (防疫白话通告) both emphasized the danger of *chuanran* (传染, transmission) of the disease via germs, which they explained as tiny bugs. They described plague as the worst of the eight notifiable epidemic diseases defined by the government. After detailing the symptoms of plague, they explained how it was spread and how to prevent it. The Vernacular Circular warned: "you have to believe the two words *chuanran*; the plague spread from Salaqi to the ten more *xian* of Baotou and Shanxi because people don't believe *chuanran*."[69] **(Figure 2.5, Vernacular circular)** The public health notices urged people to believe in the existence of germs, and explained the necessity of isolation and quarantine when family members were found to be infected.[70] They introduced many new scientific concepts to the general public. For example, "The Vernacular Circular on Plague Prevention" explained:

> 这种肺疫 因为有一种微生物 就是小虫儿 名叫配斯特菌 就是病毒 要是把病毒吸到肺里头去 一定就得这种病 取了病人的痰或是血 用显微镜一看实在是一种杆状细菌 确定无疑，这是东西各国多少专门医家研究出来的 并不是说没有凭据的空话 万不可说是天灾 以为不是人力所能挽回的.

Translation: This pneumonic plague has a microbe, that is, a tiny bug, which is called pest germ, or virus. If the virus is inhaled into the lungs, you will surely get the disease. When the patient's phlegm or blood is taken and put under the microscope, a kind of pole-shape germ is seen, without a doubt. This is the research finding of medical specialists of Western and Eastern countries, and not empty talk without evidence. Hence, you cannot say it is a natural disaster beyond human capability.[71]

Several scientific terms were used in this short paragraph, namely, 微生物/microbe, 配斯特/pest, 细菌/germ, 病毒/virus, and 显微镜/ microscope. It is obvious that modern scientific terminology was spread across Chinese society via official and non-official anti-plague and health notices, popular lectures, and vernacular writings. Among the concepts of epidemic diseases was the idea of

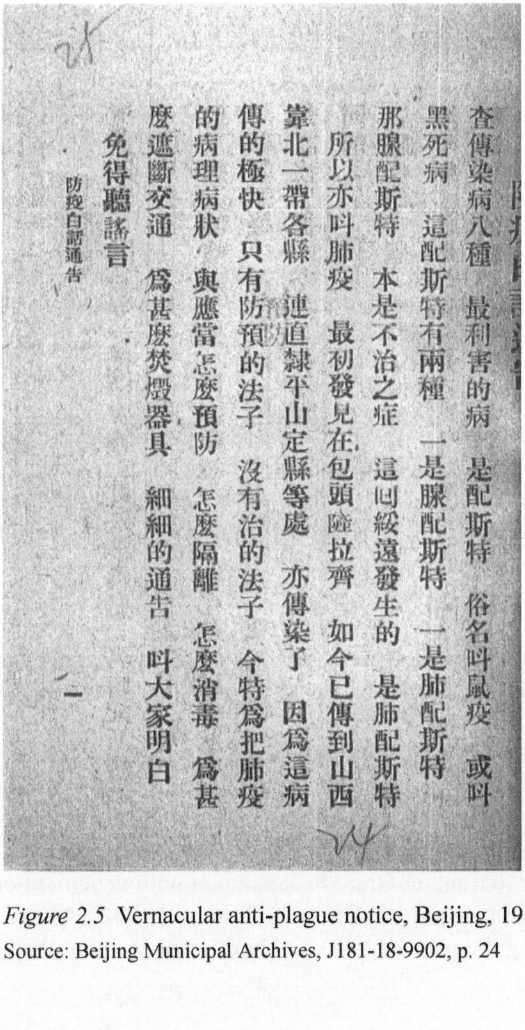

查傳染病八種 最利害的病 是配斯特 俗名叫鼠疫 或叫
黑死病 這配斯特有兩種 一是腺配斯特 一是肺配斯特
那腺配斯特 本是不治之症 這回綏遠發生的 是肺配斯特
所以亦叫肺疫 最初發見在包頭薩拉齊 如今已傳到山西
靠北一帶各縣 連直隸平山定縣等處 亦傳染了 因爲這病
傳的極快 只有防預的法子 沒有治的法子 今特爲把肺疫
的病理病狀 與應當怎麽預防 怎麽隔離 怎麽消毒 爲甚
麽遮斷交通 爲甚麽焚燬器具 細細的通告 叫大家明白
免得聽謠言
防疫白話通告

Figure 2.5 Vernacular anti-plague notice, Beijing, 1918

Source: Beijing Municipal Archives, J181-18-9902, p. 24

chuanranbing (传染病)—contagious disease, which drove home the fear of plague but made *chuanranbing* a common household word.

One of the concrete results of the government plague fight was the establishment of a Central Epidemic Prevention Bureau (later changed to National Epidemic Prevention Bureau but retained the same Chinese name 中央防疫处) in March 1919, with offices and laboratories located on the grounds of the Temple of Heaven in Beijing. The Bureau was a special government institution for the prevention and control of epidemic diseases throughout China under the Ministry of Interior. Its major functions were laboratory works that included manufacturing biological products (various kinds of immune serums, vaccines, toxins, viruses, etc.), bacteriological and chemical examinations, and research. The other function was field service of controlling communicable diseases via publicity, education and investigation. The Bureau was fully staffed by Chinese medical scientists.[72] The growth of laboratory scientific work and field activities of prevention and control during the time of political instability indicated a slow but steady progress of Chinese scientific prevention of epidemic diseases.[73] Many of the first generation Chinese public health leaders came from the Bureau, who collaborated with international colleagues and organizations.

Financially, the Bureau was controlled by an International Finance Board (as the revenue came from the Customs Service), which had six members, composed equally of three foreigners (British, French and Japanese) and three Chinese.[74] John B. Grant was invited to serve on the Board in 1924 when the board members increased from six to eight. Grant and Dr. Henry Houghton of PUMC both recommended that the International Health Board of the RF approve the invitation not because they believed Grant's serving on the Board would make the Bureau any more efficient but because it would increase his contact in the government and the medical circle in Beijing. Grant evaluated:

> The inauguration of governmental public health work in Peking in which the Board may play a part will necessitate the cooperation of the various petty factions which make up the Chinese medical world. The securing of coordination and support of these groups will be one of the outstanding difficulties to be removed before we get anywhere.[75]

Grant had been invited to serve as adviser to the Board two years before in 1922 but the IHB instructed him to decline the invitation. This time Grant made it clear that it was important to sit on the Board and the IHB gave him the green light to accept the appointment.

In July 1924, the Health Department of the Ministry of Interior of the Chinese government invited Grant to be the Honorary Health Advisor.[76] Grant thought the timing was not good and Heiser advised him not to accept the invitation because Frederick Russell, Director of the IHB, was thinking of transferring him to Japan.[77] Russell's attempt to transfer Grant to Japan met with vehement opposition from PUMC. As a result, Grant stayed on in China till 1938 when he left for India to work there during the war time. Russell and Grant often clashed over the approach to public health, as Russell focused on laboratory research whereas Grant emphasized community practice. Had Russell been successful in moving Grant out of China, the public health history of China would have to be rewritten, for Grant proved a pivotal figure in China's health modernization.[78]

When the Nationalist government established the Ministry of Health in Nanjing in 1928, the Central Epidemic Prevention Bureau (CEPB) was transferred to the Ministry of Health and became known as the National Epidemic Prevention Bureau.[79] In considering who was to lead the Bureau under the Nationalist government, Liu Ruiheng did not feel comfortable appointing Wu Liande. He wrote to Roger Greene:

> I was thinking particularly of Dr. C. E. Lim [Lim Chong-eang, 林宗杨] as a possibility to fill the directorship of the Epidemic Prevention Bureau. The work there is so very important and with the Ministry of Health and the Army Medical Service doing the publicity work, it will certainly grow into a large and important institution. . . . Dr. Grant agrees with me that Dr. Lim would be a far suitable person than Dr. Wu Lien-teh in this post.[80]

The tension between the Grant-PUMC clique and Wu Liande may have germinated during Wu Liande's work in the North Manchurian Plague Prevention Service. In 1922 when Grant attended the inauguration ceremonies of the Manchuria Medical Collage at Mukden and the Twelfth Annual Meeting of the South Manchuria Medical Society, he observed that Dr. Wu Liande was very much to the fore throughout the entire conference,

> attended by one of his junior officers, Lin. The latter always stood respectively six paces in the rear carrying a briefcase filled with Dr. Wu's Chinese edition of his last report. Whenever Dr. Wu was introduced to or met a Japanese doctor, a brief nod of the head would bring Lin to his side and Dr. Wu would autograph a copy of the report and present it to the person to whom he was talking.[81]

Grant mentioned that Wu Liande, in his conference paper on the Future of Medical Research in the Orient:

> began and ended with encomiums on the progress of Japanese science. In all, he must have specially mentioned the names of thirty or forty Japanese men of science. I previously had had occasion to borrow from Dr. Wu the last Japanese Yearbook and had noticed the blue penciling in the Who's Who of all the men of science who were mentioned.[82]

Grant thought of Wu "a very able man," despite his very great unpopularity with the Chinese. Wu Liande apparently "has recently been offered and has accepted a position as Public Health Adviser to the South Manchurian Railway, together with an honorarium of Yan 350 a month."[83]

John B. Grant and the training of public health professionals

Grant made full use of his vested privileges and responsibilities to chart a public health path in China with his own medical philosophy. Grant believed that public health was an integral part of the socioeconomic development of a society and that healthcare would be most efficiently achieved through an integration of preventive and curative medicine in a community health service. This health view was not typical of his medical and health counterparts in the United States, but more in line with the British health reformers who advocated social medicine and state responsibility for public health. Grant received his medical education at the University of Michigan (a graduate of 1917) when Victor C. Vaughan reigned as dean of the medical school from 1891 to 1920. A leading figure in American medical science and public health, Victor C. Vaughan was a reformer of medical education who "developed one of the first systematic courses on bacteriology and germ theory for medical students" and carried out reforms of medical education years before the famous 1910 Flexner report.[84] Grant continued his public health education at the Johns Hopkins University (1920–1921), where he studied with the British public health reformer Arthur Newsholme. Newsholme was instrumental in the public health movement that led to the establishment of the Ministry of Health in Britain in 1919. He emphasized state responsibility for public health. "The health of every individual is a social concern and responsibility," and "[m]edical care in its widest sense for every individual is an essential condition of maximum efficiency and happiness in a civilized community."[85] Grant was also influenced by the British public health physician George Newman, who published widely on the social problems of public health and emphasized the importance of preventive medicine.[86] Grant cited Newsholme and Newman frequently to support his ideas of a combined preventive and curative medicine, which he saw as the future of medicine and presented to the China Medical Board of the RF in his proposal for a department of public health at PUMC in 1923. Grant's belief in social medicine and state responsibility for public health may have been reinforced by his early experience of work in rural North Carolina and Chinese coal mines, where he observed first-hand the social causation of epidemic diseases.[87] If the North Carolina fieldwork taught him the frustration and ineffectiveness of disease control when preventive and curative medicine was separated, the fieldwork in Chinese coal mines made him realize the crippling prospect of public health when industrial leaders and government officials paid no attention to health issues of workers. These and later experiences in China convinced Grant of the necessity of state responsibility for public health. In designing a Department of Hygiene and Public Health at PUMC, Grant drew lessons from his fieldwork and adopted an innovative approach to public health education where integration of preventive and curative medicine was emphasized.[88] Grant would later apply his experiences in China to public health programs in other places such as India, Europe and Puerto Rico.

Grant started his public health scheme with a comprehensive survey of Beijing and its public health conditions, which included information on the city's population, education, industries, economic conditions, health organizations and activities.[89] His conclusion was not different from his contemporaries' observations that the city's main public health service was street-cleaning. He spent the next two years preparing the design of a public health education program at PUMC with a health demonstration station for teaching and community service. He envisioned the training of health professionals who would lead China's modernization with practical knowledge of health problems in real life. In December 1921, just three months after his arrival in Beijing, Grant shared with Dr. Quan Shaoqing (S. H. Chuan, 全绍清, 1884–1951), director of the Army Medical College in Beijing and a leading figure in promoting public health in China, an outline of an experimental public health station in Beijing. Grant pointed out that the experimental area should represent the average Beijing city conditions with a population of 10,000, and the ward of Dengshikou (灯市口) appealed to him because it was close to PUMC and social workers there could help advance some services of public health.[90] Quan Shaoqing became director of the Central Epidemic Prevention Bureau in 1922–1923 and was in an important position to advocate the idea of health station to Chinese authorities.

In October 1923, Grant sent the China Medical Board in New York an 80-page proposal for a Department of Hygiene with a demonstration health station. In the proposal, Grant was critical of the separation of curative and preventive medicine and was determined to avoid it in his creation of a public health curriculum at PUMC. Grant believed that "any artificial separation of curative and preventive medicine is detrimental to the efficiency of both" and that "medicine of the future" required the "establishment of this combined curative and preventive medicine in a community in . . . a real 'health station.'"[91] He emphasized that the training of public health professionals should be deeply rooted in a community where preventive and curative medicine was integrated in practice. Grant believed that the future of medicine lay in the general medical practitioner as a nucleus working with hygiene specialists in a community.[92] There was, however, no available example of such an integrated model of curative and preventive medical education or practice. Grant therefore had to experiment with his own vision of a combined practice of curative and preventive medicine at the health station. In so doing, he moved away from the "laboratory-based" model of public health education that W. H. Welch (known as the "dean of American medicine") had created at the Johns Hopkins University, and set up a "community-based" model where students directly engaged in the real public health problems in their daily routine of training.[93] In this new approach of public health education, Grant nonetheless retained the rigorous methods of scientific research, a signature feature of "the Johns Hopkins model."

The departure from the exalted Johns Hopkins' model manifested Grant's thinking rooted in the belief of medical efficiency. In designing public health education, Grant had conducted broad research on different countries of Europe and around the world. He gathered information on the experimental health stations/units being built at the time by the international health officers of the RF in different parts of the world.[94] Grant's design of the health station included medical service, disease prevention, sanitary inspection and vital statistics collection. To create such a health station in Beijing would require the approval and collaboration of local authorities. Understanding the way to conduct business in China, Grant made friends with Chinese leaders in the medical and governmental circles through personal connection, professional affiliation, and leadership of medical associations.

Instead of presenting his ideas directly to Chinese officials, Grant chose to work behind the scenes with Chinese medical leaders who were keen on promoting public health. He encouraged them to take the ideas to government officials. In the early 1920s, China had no central health administration but two government-run public health institutions—the North Manchurian Plague Prevention Service and the Central Epidemic Prevention Bureau. These two pioneering government institutions of public health conducted scientific research for the prevention and treatment of epidemic diseases such as plague, smallpox, cholera, rabies, scarlet fever and so on.[95] Medical scientists at these institutions actively promoted public health education and worked with such organizations as the YMCAs and the Council on Health Education in health campaigns.

The interest of medical scientists in public health and the absence of a central health administration presented opportunities to shape the future of Chinese health system. To Grant, the Department of Hygiene and Public Health of PUMC should play a pivotal role in the development of public health in China. However, political chaos and instability of China in the 1920s complicated the scheme. The nationwide anti-imperialist movement that aimed to achieve national sovereignty and unity since the May Fourth Movement set the context in which the RF officials had to act cautiously in dealing with Chinese nationalist sentiment. Grant wrote to the New York headquarters: "at the present stage of the history of this country direct administration [by the PUMC] of such a demonstration [station] is in my opinion a rather bad thing to do . . . such work should ostensibly be carried out under Chinese supervision."[96] He encouraged his Chinese colleagues to take initiative publicly in the matter of establishing a demonstration health station. In the meantime, Grant strategically took a seat on the International Finance Board of the CEPB to keep up important contacts and to secure the support of key members of the central government in Beijing.[97] These strategies characterized Grant's working-style in China throughout the years.

Grant's work with leading Chinese public health advocates paid off in the end. Fang Qing (Fang Ch'in, 方擎, Shih-san Fang, 方石珊, 1884–1968), who was director of the CEPB, submitted a petition to the chief of Beijing Metropolitan Police, Zhu Shen (Chu Shen, 朱深) in May 1925, for "the establishment of a Station [sic] in the Second-inside-left District in Peking for the experimentation of public health measures in co-operation with the district police authorities."[98] Zhu Shen favored the petition and appointed Fang Qing as Director of the station with full responsibility of selecting and appointing officers and devising means to secure necessary equipment and facilities.[99]

The Second Inner Left District occupied the central east section of the inner city of Beijing (Dengshikou area) with a population of approximately 56,000 at the time. In 1928 when the Nationalist government was established in Nanjing, Beijing was renamed as Beiping and its districts re-arranged. As a result, the Experimental Area was re-organized into a larger First District, with the population increased to approximately 100,000. In the ward of experimental area, about half a mile from the PUMC was an old temple located at 12 Neiwubu Jie (内务部街), which the city government converted into the administrative office and clinic of the station.[100] On September 1, 1925, the station began to operate with four divisions, with all but one being headed by the leading men of the CEPB. T. F. Huang (Huang Zifang, 黄子芳) was chief of Sanitation Division, H. K. Hu (Hu Hongji, 胡鸿基, not of CEPB) chief of Vital Statistics, P. Z. King (Jin Baoshan, 金宝善) chief of Medical Services, and C. L. Wang (Wang Changling, 王长龄) chief of Communicable Diseases. John B. Grant took no official title but served as the Superior Advisor.[101] As the work of the division of vital statistics involved the investigation of cause of death and communicable diseases, the two divisions were soon merged. Two more divisions were added in 1930: one was public health visiting and the other was general administration. Work of the station was divided in the following manner. The Sanitation Division investigated sanitation of water, foods, latrines/flies, home hygiene such as delousing and general cleanliness, street cleanliness, and public health education. The Division of Vital Statistics and Communicable Diseases collected statistics of births and deaths, population, cause of death, and communicable diseases. The Division of Medical Services covered school health, industrial health, public health nursing, maternity health, infant health and medical clinic services. The Division of Public Health Visiting made health visits to schools, factories, homes, maternal and children's health cases. The Division of General Administration was responsible for correspondence, library, business and accounting, health publication (including monthly, quarterly and annual reports), health education (including distribution of health literature and posters and giving health talks and lectures), cooperation with other agencies, and all other administrative matters.[102]

The full name of the station was the Public Health Experimental Station of the Metropolitan Police Department of Beijing [京师警察厅试办公共卫生事务所]. In reality, the station was a collaborative project of the Beijing Metropolitan Police and the Peking Union Medical College, with the assistance of the CEPB.[103] Financially, the Beijing metropolitan government contributed 40 percent to the health station while the PUMC contributed 60 percent.[104] The station constituted "the <u>practice</u>, <u>investigation</u> and most of the <u>teaching</u> fields for the work of Hygiene."[105] Grant and his associates considered the station a "social laboratory" to train public health professionals and medical students of PUMC as well. The goal was to acquaint students of medicine and nursing with the existing conditions of sanitation and illnesses in China and the necessary public health measures to deal with them. In 1928, all medical students at PUMC were required to take a three-week internship at the station in their 4th year. In the

1930–1931 academic year, a total of 64 medical students received public health training at the station varying from three months to a year.[106]

Public health visiting was an essential element in the training of medical and nursing students in school hygiene, industrial health, community health, maternal care and child welfare, and home hygiene. Originally, it was called public health nursing, copying the American public health nurses. Grant specifically pointed out the importance of public health visiting to the station:

> The immediate objective of the Health Center is to introduce as efficient a system of public health nursing as possible, adapted to Chinese conditions. The success or failure of this, we believe, would be reflected in the success or failure of the Health Center as a whole—to a greater extent perhaps than any other phase of the work.[107]

But there were no public health nurses in China and Grant was anxious to hire someone from the United States who could provide leadership in creating a curriculum of public health nursing for both didactic and field-work purposes. He recommended that public health nursing be located in the Hygiene Department and then transfer to the School of Nursing after its fieldwork passed the experimental stage at the health station.[108] As both nursing and medical students made public health visits, it was clear that they should be called public health visitors instead of public health nurses. Public health visitors were trained in techniques to deal with medical, surgical, obstetrical, and pediatric patients. They became familiar with the patient and the family through visits and knew the steps taken in dealing with the patient's problems. They also provided health instruction and home hygiene classes, organized health club meetings, and referred patients to clinics and doctors.

Sanitary inspection was another area for medical interns to practice their classroom knowledge in the community. Students would go with sanitary inspectors and write reports on the conditions of each house, paying special attention to the conditions related to gastro-intestinal diseases and measures taken to spread health knowledge. Emphasis on the prevention of gastro-intestinal diseases during sanitary investigation demonstrated the integration of sanitary control with communicable disease prevention. Students' reports included these main components: (1) sanitary surveys of homes, public wells, and public latrines; (2) epidemiological investigation of causes of death and preventive follow-ups to deal with communicable diseases; (3) analysis of statistical data; and (4) conferences on methods of sanitary inspection and epidemiological investigation of the causes of death. Students were encouraged to make suggestions on how to solve the problems they encountered during the inspection.[109]

Sanitary control, vital statistic collection, and tensions in the community

The health station began sanitary inspection and vital statistics collection in September 1925. Three police officers were assigned as sanitary inspectors to check on the sanitary conditions of each house in the ward twice a month. Each of the three men inspected about 200 houses a day, covering many things such as conditions of flies in residential houses, conditions of public water closets (W.C.), removal of dirty water and refuse, and conditions of drinking water. One of the main purposes of inspection was to reduce the breeding of flies and bad smells. The Monthly Report for September 1925 showed a list of details of the inspection:

> Surrounding of the house: dirty, average, clean
>
> Courtyard: dirty, average, clean
>
> Total rooms and bedrooms
>
> Floor: earth, broken bricks, bricks, cement, wood
>
> Ceiling: paper, plaster
>
> Wall: earth, bricks, wood,
>
> Window: paper, wood, glass
>
> Screen: cloth, iron screen
>
> Air ventilation: insufficient, average, sufficient
>
> Lighting: candles, oil lamp, electricity
>
> W. C.: old-style, half-western, western, dirty, average, clean
>
> Latrines: earth pit, jar, bricks, basin, bucket
>
> Sewage: hidden, open
>
> Flies-breeding: yes, no
>
> Mosquitoes-breeding: yes, no
>
> Rat: yes, no
>
> Bad smell: yes, no
>
> Drinking water: carry-water, well, running water
>
> Food: storage—cold cupboard, screen cover, cold storage—ice box, cold room, condition—fresh, old, rotten
>
> Individual body appearance: clean, tidy, not clean
>
> Animals: pigs, cows, horses, donkeys
>
> (Source: Monthly Report for September 1925, Beijing Demonstration Health Station, folder 465, box 66, RG IV 2B9, CMB Inc., RAC)

With so many things to inspect, it was not likely that the inspectors would be thorough with their work. In fact, the three policemen lacked professional training in public health work when they were assigned to do the job. Residents in the community did not welcome the inspection, viewing it as intrusive and disruptive. Nonetheless, when problems were found, follow-up actions were taken. For instance, inspection of drinking water revealed that the city water was polluted and unsanitary. The station sent a memorandum to the police chief asking him to advise the water works company to improve water sources. It even had the memorandum published in the city's leading newspapers to warn the public of the problem. Naturally, public health work like this caused tensions between the station and the city's businesses.

Statistical collection of births and deaths and the causes of death also began in September 1925. Causes of death were classified according to 20 categories of diseases, in addition to information on sex, treatment and economic status of the dead.[110] Only 74 deaths (40 male, 34 female) were reported in September. Among the causes of death, dysentery (16) and tuberculosis (21) stood out. Economic status of the dead was categorized as destitute (8), poor (45), average (18), and rich (3). Medical treatments received by the dead were distributed as follows: no treatment by Chinese and Western doctors (19), treatment by Chinese doctors once and more (41), treatment by Western doctors once and more (14). Communicable diseases reported in the ward by hospitals, the station, or doctors (Chinese and foreign) in September included typhoid (2), smallpox (1), measles (1), diphtheria (1), likely cholera (11, reported by Chinese doctors), dysentery (17), scarlet fever (1, reported by a foreign doctor).[111] In light of the ward population, the numbers of deaths and sick cases were unusually small. The report also showed that the majority of the sick sought Chinese medical treatment.

Families were asked to report deaths and births with certificates issued by the attending physicians. Among the 74 reported deaths, only two had doctors' certificates. Many deaths were not certified by any doctors, most probably due to poverty and ways of life. The number of reported births was 20 in September. This was an anomaly because the general rule was "the rate of the birth should excess [sic] the rate of death in every country."[112] Feeling frustrated, the station staff sought to collect death statistics by finding out how many coffins were ordered during the month by whom and from where. This method helped a bit with death statistics, but the data of births were not easy to come by. Consequently, sanitary inspectors were instructed to inquire about births and deaths when they inspected each house. They also investigated whether any individual had gotten contagious diseases. With the mechanism of house-to-house inquiry, the numbers of births increased by 20 percent compared to the previous month, but the data were still far from complete. The number of births was only a bit over half of the number of deaths collected in November, an anomaly that meant many births were not reported or found.[113]

The economic and medical conditions revealed during the sanitary inspection indicated that it was difficult to institute an effective system to collect vital statistics. Birth and death registration remained far from complete by depending "upon the volition of the individual families concerned. The same problem remains to be solved for registration of infant deaths." The station had "to work out the most satisfactory system under existing circumstances."[114] Birth reports used to be obtained mainly by sanitary inspectors but that proved to be unsatisfactory. In 1927–28 the station began to use community governance as a mechanism to register births, educating the public on the importance of birth registration.

Sanitary inspectors began to separate residences from shops in November 1925, to find out if each place had a water closet, and to report any refusal to let in the inspectors. Among the 1169 shops they inspected, 846 did not have water closets and 16 shops "showed unwillingness to let in the inspectors because of misunderstanding. Among the 5458 residencies, 300 houses had no water closets, and 157 were not inspected."[115] Apparently there was non-cooperation among the residents and shopkeepers, though the report did not specify why people did not let in the inspectors. It was possible that people refused the inspection for reasons of privacy, pride, suspicion and distrust. Nowhere in the station's various reports was it mentioned that residents sought help from or offered cooperation with the inspectors. Even when free lime powder was offered to clean their water closets, residents still made it difficult for the inspectors to do their work.[116] From the modernizers' point of view, the community resistance was ignorance and backwardness; but for the residents, the inspection was invading their family life and private space. Modern public health work had violated the sacred family space and social norms of daily life. The traditional boundary of the public and the private was clearly broken by the sanitary inspection. With the introduction of modern health practices into the community, residents experienced profound social disruptions to their traditional ways of life, social relations, and means of living. Yang Nianqun has analyzed the deeper social implications and disruptions in the statistical collection of births and deaths.[117]

In the first year, the immediate purpose of the house-to-house inspection was to take measures against flies-breeding and to check on the registration of births and deaths and the notification of communicable diseases. In the second year, sanitary inspectors continued the collection of vital statistical data and the spread of sanitary and health information. They also distributed free tickets for children to take smallpox vaccines at the health station.[118] By these measures, sanitary inspection became a comprehensive program that conducted checks on the cleanliness of premises, collection of vital statistics, notification of communicable diseases, and steps of disease control.

The three sanitary inspectors, who were ward policemen, proved disappointing in their work. John B. Grant wanted them trained as efficient sanitary inspectors as well as efficient educators regarding flies prevention and gastro-intestinal disease control.[119] Grant emphasized the importance of professional training:

> The training course which is now established must be regarded as one of the essential duties to be carried out by the officers of the Station. . . . The efficiency of extension of public health to the whole city will be dependent upon sanitary inspectors. The latter to do intelligent work will have to be trained. . . .[120]

But things did not seem to improve even after serious efforts were made to train the three policemen. Grant complained: "The three men . . . could not learn to ride on the bicycle or remember a few simple instructions despite many months of training. Various duties assigned to them have been performed in a most haphazard and unreliable fashion."[121] The true cause of this frustration seemed to lie in the station's relation with the metropolitan police of Beijing. Grant wrote:

> activities of the Health Station were found unwelcome by both the Sanitary Bureau, which was the official Sanitary authority for the city, and the local Police, who had direct responsibility over the sanitation in the Ward. A policy of non-cooperation has been kept up by the police authorities referred to above; and insomuch as the Station itself lacked real police authority which is essential in carrying out sanitary reforms, progress in the Division [of Sanitation] has been severely hampered.[122]

The station repeatedly requested, to no avail, to have the three men replaced with better and younger men. "The attitude of the sanitary officials in the Central Police Headquarters and the police officials of the Ward towards the Health Station, was due no less to the ignorance of these officials than to the anomalous position" of the station, which was "directly under the [police] Superintendent and not an integral part of existing health machinery."[123] Clearly, there was competition for the control of public health work between the city police and the station. The police had long been the authority over public health work in China. The station, particularly when it initiated Western standards and methods of public health work, threatened the routine of police work and challenged the competency of the police. Chinese nationalist sentiment could easily be aroused when the operation of the station, identified with the foreign institutions of the RF and PUMC, was conducted with the scientific authority over public health matters. In 1928, a municipal department of health was established in Beiping (Beijing was called Beiping during the Nationalist era) after the Nationalist government was established, and the working relation between the station and the police was improved with previous obstacles removed.

Before the health station was established, Beijing police had conducted health administration, in regard to street cleaning, night soil removal, and supervision of the city hospitals. Anti-fly measures were a major component of sanitary improvement and disease prevention in the city. The public was educated that flies spread diseases, causing horrific epidemics like cholera, typhoid, and dysentery. Surveys of flies had been conducted by the city police and the Central Epidemic Prevention Bureau over the years. A report of surveys in the First Right Outer District in May 1925 was published in August by the metropolitan police. The report recommended methods to kill flies that were easy to carry out voluntarily by the residents without the interference of government officials. Residents and night soil collectors were encouraged to clean and empty latrines once a week and to add disinfectant to the latrines. It was recommended that cleaning methods should take into account that the fertilizing effect of night soil be retained and not to harm agricultural production. Green sodium (青酸钠) was recommended as the appropriate disinfectant. The method was to mix one unit of green sodium with a hundred units of water when applied to cleaning the latrine. People were warned not to inhale green sodium for sake of safety. Night soil factories and night soil carts were considered dangerous places of flies-breeding, but city police and health officials could not find a satisfying solution in dealing with them without stopping their business. Therefore, it was decided that night soil carts were not allowed to stay on the streets except outside public toilets.[124] In contrast, the anti-fly campaigns of the health station provided free lime powder as disinfectant for public and private toilets, without considering the farming use of night soil. Public W.C. cleaners were asked to remove feces at least twice a day and dust lime powder after cleaning. Police officers were assigned to inspect the work of W.C. cleaners. Lime powder was also poured into the water closets of residential houses and shops in the ward. A special form of certificate was created to register the number of times lime powder was used in each house every month.[125]

Awards and punishments were used to encourage the toilet cleaners to do a good job, but only two persons received awards in September and October. In November, three persons received awards—a sort of progress. In the fall months of 1926, the station attempted to enforce daily cleaning and dusting of lime powder into the 600 odd private latrines, but it had to give it up "as a result of the refusal of the Ward police to cooperate."[126] Grant did not explain why the ward police refused to cooperate with the program, but it was possible that they faced resistance from the owners of private latrines. There were serious economic concerns involved and the owners were hurt by the station's forceful sanitary measures in the community. Night soil was a profitable business in the agricultural society of China. Families received money from the night soil collectors, who in turn would earn money by selling their collection to the night soil factories. If the latrine was cleaned twice daily and dusted with lime powder, it not only required resources to do the cleaning but also destroyed the collection of night soil and its trade. It was an economic loss of the household, the collector, and the factory; and more devastating to the entire agricultural farming. A comparison of the station's rigorous sanitary control with the police's gentle recommendation of toilet cleaning revealed a fundamental change in methods and consideration. Chinese police preferred to let people do the sanitary cleaning themselves, whereas the health station exercised coercive measures of public health work. Previously, there were concerns for the farming use of night soil, now there was none. Chinese society had long practiced the eco-recycle system of night soil management, but that system was considered incompatible with the modern public health standards introduced by the station from the industrial West.

The station made efforts to educate residents about sanitation and public health. It bought numerous copies of public health materials from the Council on Health Education, including booklets, pamphlets and pictures, and distributed them to residents and patients. It even exhibited models of children's clothes and beds in the hall of its headquarters to show people how to care for their babies.[127] The station worked with the CEPB to use illustrative posters and lectures to demonstrate how to prevent fly-breeding, screen against flies and conduct personal hygiene. It also cooperated with the YMCA's week-long campaigns to get people involved in public health activities of killing flies, attending lectures and demonstrations, and distributing printed materials against flies.[128] The station built 14 new "sanitary public latrines" in the ward to meet the sanitary needs of the community.

The health station area underwent a re-organization during the new arrangement of Beiping city districts in 1928. The station area was expanded as the First District of Beiping and the population increased to about 100,000. According to the census of May 1929, the district had 97,877 people, with 63.2 percent male and 36.8 percent female due to large numbers of male apprentices, students and workers. Families were required by the Nationalist government law to report births and deaths to the police. With this mechanism, the station estimated that death reports were 95 percent complete, but birth reports still had considerable inaccuracy. In 1929–1930, crude birth rates and death rates were 18.0 and 17.2 per 1000 respectively.[129] But corrected birth rates and death rates were 24.5 and 22.5 per 1000 respectively. The fertility rate was 96.3 per 1000 females from 15 to 45 years old.[130]

The introduction of public registration of births, deaths and causes of diseases initiated a fundamental change in the Chinese tradition of family recording of births and deaths, and made the private life of family matters public knowledge. Sanitary inspection and communicable disease control brought about new requirements for and transformation of health behavior among the residents. In 1930, the communicable disease control program included "diagnosis, reporting, investigation, isolation, care of contacts, disinfection, active immunization and health education. Nine diseases, namely, smallpox, diphtheria, scarlet fever, cholera, plague, epidemic cerebro-spinal meningitis, typhus, typhoid, and dysentery are reportable." "Dysentery, scarlet fever, diphtheria and typhoid are among the most prevalent acutely communicable diseases in the Area [of the health station]; smallpox is not so prevalent and is decreasing."[131] Vaccination apparently reduced the cases of smallpox disease. Once a communicable disease was reported, it would be investigated by either a physician or a public health nurse. Isolation in the hospital or at home was advised in all cases; and immunization against smallpox, diphtheria and typhoid was increasingly carried out. Due to the stigma associated with communicable diseases and fear of isolation and family separation, reporting of communicable diseases was still limited.

The public had doubts about Western medicine and its practice. Even when a free medical service was offered at the station medical clinic, many residents did not go to take advantage of the service. Very few sought treatment for the widespread communicable diseases such as dysentery, scarlet fever, smallpox, plague, cholera and diphtheria, as the Clinic Report of 1926–1929 did not show any of them. The Report showed some trends of public behavior towards the clinic service, however. For instance, the number of people who sought medical help about tuberculosis was surprisingly small, with 54 in 1928 and 73 in 1929. In comparison, more people sought medical service for trachoma, with 254 in 1928 and 307 in 1929. More children went to the clinic for medical service than adults. Among pregnant women, more went for antenatal help than for post-partum service. The lack of interest in using the free medical service at the clinic may also be attributed to the way the residents viewed PUMC, a foreign institution. Chinese nationalist sentiment was strong in those years with the movement to reclaim Chinese sovereign rights and national unity. Mistrust of Western medicine, coupled with the alienation of PUMC as a foreign institution, contributed to the lack of interest among residents and the indifference of the community to health programs and medical services.

Of national significance was the use of the health station's data to formulate a "Tentative Appraisal Form for Health Work in Cities in China."[132] The Nationalist health authority adopted the form as the standard for vital statistical collection and analysis. The station staff frequently published their studies of the ward population in the *National Medical Journal of China* and the *Chinese Medical Journal*, the two top medical journals in China.[133] Their studies of communicable diseases, industrial health, and school children's health, in addition to general public health, shaped the professional research methods and public health development on the national level.

Maternal care and midwifery training

Maternal care was an extremely challenging issue of public health when tetanus neonatorum and smallpox were the two leading causes of death in China. Both diseases, however, were easily controllable. In 1925 when Grant and Marion Yang (Yang Chongrui, 杨崇瑞, 1891–1983) visited a village of 1200 people near Beijing, they found the place "had 80 percent mortality over a ten year period of all infants born," solely because of the dirty habits of one single village midwife. Not knowing the real cause of death, a villager said that he lost all of his six sons in the first week of life from "wind" disease.[134] The village was an extreme case, but it revealed the terrible conditions many women experienced when birth delivery was handled by an unhygienic self-taught old-style midwife. An aseptic procedure would have saved many children and mothers' lives. The government had issued regulations on midwifery as early as 1913, but apparently little enforcement of the law was carried out.

The terrible situation of the village prompted Grant to propose the establishment of midwifery training and control by the Metropolitan Area Government of Beijing in 1926. He wrote to Victor Heiser, head of the RF's International Health Board (IHB), that the Beijing government was interested in creating a midwifery division in the health department with a midwifery training school. The plan was to have each of the 20 *xian* (county) of Beijing area "support a student, who upon graduation would be obliged to serve the county for a period of years." "The graduates of the first two or three years would have to combine teaching with delivery duties while visiting the villages in their county."[135] Grant informed Heiser that Professor Maxwell of Obstetrics Department of PUMC had drawn a six-month course curriculum, and Dr. Yang Chongrui of the Health Station and the Hygiene Department would be the chief administrator of the school. Grant told Heiser that Yang Chongrui "would hold a concurrent position in the Metropolitan Area Health Department. Our hopes for her is [sic] that she would eventually find the work sufficiently time-consuming to go entirely into government service."[136] Grant sought the cooperation of the IHB in this project by suggesting that IHB provide 10,781 Mexican dollars for the purchase of equipment and the remodeling of the premises the Beijing government would provide. Roger Greene and Henry S. Houghton were supportive of Grant, but Heiser and Russell were more conservative and hesitant. They felt the time was not right and it was not wise to commit the RF to the plan, though they expressed appreciation of Grant's work and encouraged future proposal. As expected, Grant continued working on the midwifery training proposal by re-submitting it till he received favorable consideration from the China Medical Board. In 1928, the Beijing Midwifery School opened, with Yang Chongrui as director. In 1929, the National Health Administration of the Nationalist government appointed a Midwifery Commission with Yang Chongrui as chairman, and the Beijing Midwifery School was renamed as the First National Midwifery School.[137]

Grant regarded Yang Chongrui "an outstanding Chinese woman of ability."[138] He encouraged and guided Yang in the pioneering path of modern midwifery training in China, by sending her to the Johns Hopkins University for advanced training in obstetrics and midwifery and to Europe to observe midwifery training in different countries in 1925–1926. Roger Greene also thought Yang Chongrui a remarkable woman when he wrote to John D. Rockefeller, Jr. about her extraordinary efforts to launch a national movement for midwifery training for the improvement of maternal and child welfare.

> I am the more pleased with this result since there were times when she was discouraged and would have gone into private practice if it had not been for the patient and persistent efforts of Dr. Grant, our Professor of Public Health, to show her the great opportunity for usefulness which her midwifery program opened up.[139]

Yang Chongrui was a Beijing native, born in Tongxian (通县), a county of Beijing. She received her M.D. from the Union Medical College in 1917. She worked in the Tianjin Women and Children's Hospital and the Department of Obstetrics of PUMC before she went to America for advanced studies. She joined the Hygiene Department and the Health Station in 1926 and became the Director of Medical Service Division and Lecturer of Public Health. She worked with Lily Tseng in teaching and training midwives with emphasis on aseptic tools and procedures. Courses offered for the training of midwives included a two-month course for old-style midwives, a six-month course for young and modern midwives, and a two-year extensive course for high school graduates who would become leaders in midwifery training programs across the country. During the Nationalist era, modern midwifery training and services spread in major cities, but barely touched rural China. Yang Chongrui tried to set up a pilot program in Dingxian with a modern doctor of obstetrics and a trained nurse, but it did not work. The rural people, who were used to the delivery help from older women with personal birth experiences, did not accept a young city girl of twenty-something as a trusted midwife, and a physician of obstetrics was a luxury as abnormal cases of labor were very few, according to C.C. Chen (Chen Zhiqian, 陈志潜, 1903–2000).[140] The modern physicians and nurses from big cities appeared to rural people strange and suspicious as outlandish aliens in white uniform. Even when a labor emergency occurred, the poor transportation conditions in rural village made it difficult, if not impossible, for the doctor to arrive in time to provide help. Their service also cost a lot, compared with the token type of payment villagers made to granny midwives. In Dingxian, C.C. Chen started training local natives—the young relatives of village granny midwives, but he failed to get their commitment to midwifery despite his continuous attempts.

Infant mortality was often blamed on the ignorant unhygienic handling of delivery by old-style granny midwives (*jieshengpo*, 接生婆). Hence, attention was turned to the emphasis of scientific midwifery training with modern aseptic knowledge. In reality, the majority of babies in China were delivered by relatives who had birth experience and knew personally what to do at a baby's birth. For instance, field investigations indicated that as high as 88 percent of births were not attended by any midwife, old or new type, in the Dingjia rural district of Bishan county of Sichuan province.[141] This finding, in addition to Dingxian experience, shed light on the wrong assumption of Nationalist health authorities that was accepted by existing scholarship that high infant mortality was caused by granny midwives. Birth was a very private and family matter of the female members who had passed on the birth knowledge from mothers to daughters and the experienced women to the new mothers. The high cost associated with the service of modern midwifery made modern midwives affordable only to the middle class in cities. Infant mortality was much higher in rural areas than in urban cities because of other reasons as well.

Health stations in urban and rural China

Yan Fuqing (F. C. Yen, 颜福庆, 1882–1970) and his colleagues at Shanghai Medical College (SMC) created a Wusong (吴淞) Health Demonstration Area in July 1928 for teaching and training public health students. The Wusong station, which was a rural area of Shanghai, was clearly modeled after the Beijing health station with similar medical and public health services.[142] It was the first rural health demonstration station, established earlier than the well-studied Dingxian rural health program, but has been largely neglected by scholars. Several prominent public health advocates sat on the faculty of SMC, including Hu Xuanming (胡宣明), Huang Zifang, and Zhang Wei (张维). Hu Xuanming was in charge of the station, where all SMC medical students were required to intern for a month. Their internship included conducting public health education and clinical treatment that combined with disease prevention, sanitation, maternal health and dental hygiene. In 1929, the Health Bureau of Greater Shanghai joined the college as a partner in the operation of Wusong station. Unfortunately, Japanese bombing totally destroyed the station in January 1932.[143]

More rural health demonstration stations and programs were established in 1929, namely, Xiaozhuang (晓庄) of Nanjing, Dingxian (定县) near Beijing, and Gaoqiao (高桥) of Shanghai. Xiaozhuang started as a Rural Normal School experiment in 1927 led by Tao Xingzhi (陶行知, 1891–1946). Tao and Yan Yangchu

(James Yen, 晏阳初, 1890–1990) were the founders of the Mass Education Association of China (中华平民教育促进会) that aimed to reconstruct rural life by improving literacy and economic development. Their organization gained the support of progressive intellectuals, local officials and landed gentry, with partial funding from the Milbank Memorial Fund in the United States.[144] Both Tao and Yan were educated in the United States and influenced by the progressive education movement in the United States that emphasized public education as a means of social progress. Tao was a 1917 graduate of Teachers College, Columbia University, whereas Yan was a 1918 graduate of Yale University. At Columbia, Tao determined to bring public education to China:

> I was convinced that no genuine republic could exist without a genuine public education. . . . I shall go back to cooperate with other educators to organize an efficient system of public education for our people so that they, following the steps of the Americans, will be able to develop and maintain a genuine Democracy which is the only realisable [sic] utopia of justice and liberty.[145]

Tao also thought that peasant health was important for rural development. He wrote to the editor of *Binying Weekly* (《丙寅医学》周刊):

> Health is the starting point of life. Rural education should emphasize health protection. Primary schools and kindergartens should consider health as the most important part of education. If a child cannot live long and remain healthy, what is the use of education?[146]

Chen Zhiqian (C.C. Chen) served as editor of *Binying Weekly* when he was a student at PUMC. He had great respect for Tao's educational efforts to reform rural life. When he graduated from PUMC in 1929, he was invited by Tao to come and organize a rural health program. Chen accepted the offer as Chief of the Xiaozhuang Rural Health Demonstration Program and began what he called the "early milestone" of his career.[147] He and his brand new wife Wang Wenjin (王文瑾) immediately opened a clinic at Xiaozhuang—he worked as the doctor and his wife the nurse—to treat patients. In teaching rural students, Chen followed Tao's idea of integrating education in real life with demonstration and participation. Locals observed and participated in the treatment and prevention of diseases, such as the successful ridding of ringworm of the scalp that had plagued the children constantly. Chen wrote lectures on the fundamentals of modern medicine and used them in the evening classes for men and women. His emphasis was on prevention, and the students, who were the future teachers in the village, enjoyed the health knowledge as it enabled them to solve real problems in life. Chen also trained village teachers in the fundamentals of first aid, smallpox vaccination, hygiene, and sanitation. He recalled years later: "Xiaozhuang may have germinated the ideas I developed subsequently at Dingxian to train village health workers to take on some of these relatively simple tasks."[148] It was at Xiaozhuang that Chen observed that villagers, once trained, were a great force in spreading public health information and service. In April 1930, the Nationalist government shut down Xiaozhuang and arrested Tao after his students demanded the socialization of facilities and Tao criticized Jiang Jieshi, the leader of the Nationalist government. Chen Zhiqian left Xiaozhuang and took a RF fellowship to study public health at Harvard University upon the recommendation of Grant.[149]

Xiaozhuang was also an inspiration for Liang Shuming (梁漱溟, 1893–1988), the philosopher scholar and, in Guy Alitto's words, the last Confucian of China, who created the rural reconstruction experimental area in Zouping (邹平) county of Shandong province.[150] Liang visited Xiaozhuang in 1928 and investigated rural reconstruction experiments in different provinces such as Jiangsu, Hebei, and Shanxi before he started his own design of rural education and health programs in Zhouping in 1931.

Health improvement was an integral part of mass education and rural reform movement led by Chinese progressive intellectuals in the 1920s–1930s. Their goals were to change rural China via mass education, hygiene and health improvement, and economic development. The Beijing health station was taken by many as the prototype to conduct hygiene and health reform. When Chen Zhiqian completed his advanced study of public health in America and Germany in 1931, he was offered the position of Director of Rural Health Department in Dingxian. Yan Yangchu and his associates had started the Rural Reform and Mass Education Movement (MEM) in Dingxian in 1926.[151] Like Tao Xingzhi, Yan emphasized education as a means to change rural China, but he soon realized that education alone, without addressing poverty, disease, and agricultural economy, would not solve rural problems. The MEM, therefore, was broadened into a multi-facet rural reconstruction program that integrated public health, transportation, cooperatives, agricultural improvement, and literacy education. Grant was impressed with the MEM and invited Yan to come and speak to his students at PUMC. Chen Zhiqian, being a student in the audience, was mesmerized by Yan's charisma and persuasion, and his calling for the students to work with MEM. Grant's own view on rural health in China also began to change because of the MEM. In his early days in China, Grant thought rural public health "entirely impracticable."[152] By 1927 he had changed his mind and was seriously working with Yan Yangchu to extend the idea of a health station to Dingxian and use it as a training ground for PUMC students. Moreover, Grant wanted to spread health stations in rural and urban locations as pilot experiments to achieve two major goals—the study of local health conditions and the delivery of a healthcare service to local people.

Grant recommended his student, Yao Xunyuan (姚寻源), to lead the Rural Health Department in Dingxian in 1929. Yao was a 1925 graduate of PUMC and was thought a good fit for the position because he came from rural background. Yao, however, centered his work on curative medicine by undertaking clinical work and building a small hospital in Dingxian. Two years later he received a fellowship for advanced public health study abroad and left Dingxian. Chen Zhiqian succeeded Yao as the director of the Rural Health Department in Dingxian. His approach to rural health problems differed drastically from Yao Xunyuan's.

A true disciple of John Grant's philosophy of combined practice of curative and preventive medicine, Chen emphasized prevention with curative medicine. Equipped with Xiaozhuang experience and advanced public health training in America and Europe, Chen dedicated himself to rural health with innovative ideas of practice and achieved extraordinary results. One of his significant innovations was the training of local youth as health workers to provide service to their fellow villagers. The intrinsic trust of one's own by the villagers made a huge difference in facilitating local health cooperation. Village health workers, though a new phenomenon, were not the outsiders villagers tended to hold in suspicion and distrust. The other outstanding innovation was the organization of a village-based three-tier health network that connected the village with the *xian* (county) health center/station and district substation via the village health worker. This organizational structure of health network conveniently overlapped with the rural administrative structure. Chen's organizational scheme was similar to what Grant did with the Beijing health station, the size of which overlapped the city ward/district of Beijing. More importantly, Dingxian health programs were well integrated in a general rural reform movement of education and agricultural improvement. Dingxian's success provided the Nationalist government with ideas of how to design rural health (see chapter 3). Unfortunately, Japanese aggression in north China forced the closure of Dingxian in 1936, and the MEM moved south. Scholars have been fascinated with the Dingxian experience with a variety of studies.[153]

The Gaoqiao health station has been understudied, but it deserves more scholarly attention. The station was originally planned and recommended to the RF by Grant and Hu Hongji, the Health Commissioner of Shanghai. It was one of two health demonstration units to be established in Shanghai, the other being an urban school health station. Hence, Gaoqiao health station started as a collaborative project between the Health Bureau of Greater Shanghai and the demonstration program of the RF's International Health Division.[154] The school health demonstration station was to educate young students about hygiene and health and to provide a medical service.[155] The two health stations were supposed to start on January 1, 1929, but due to lack of personnel, the school station did not start until April 1 and the rural station July 1 that year. Grant was so desperate to have Li Ting-an (李廷安, 1899–1948) return from Harvard to lead the Shanghai demonstration stations that he tried to rush Li's studies by cabling the New York office: "Try your best to arrange with Edsall earliest possible completion requirements for degree Li Ting-an local situation demands immediate return."[156] But Li Ting-an did not return until late February 1929. Jin Baoshan had to be placed in Shanghai to take care of the two demonstration stations with special attention to the rural station while Li Ting-an assisted Jing upon his return and directed the school station. Jin was later called upon to serve the newly established Ministry of Health in Nanjing, leaving Li Ting-an in charge of both stations.[157] Li Ting-an, however, spent only nine months running the two stations in Shanghai before he went to Beijing to work with Grant and served as the Chief Medical Officer of Beijing First Public Health Demonstration Station.[158]

Gaoqiao was a better-than-average Chinese rural town, having various small businesses and merchants with a 40 percent literacy rate (cf. 10 percent of national literacy rate). Sitting on the east bank of the Huang Pu River and south bank of the Yangtze River, 12 miles from the city center, Gaoqiao occupied more than two hundred square *li* (one *li* is half a kilometer) with 200 villages and a town of a population of 33,959 in 1929. A large village had 200–300 families of 1000 people while a small one only 2–3 families of 10–20 people. The following factors were the main reasons for choosing Gaoqiao as the demonstration area: (1) rural but close to city center, with better economic and literate conditions, (2) political and administrative stability, (3) good cooperation between locals and police, and (4) the medical school of the Central University on the opposite side of the river could make good use of it for teaching purposes.[159] The Gaoqiao station was also destroyed by the Japanese when they started the full-scale invasion of China in 1937.

Major activities of the Gaoqiao station were medical services, though it followed the model of Beijing health station in collecting vital statistics, preventing communicable diseases, and conducting popular health education. The first quarterly report showed that gastrointestinal diseases, malaria, rabies, tuberculosis, syphilis, smallpox, leprosy, puerperal sepsis and infections of the newborn were prevalent in Gaoqiao. The station ran a daily medical service of those functions: 8 a.m.–10 a.m. surgical clinic, 10 a.m.–12 p.m. medical clinic, and 2 p.m.–4 p.m. gynecological obstetrical and pediatric clinic. A total number of 1281 patients were treated at the clinic in the first quarter, though there was a general lack of interest among the locals.[160] Different from Dingxian, Gaoqiao station did not train local villagers but relied on urban outsiders to provide a medical service, which may explain the lack of local interest. Villagers, who tended to distrust outsiders, distanced themselves from the modern medical men and women in white uniform with an urban attitude.

Gaoqiao was a relatively large area and travel to the clinic was not easy for locals. In order to reach out to the villagers, the station developed a "traveling clinic," which operated under the subdivision of infectious disease control. It was probably the first mobile clinic in China.[161] (**Figure 2.6 Traveling clinic**) (cf. the medical kit of barefoot doctors in the 1960s–1980s in chapter 4.)

> The main idea for having this clinic was to give smallpox vaccination to those villagers of the district who for various reasons were not able to attend the health center clinic. It consisted of two wheel-barrows, carrying a staff of three [a doctor, a public health nurse and a sanitary policeman . . .] was equipped with a bag containing vaccines, knives, antiseptics, other necessary medical supplies and health pamphlets.[162]

The divide between the urban modern health persons and the locals was portrayed by the image of Figure 2.6 where instead of walking the doctor, the nurse, and the sanitary policeman were carried by local peasants on the wheel-barrows. In 1929 the traveling clinic made 14 trips and vaccinated 634 individuals.[163] These were

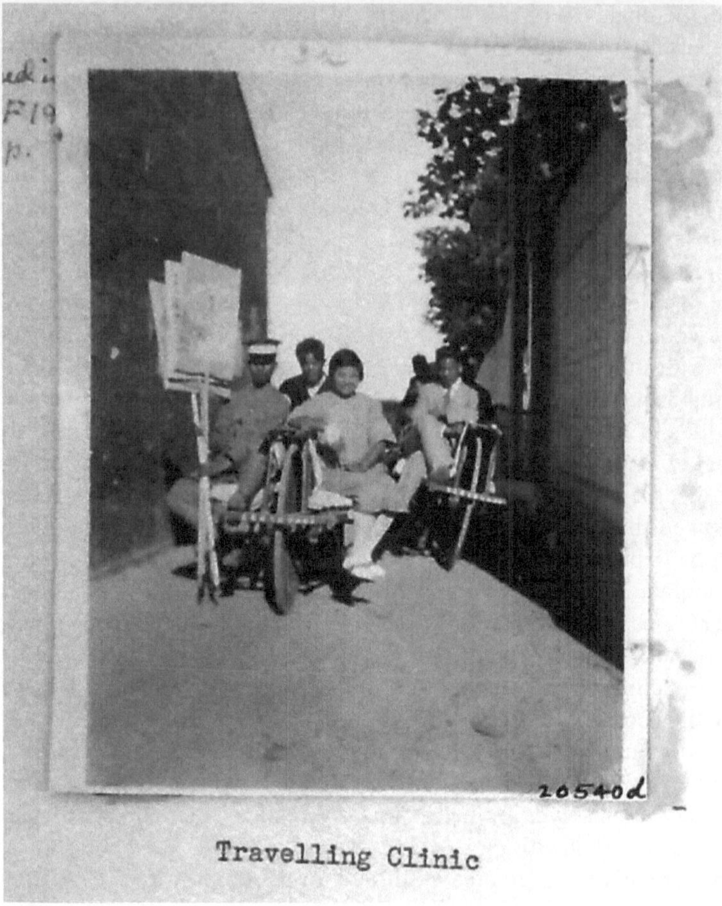

Figure 2.6 Traveling clinic, Gaoqiao, Shanghai, 1929
Source: Folder 2742, box 220, Series 601J, RG5.3, RF., RAC

rather small numbers out of a population of 34,000 in Gaoqiao. But the number of treated patients slowly increased at the clinic with the outreach effort. The last quarter of 1930 saw the numbers of patients at the clinic increase to 2488, with 582 for medical, 1758 for surgical, 81 for pediatrics, and 67 for gynecological and obstetrical treatment.[164] Despite the progress, villagers largely remained suspicious of the city health authorities who brought them Western medicine.

The idea of developing health stations was incorporated into the scheme of developing a national health system after the Nationalist government established a Ministry of Health in October 1928. Individual health stations were created as pilot program for local health development, but most of them were initiated and run by local and private organizations and individuals. At least 17 health centers/stations were established in rural China during 1929–1934, and they were located in six coastal provinces of Hebei, Shandong, Anhui, Jiangsu, Zhejiang and Guangdong, and two cities of Beijing and Shanghai.[165] Municipal health commissions and bureaus were established in major cities across eight different provinces of Anhui, Zhejiang, Fujian, Hebei, Hubei, Jiangxi, Jiangsu, and Guangdong during 1924–1931. In order to evaluate the health practices of these centers/stations and their impact on the health of local population, a survey was conducted by the National Medical Association of China and published in 1934.[166] The report concluded that the majority of rural health stations were ineffective and limited in providing health service to rural population.

> All of them undertake curative work; next to curative work in importance is the control of communicable diseases, which has frequently been the cause for the establishment of the center. The less frequent activities are public health publicity, school health, maternity and child health, sanitation and treatment of opium addicts. Industrial health and vital statistics are very minor activities in all of the centers. Seven centers are reported to serve as training centers for public health officers or medical students, or both.[167]

In the meantime, another survey was conducted on urban public health practice.[168] The urban health situation bore similar features to rural health centers in many aspects, but the report on urban health detailed the leading causes of morbidity and mortality, namely, gastrointestinal diseases, tuberculosis, malaria and tetanus. They were all controllable diseases, but none of the surveyed cities took:

> systematic steps for their control. . . . Only 5 out of the 19 cities have attempted to give free smallpox vaccination. Cholera vaccination was not extensively practiced. . . . Immunization against diphtheria and scarlet fever was not mentioned. No measure was described for the control of venereal diseases or tuberculosis. . . .no facilities for obstetrical service and child health work.[169]

Local authorities claimed that poverty was the reason for inadequate health measures. The authors of the urban health report did not agree. They argued that the "chief requirement for the establishment of modern health administration appears to be competent technical personnel rather than finance." [170]

The emphasis on technical expertise had been a constant concern of Grant, who lamented the lack of technical persons to work with health stations.[171] In order to increase the number of public health professionals and to enhance their technical knowledge, he suggested the creation of two tracks of training. One was a lower level training program to be taught in Chinese, and the other was an advanced program to be taught in English. He sought every opportunity to train and recruit the best talent for public health work. In addition to sending Chinese students and medical doctors to the United States and Europe for advanced public health training, he looked into Chinese students who were studying at American medical schools to find out who might be interested in public health work, especially those at the medical schools of Harvard University, University of Chicago, University of Michigan, and the Johns Hopkins University.[172] Grant introduced ideas and institutions that were essential for the development of a Chinese national health system in the 1930s.

State medicine and national health

Training of public health professionals and development of health demonstration stations were happening simultaneously with the scheme of building a national health system in China. As early as 1923, Grant requested the RF's New York office to send him material on the organization of ministries of health of different countries, "for the possible use in the establishment of a ministry of health in China." The RF's information director sent Grant "a list of the laws and other material" regarding the organization of health ministries in countries of Czechoslovakia, Cuba, Poland, Yugoslavia, Nicaragua, Brazil, and France.[173] In the early 1920s, chaotic political situation and lack of funds were often cited as the primary reasons for the Chinese government's inactivity in expanding public health work. Grant did not believe it. He thought that the major obstacle was essentially officials' "lack of any conception of what Governmental Public Health is."[174] He and his Chinese associates prepared a pamphlet in Chinese on public health in order to educate the officials in Beijing.[175] Grant sent a pamphlet on rural public health to Xue Dubi (Hsueh Tu-pi, 薛笃弼, 1890–1973), who served at the time as governor of Beijing metropolitan area (京兆尹, equivalent to mayor of Beijing) when Xue showed interest in public health.[176]

In an effort to obtain funding, Grant worked with his British associates in the attempt to persuade the British government to allow a significant portion of the British Boxer Indemnity to pay for public health in China (after all, the British started the opium epidemic in China), but that effort did not materialize.[177] Roger Greene and John Grant had regular conversations with the medical officer of the British Legation in China, Dr. G. Douglas Gray, regarding the creation of a Ministry of Health in China. Gray suggested focusing on the intensive training of good men for public health.[178] He told Huang Zifang:

> In my opinion the best way to go about it is to consolidate P H work round a central focus either at Peking or Shanghai, preferably the former, making a model station from which graduate students would learn the proper way of working and then return to their various cities and establish Municipal Public Health. Then when China becomes purged of its present misrule and has a National Government you could link up these municipal schemes and weld them into a National service comprising not only municipal schemes but also a maritime quarantine service.[179]

These ideas were exactly what Grant and his associates were working on, especially in the efforts of developing modern health bureaus in major cities like Beijing, Tianjin, and Shanghai. Political stability seemed to have arrived when the

Nationalist government was established in Nanjing after the Northern Expedition.[180] But misrule was not purged with the arrival of the new government, as different political forces vied for control. The creation of a Ministry of Health in 1928 demonstrated the lobbying power of modern medical elite and the intense competition among different political and medical factions, which is discussed in chapter 3.

At the annual conference of the National Medical Association of China on January 27, 1928, Grant delivered his speech on state medicine as the logical health system of China.[181] In evaluating China's health conditions, he pointed out that China faced two immediate medical needs: "First, to control the causes of an excess mortality resulting in not less than 4 million unnecessary deaths a year. Second, to offer palliative medical facilities" for millions of Chinese who fell ill because of its absence.[182] Grant estimated that the daily illnesses in China amounted to "some sixteen million cases a day and now inadequately met by one-fortieth the requisite number of physicians and one-sixtieth the number of beds set as a standard for communities with only half the morbidity of China."[183] Grant, of course, was talking about modern Western medicine in China, excluding Chinese medicine in his account. Grant believed that China had to take care of the health of its citizens under a national health administration. What kind of health system should China have in order to effectively protect its entire population? The answer was state medicine, Grant emphasized.

State medicine means state responsibility for the health of the people. Influenced by the British public health philosophy and practice that took shape since the mid-nineteenth century, Grant believed that the government had the responsibility to care for the health of its citizens. He sought every opportunity to convey this idea to Chinese leaders. In a pamphlet on public health for Chinese officials, Grant pointed out:

> Gladstone, the great English statesman, is responsible for the statement that 'the first duty of government is a safeguarding of the health of its citizens.' A study of the present important position of public health in any efficient government of the leading nations of the world shows an appreciation of this statement.[184]

Grant mentioned four major divisions of a governmental public health administration—municipal, rural, provincial and national. He thought the importance of rural public health was obvious to a big agricultural country like China. Looking at what was being done in other large agricultural countries such as Russia and India, Grant felt the urgent need for China to pay attention to this issue.[185] Summing up the health practices across the world, Grant explained that there were two types of medical systems: one was private run and the other was government run. He cited different countries such as England, Russia and Australia to support his point that most Western nations had developed a health system along the lines of partially governmental and partially private. Given China's particular conditions, such as large population, low-level socioeconomic development and limited medical personnel and facilities, Grant believed the logical health policy for China was state medicine.[186]

Grant analyzed that under private medicine there would be "a haphazard and inefficient distribution of curative facilities" with two outstanding deficiencies: (1) rural areas would be insufficiently served; and (2) in urban cities some districts would have *unjustified* concentration of hospitals with duplication of expensive equipment, causing the disadvantage of other districts being inadequately served. Furthermore, under private medical system, there would be:

> an unequal availability to each class of population of medical science. The rich will command the best of medical service, the poor will have it made available through charity clinics and the large middle class will be unable to afford either.[187]

In light of this analysis, Grant thought that state medicine—the entirely governmental responsibility for medical service for all people—was suitable for China, because state medicine "would make certain outstanding benefits compulsory" and "ensure an adequate position for Hygiene in General Education."[188]

In terms of implementing state medicine, Grant believed that, first, it had to secure efficient health workers. "Such personnel should equal in training and administrative ability the best medical men in the world." It was imperative that "political leaders appreciate that medical affairs are non-partisan and scientific in nature . . . that personnel was chosen on merit alone." Second, "the most important would be the establishment of a centralized medical authority with power to execute the adopted policy on a nation-wide scale."[189] Grant published his speech on state medicine a month later in the *National Medical Journal of China*. His call for state medicine set in motion a continuing debate among Chinese medical professionals in the next two decades. Articles on state medicine appeared in professional journals as well as popular magazines. Chinese medical leaders supported the idea of state medicine but they seemed to understand the concept differently. Some focused on the health service for all—rich and poor, rural and urban; while others emphasized a centralized health administration system. Gao Xi's examination of the state medicine debate indicated that the connotations of state medicine shifted from the original "health service for all" to a bureaucratic adoption of "centralized medical system" in the 1930s–1940s when Chinese health professionals searched the means to deliver state medicine.[190] Grant's definition of state medicine actually meant both health service for all and the establishment of a national health administrative system as two sides of a coin.

The promotion of state responsibility for public health was an international trend in the 1920s through the 1940s, spearheaded by the League of Nations Health Organization (LNHO). Grant had extensive working relations with leaders of the LNHO, such as Ludwik Rajchman, Berislav Borcic and Andrija Stampar, all of whom came to work in China to help build a national health system under the Nationalist government.[191] (See chapter 3.) The LNHO helped health reforms in many countries, of which China was one. In fact, one of the most important functions of the LNHO, as Iris Borowy pointed out, was to help set up a national health system when requested by a particular country.[192]

Conclusion

China witnessed a fundamental shift from the traditional culture to a dynamic cultural rejuvenation of science during the New Culture and the May Fourth Movements. The cultural re-orientation guided by the belief in science profoundly informed the social and political revolutions led by the political parties of Guomindang (GMD) and Chinese Communist Party in the twentieth century.[193] In the iconoclasm of traditions, science gained "cultural authority" to guide Chinese intellectuals and revolutionaries in their search for national identity and order. The concept of science, a key element of modernity that spread along with the global expansion of the West, came to signify the advancement and superiority of the modern West over the traditional societies of the rest. When Chinese intellectuals emulated the West in the effort to make China modern and strong, they embraced science as the driving force for national renaissance. Science became the touchstone of rationality and truth and the engine of progress to empower the nation. Chinese intellectuals used science in public discourse to shape and legitimize the modern nation they sought to create. In the national renaissance, science came to "anchor the entire edifice of modern culture, identity, politics, and economy."[194]

Members of the Science Society of China, who dominated every discipline of learning, put into practice the slogan of "saving the country with science." In the cultural assimilation of Western knowledge and the practice of science, science was disseminated not only in technical terms but also used in the political rhetoric and debate of China's social and political transformations. Writers and essayists embraced science and helped shape a pro-science culture through their praise of science and modernity and their attacks on Chinese traditional values and social norms.

Western medicine, which was revolutionized by bacteriology, immunology and the germ theory, spearheaded the scientific thrust of cultural modernization of China. The Rockefeller Foundation dedicated its modern medical enterprise—PUMC—as the American vanguard of medical science to transform traditional China into a modern nation. The Chinese government welcomed PUMC as "a monument to the progress of modern medical science in China."[195] Chinese leaders regarded the medical philanthropy of the RF as a demonstration of universal love and altruism that had been part of Chinese belief that "a physician is the Minister of Love and Humanity; his virtue dispenses benevolence, his knowledge brings healing."[196] The RF, however, did not establish the American outpost of medical science to benefit the masses but to produce a small number of elite to lead China. Western-trained Chinese intellectuals, in contrast, differed from the medical leaders of the RF in that they promoted vernacular writing and popularization of science among the masses. They believed that the Chinese masses had to grasp science and modern ideas to change their own world outlook if China was to transform into a modern nation.

The significant influence of PUMC in China lay not in bringing the modern medical benevolence to the Chinese masses but in the training of medical leaders to shape China's medical education and health administration. The PUMC produced 321 medical doctors in 20 years (1924–1943) and 279 nurses in 25 years (1924–1950) when China had more than 500 million people in urgent need of medical care.[197] The PUMC students, who learned modern knowledge of medicine in English, gained prestige and pedigree, but they were a small group of elite professionals distanced from the Chinese masses. Except for Chen Zhiqian who devoted himself to rural health, few of them dedicated their lives to the medical service of ordinary Chinese. The majority went into the service of government, conducted medical research and teaching, provided hospital leadership, or carried a profitable private medical practice in major cities.[198] Their leadership in medical education and health administration, however, profoundly influenced China's modern medical education and health policies. The PUMC circle, as chapter 3 shows, dominated the leadership of the Ministry of Health and local health bureaus of the Nationalist government.

John B. Grant was inseparable from the origin of public health profession and the creation of a national health system in China. In his 20 years of work in China, Grant collaborated with his Chinese colleagues, making significant contributions to the training of public health professionals and the building of health institutions. When the Nationalist Government established a Ministry of Health in 1928, the PUMC public health professionals formed the key cadre of the administration, many of whom were either Grant's former students or his colleagues at PUMC. Through health stations, Grant advocated and tested his vision of the combined practice of curative and preventive medicine in a community as the best efficient delivery of healthcare. He accomplished his ultimate career ambition in China by helping the Nationalist government create a modern health administration system of state medicine. He and his Chinese colleagues did not imitate dogmatically the existing systems of other nations but tried to build their own creatively and intelligently to avoid the mistakes and detours that others had gone through.[199] In his dealings with Chinese professionals and government officials, Grant was sensitive to Chinese sentiment during the politically tumultuous years of the Chinese nationalist movement. His confidence in Chinese themselves in carrying out medical and health tasks proved to be vitally important to his many successes. Chen Zhiqian commented that Grant "believed that no one was better suited to solve China's grievous problems than the Chinese themselves."[200]

Grant was a champion for medical efficiency based on the technical expertise of public health professionals.[201] However, he began to realize the limits of technical expertise in solving public health problems after learning about the programs of the Rural Reform and Mass Education Movement in China. He initiated the cooperation between PUMC and the Mass Education Movement in Dingxian and emphasized the importance of rural public health training for PUMC students.[202] The exceptional accomplishments of Dingxian demonstrated that the public health program had to be integrated into a broader socioeconomic reform movement in order to succeed. Grant used critical evaluations to assess the Beijing health station in order to improve the teaching of public health. The 1932 study of the station found deficiencies in several areas, such as the communicable disease control and sanitation control.[203] The interfering measures of the modern public health mechanism, which led to tensions and resistance in the station community, demonstrated the authority of modern health measures in redefining the healthy individual and sanitary environment, and the difficulty in transforming the populace from traditional to modern mode of life without changing the socioeconomic conditions. Nonetheless, the work of the health station laid the groundwork for national standards and methods of public health and vital statistics collection and analysis in China.

The ideas and institutions of Western medicine and public health secured their legitimacy in Chinese society on the basis of science, but at the expense of Chinese medical knowledge. Modernizers denied the value of Chinese medicine on both medical and political grounds. Although there was a huge gap of mentality between modern intellectuals and traditional masses in view of Western medicine, the intellectuals made conscientious efforts to disseminate Western cultural concepts and educate people about science and democracy. Starting in cities, Chinese intellectuals, acting much like their counterparts in the West, organized popular lectures on modern education and social development, on modern political ideas and national revival, and on medical science and epidemic prevention. When plague epidemics broke out, government and civic organizations circulated vernacular health notices to explain diseases and methods of prevention. Newspapers and magazines became a main communication channel from the government to the people when they published government health regulations and reported disease prevention notices. Modern concepts, such as germ/*jun* (菌) and microbe/*weishengwu* (微生物), were popularized to the people in colloquial language. People learned the ideas of disease transmission (*chuanran*, 传染) and the methods of disease prevention (*yufang*, 预防). Germ theory was, thus, popularized among the people without the pain of theorization. The idea of disease prevention fundamentally re-oriented the understanding of disease causation and gave rise to the new emphases on hygiene and sanitation as methods of keeping people healthy. Popular understanding of *weisheng* as hygiene, sanitation and public health, was promoted by a variety of organizations, such as the Council on Health Education, Central Epidemic Prevention Bureau, North Manchurian Plague Prevention Service, the YMCA, in addition to media, educational and social institutions, and the government.

Scientific understanding of diseases prompted scientific understanding of the human body. Students were taught the latest Western interpretation of human body at schools and were encouraged to study modern medicine as life work in the modernization of their country. Medical supplements of newspapers and pharmaceutical advertisements further popularized the new concepts of disease and human body to the general public. Intellectual attention to the human body underwent a transition from the focus on its social importance in national survival to the scientific analysis of its chemical components. The human body was now scientifically analyzable and quantifiable in terms of its chemical percentages.

Western medicine and science helped market to Chinese people the ideas of national strength and the dreams of modern progress. Western medicine came to dominate the thinking of both the Nationalist and the Communist health modernizers, though the Communists valued the usefulness of Chinese medicine more than the Nationalists.

Notes

1 D. W. K. Kwok, *Scientism in Chinese Thought, 1900–1950* (New Haven: Yale University, 1965); and Ralph C. Croizier, *Traditional Medicine in Modern China: Science, Nationalism, and the Tensions of Cultural Change* (Cambridge, MA: Harvard University Press, 1968).

2 Peter Buck, "Western Science in Republican China: Ideology and Institution Building," in *Science and Value: Patterns of Tradition and Change*, eds. Arnold Thackery and Evertt Menddelson (NY: Humanities Press, 1974), 159–184; and "Order and Control: the Scientific Method in China and the West," *Social Studies of Science*, vol. 5 (1975), 237–257.

3 Gyan Prakash, *Another Reason: Science and the Imagination of Modern India* (New Jersey: Princeton University Press, 1999).

4 On the numbers of Chinese students in America, see Y. C. Wang, *Chinese Intellectuals and the West, 1872–1949* (Chapel Hill: The University of North Carolina Press, 1966), 510–511. See also Hongshan Li, *U.S.–China Educational Exchange: State, Society, and Industrial Relations, 1905–1950* (New Jersey: Rutgers University Press, 2008).

5 Saito Keishu argued that Japan not only became the place where Sun Yat-sen organized his Revolutionary Alliance and trained revolutionary leaders among the students, but also was the source where Chinese modernizers found Japanese translations of Western books. They translated them into Chinese, introducing many alien Western concepts via Japanese translations. These terms and phrases included *shijie guan* (世界观, worldview), *yishi xingtan* (意识形态, ideology), *zhuyi* (主义, ism), *ziran kexue* (自然科学, natural science). Japan somewhat provided a short-cut for the Chinese to learn from the West at the turn of the twentieth century. Saito Keishu, *Zhongguo ren liuxue riben shi* [History of Chinese Studying in Japan], trans. Tan Ruqian and Lin Qiyan (Hong Kong: Chinese University Press, 1982). In contrast, Chinese students in the West contributed more to natural sciences and the ideology of scientism and Communism in China.

6 Weili Ye, *Seeking Modernity in China's Name: Chinese Students in the United States, 1900–1927* (Stanford University Press, 2001); and Vera Schwarcz, *The Chinese Enlightenment: Intellectuals and the Legacy of the May Fourth Movement of 1919* (Berkeley, CA: University of California Press, 1990).

7 Wang Qisheng, *Zhongguo liuxuesheng de lishi guiji* [The Historical Trend of Chinese Students Abroad, 1872–1949] (Hubei jiaoyu chubanshe, 1992), 288.

8 The nine founding members of the society included Hu Mingfu, Zhao Yuanren, Zhou Ren, Bing Zhi, Zhang Yuanshan, Guo Tanxian, Jin Bangzheng, Yang Xingfo and Ren Hongjun. All were Boxer Indemnity fellows except Ren Hongjun and Yang Xingfo who were revolutionaries, having worked as aides to Sun Yat-sen in the 1911 revolution (see Wang Qisheng, 288; and Wang Zuoyue, 300).

9 *Kexue* [科学, Science], vol. 1, no. 1 (Shanghai: The Science Society of China, 1915), 7.

10 By superstition they meant Chinese traditional beliefs and customs associated with folk religions. The subject was discussed by Prasenjit Duara in his article, "Knowledge and Power in the Discourse of Modernity: The Campaigns against Popular Religion in Early Twentieth-Century China," *The Journal of Asian Studies*, vol. 50, no.1 (1991), 67–83.

11 Benjamin A. Elman, *A Cultural History of Modern Science in China* (Cambridge, MA: Harvard University Press, 2006), particularly chapter 4 and appendixes.
12 Huang Zhizheng, "Dissemination of Science by Chinese Students in America during the May 4th Era," *Jindaishi yanjiu* [*Studies of Modern Chinese History*], vol. 50, no. 2 (1989), 17–40.
13 D.W.Y. Kwok, *Scientism in Chinese Thought*, 15.
14 The Science Society of China, *The Science Society of China: Its History, Organization, and Activities* (Shanghai: Science Press, 1931).
15 Wang Zuoyue, "Saving China through Science: the Science Society of China, Scientific Nationalism, and Civil Society in Republican China," *Osiris* 33 (2002), 291–321; Jia Sheng, "The Origins of the Science Society of China, 1914–1937," Ph.D. diss. (Cornell University, 1995); David C. Reynolds, "The Advancement of Knowledge and the Enrichment of Life: The Science Society of China and the Understanding of Science in the Early Republic, 1914–1930," Ph.D. diss. (University of Wisconsin—Madison, 1986); and Peter Buck, *American Science and Modern China* (Cambridge University Press, 1980). Buck presented a problematic account, claiming that the Science Society of China accomplished little in institution-building and research in China. He also held the view that few Chinese scientists properly understood science.
16 Wang Qisheng, *Zhongguo liuxuesheng*, 290–293.
17 Jia Sheng detailed the story in chapter 4 of his dissertation, "The Origins of the Science Society of China, 1914–1937."
18 Science popularization is an important theme of science education in modern China, and yet, it is still an understudied subject, as it is in the West. See Roger Cooter and Stephen Pumfrey, "Separate Spheres and Public Spaces: Reflections on the History of Science Popularization and Science in Popular Culture." *History of Science*, vol. 32 (1994), 237–267.
19 Croizier, *Traditional Medicine in Modern China*, 70–80.
20 A letter of August 25, 1928, quoted in Jiang Shaoyuan, "Zhongguo ren dui yu xiyang yiyao he yixue de fanying [Chinese reaction to western drugs and medicine]" *Gongxian*, vol. 4, no. 3 (1928), 23. (See Croizier, 252, footnote 22.
21 Croizier, *Traditional Medicine in Modern China*, 77.
22 For the major challenges to Chinese medicine, see Zhao Hongjun, *Jindai zhongxiyi zhenglun shi* [*History of the Debates between Chinese and Western Medicine*] (Hefei: Anhui kexue jishu chubanshe, 1989); and Sean Xiang-lin Lei, *Neither Donkey Nor Horse*.
23 Chang Tsung-liang, " 'Old Style' Versus 'Modern' Medicine in China," *Medicine as a Life Work Campaign, First Prize English and Chinese Essays of the 1926 National Essay Contest* (Shanghai: Council on Health Education, 1926), 5–8.
24 Croizier, *Traditional Medicine in Modern China*, 76.
25 Franklin C. McLean to Roger S. Greene, 19 January 1917, folder 65, box 6, Series 1, RG4, RF, RAC.
26 *The Reminiscences of Dr. John B. Grant*, Columbia University Oral History Project (Oral History Research Office, Columbia University, 1961), 140–41.
27 Peter, Annual report, 1916.
28 *The Rockefeller Foundation Annual Report*, 1921, 307.
29 Chieko Nakajima, "'Healthful Goods': Health, Hygiene, and Commercial Culture in Early Twentieth-Century Shanghai," *Twentieth Century China*, vol. 37, no. 3 (October 2012), 250–274.
30 Edgar Snow, *Red Star over China* (New York: Grove Press, 1968), 147.
31 Stuart R. Schram, *The Political Thought of Mao Tse-tung* (New York: Praeger Publishers, 1971), 153–160. Mao Zedong published this article titled "A Study of Physical Education," in *New Youth* [新青年], vol. 3, no. 2 (1917), 1–11 under the pseudonym "twenty-eight stroke student [二十八画生]," the number of strokes of his name.

32 Shigehisa Kuriyama, *The Expressiveness of the Body and the Divergence of Greek and Chinese Medicine* (New York: Zone Books, 1999), 8–11.
33 Fritz Kahn, *Der Mensch als Industriepalast* (Man as Industrial Palace) (Kosmos Verlag, 1926). See also Uta von Debschitz and Thilo von Debschitz, *Fritz Kahn: Man Machine Maschine Mensch* (Springer Vienna Architecture, 2009).
34 See images at http://www.nlm.nih.gov/hmd/chineseposters/understanding.html
35 https://www.nlm.nih.gov/hmd/chineseposters/images/1200/DSC_4003.jpg.
36 https://www.nlm.nih.gov/hmd/chineseposters/images/1200/DSC_4085.jpg.
37 Sherman Cochran, "Marketing Medicine and Advertising Dreams in China, 1900–1950," in *Becoming Chinese: Passages to Modernity and Beyond*, ed. Wen-hsin Yeh (Berkeley, CA: University of California Press, 2000), 62–97
38 China Medical Commission of the Rockefeller Foundation, *Medicine in China* (New York: the Rockefeller Foundation, 1914).
39 *Addresses and Papers, Dedication Ceremonies and Medical Conference, Peking Union Medical College. September 15–22, 1921, Peking, China* (Concord, New Hampshire: Rumford Press, 1922), 12–13.
40 Raymond B. Fosdick, *The Story of the Rockefeller Foundation* (New York: Harper and Brothers Publishers, 1952), 25.
41 Noel H. Pugach, "Standard Oil and Petroleum Development in Early Republican China," *The Business History Review*, vol. 45, no. 4 (Winter, 1971), 452–473. The Rockefellers and Standard Oil were household names to many Chinese in the early twentieth century.
42 *Addresses and Papers, Dedication Ceremonies and Medical Conference*, 3.
43 *Addresses and Papers, Dedication Ceremonies and Medical Conference*, 4.
44 Mary E. Ferguson, *China Medical Board and Peking Union Medical College: A Chronicle of Fruitful Collaboration, 1914–1951* (New York: China Medical Board of New York, Inc., 1970), 23–25.
45 Information on the transition of the school can be found in the collection, *Addresses and Papers: Dedication Ceremonies and Medical Conference, Peking Union Medical College, September 15–22, 1921*.
46 Mary E. Ferguson, *China Medical Board and Peking Union Medical College,* 25.
47 Welch, Diary # 1, 83, quoted in Mary Bullock, *An American Transplant* (Berkeley, CA: University of California Press, 1980), 41.
48 Welch, "North China," 17, quoted in Bullock, *An American Transplant*, 42.
49 John D. Rockefeller, Jr., "Speech at the Dedication Ceremonies of Peking Union Medical College, 1921," in *Addresses and Papers, Dedication Ceremonies and Medical Conference,* 65–66.
50 Welch, Diary #2, 30, quoted in Bullock, *An American Transplant*, 42.
51 Bullock, *An American Transplant*, chapter 2, 24–47.
52 Eric Andrew Stein, "Hygiene and Decolonization: The Rockefeller Foundation and Indonesian Nationalism, 1933–1958," in *Science, Public Health and the State in Modern Asia*, eds. Liping Bu, Darwin Stapleton and Ka-che Yip (Routledge, 2011), 53.
53 Roger S. Greene to M. K. Eggleston, August 27, 1926, folder 899, box 124, CMB Inc., RAC.
54 Paul Monroe, "Education and Nationalism," folder title "Speeches and papers, 1926–1936, box 6B, RG 28. Monroe Papers, Teachers College Special Collections, University of Columbia, New York.
55 On American self-image in China in early twentieth century, see Ariane Knüsel, *Framing China: Media Images and Political Debates in Britain, the USA and Switzerland, 1900–1950* (Ashgate, 2012), 46–62.
56 Frederick L. Gates, "Hankow and Changsha," January 1916, p. 7, Simon Flexner Papers. Quoted in Bullock, *An American Transplant*, 40 and footnote 39.
57 Ferguson, *China Medical Board and Peking Union Medical College*, 45.

58 John Z. Bowers, *Western Medicine in a Chinese Palace: Peking Union Medical College, 1917–1951* (Philadelphia: Josiah Macy, Jr. Foundation, 1972), 142–143.
59 Paul C. Hodges to L. C. Goodrich, September 11, 1922, attachment to L.C. Goodrich to R.S. Greene, September 13, 1922, folder 968, box 134, CMB, Inc. RF, RAC.
60 "Activities of the China Medical Board," in *Addresses and Papers, Dedication Ceremonies and Medical Conference,* 4.
61 Richard M. Pearce, March 7, 1921, folder 1802, box 78, series 1, RG 4, RF, RAC.
62 Ibid.
63 Ibid.
64 Memo, "The Purpose of the Founding of the Chair of Hygiene," Sept. 26, 1921, folder 525, box 75, series 2B9, RG IV, CMB Inc., RAC.
65 The 1917–1918 plague is a less researched topic compared with the 1910 plague. Current studies include Cao Shuji and Li Yushang, "The Impact of Plague Epidemics on Modern Chinese Society," in *Natural Disasters and the Social Historical Structures in China* (Fudan University Press, 2001); and Cao Shuji, "National and Local Public Health—A Study Centering on the 1917–1918 Pulmonary Plague," *Zhongguo Shehui Kexue* [*Social Sciences in Chin*], no. 1 (2006), 178–190.
66 *Dagongbao* published the Regulations on Infectious Diseases on March 14, 17 and 18, 1916.
67 Wu Liande recalled that he was beaten by the relatives of the two plague victims when he was dissecting the bodies for examination, because he did not get their approval beforehand. He and his colleagues, on another occasion, had their vehicle burned by local people and officials. See "Plague Prevention Incident in Fengzheng, People against Dissection," *Dagongbao*, January 14, 1918. In another extreme situation, an American medical missionary gunned down two locals and injured one during the plague control, causing an upheaval of the local people against them. See *Dagongbao*, March 2, 1918.
68 Health Department of Beijing Police Bureau, J181-18-9902, p. 18, Beijing Municipal Archives.
69 Ibid., 27.
70 Ibid., 17–40.
71 Ibid., 25.
72 Central Epidemic Prevention Bureau, *First Annual Report*, December 1, 1922 to November 30, 1923 (Beijing, 1923), 1–6.
73 National Health Administration and Central Field Health Station, *National Epidemic Prevention Bureau: A Report, Being a Review of Its Activities from Its Foundation in March 1919 to June 1934* (Beiping, China, 1934).
74 Central Epidemic Prevention Bureau, *First Annual Report*, 7.
75 Grant to Heiser, letter, December 29, 1924, folder 601, box 202, series IHB/D, RG5, RAC.
76 Invitation letter to Grant from the Health Department of Interior Ministry [内务部卫生司], July 16, 1924, 1001-1-6, Second National Archives, Nanjing.
77 Correspondence of Grant and Heiser over health advisor, August 20–September 25, 1924, folder 601, box 202, series IHB/D, RG 6, RAC. It was not clear whether Grant actually declined the invitation, but he acted much like an advisor by giving Chinese government suggestions on public health matters.
78 On the relations between Russell and Grant, see Socrates Litsios, "Selskar Gunn and China: The Rockefeller Foundation's 'Other' Approach to Public Health," *Bulletin of the History of Medicine*, vol. 79, no. 2 (2005), 295–318, esp. 306–309.
79 National Health Administration, *National Epidemic Prevention Bureau*, 2.
80 Liu Ruiheng to Roger S. Greene, June 4, 1929, Liu Ruiheng papers, PUMC archives, # 2144, Beijing Xiehe Medical University, Beijing.
81 Grant to the Director, October 7, 1922, H. S. Houghton Journal, 1921–1924, PUMC archives, #159, Beijing.

82 Ibid.

83 Ibid. The South Manchuria Railway (南满铁路) was operated by the Japanese.

84 Howard Markel, "Victor C. Vaughan," *JAMA* 283 (7), February 16, 2000. For more on V. C. Vaughan, see H. W. Davenport, *Victor Vaughan: Statesman and Scientist* (Ann Arbor, MI: Historical Center for the Health Sciences, 1996. Monograph No. 4.); V.C. Vaughan, *A Doctor's Memories* (Indianapolis, IN: Bobbs-Merrill Publishing Co., 1926); and John Duffy, *The Sanitarians: A History of American Public Health* (Urbana-Champaign, IL: University of Illinois Press, 1992).

85 John M. Eyler, *Sir Arthur Newsholme and State Medicine, 1889–1935* (Cambridge, UK: Cambridge University Press, 1997), 362. On state medicine, see Newsholme, *Medicine and the State: The Relation between the Private and Official Practice of Medicine with Special Reference to Public Health* (London: George Allen and Unwin, 1932; Baltimore: Williams and Wilkins, 1932).

86 Conrad Seipp, "Introduction," in *Health Care for the Community: Selected Papers of Dr. John B. Grant* (Baltimore, MD: Johns Hopkins University Press, 1963), xiii–xiv. Newman and Newsholme were professionally rivals but Grant was non-partisan and found the ideas of both men making sense.

87 Biographical files of John B. Grant, RF. RAC. For Grant's fieldwork in American South and at the Pingxiang mines in China, see Bullock, *An American Transplant*, 135–138.

88 The name of the department was changed to Department of Public Health and Preventive Medicine, and then to Department of Public Health. On Grant's public health education, see Liping Bu, "Beijing First Health Station: Innovative Public Health Education and Influence on China's Health Profession," in *Science, Public Health and the State in Modern Asia*, eds. Liping Bu, Darwin H. Stapleton and Ka-che Yip (London: Routledge, 2012), 129–143.

89 Grant, "Report on a General Health Survey of Peking, China," February 1922, PUMC archives, # 393, Beijing.

90 Grant to S. H. Chuan, December 9, 1921, folder 1803, box 78, series 1, RG 4, RF, RAC.

91 Grant, "A Proposal for a Department of Hygiene for Peking Union Medical College," 1923, 42, folder 531, box 75, series 2B9, RG IV CMB Inc., RAC.

92 Ibid., 26. It was ironic that preventive and curative medicine completely diverged in America, while in China the government made prevention the first priority of medical policy during the 1950s–1980s.

93 Public health education at the Johns Hopkins University later incorporated community work in the training of public health professionals.

94 On the health stations and units by the IHB, see John Farley, *To Cast out Disease: A History of the International Health Division of the Rockefeller Foundation, 1913–1951* (New York: Oxford University Press, 2004).

95 National Health Administration and Central Field Health Station, *National Epidemic Prevention Bureau*; and Carsten Flohr, "The Plague Fighter: Wu Lien-teh and the Beginning of Chinese Public Health System," *Annals of Science*, vol. 53 (1996), 361–380.

96 Grant to Heiser, January. 13, 1922, folder 1803, box 78, series 1, RG 4, RF, RAC.

97 Memo, Houghton to Greene, December 27, 1924, folder 525, box 75, series 2B9, RG IV, CMB Inc., RAC. The staff at the CEPB included Chinese leaders in the field of medical science and public health, such as Fang Qing, Robert Lim, Quan Shaoqing, Jin Baoshan, and Huang Zifang.

98 *National Epidemic Prevention Bureau,* 107–108.

99 Ibid., 109.

100 Ting-an Li, Director, "The Health Station of the First Health Area, Beiping,"1930, 4, folder 366, box 44, series 601, RG1, RF, RAC.

101 "Health Station—First Quarter Review," December 24, 1925, 1, folder 465, box 66, series 2B9, RG IV, CMB Inc., RAC.

102 Ting-an Li, Director, "The Health Station of the First Health Area, Beiping," 1930, 7; and "Monthly Report" of the station, September and November 1925, folder 465, box 66, RG IV 2B9, CMB Inc., RAC.

103 The health station was originally called Public Health Experimental Station, Metropolitan Police Department, Peking [京师警察厅试办公共卫生事务所]. After it showed some satisfactory results, the word "experimental" was dropped in 1926 and the station was called Public Health Station, Metropolitan Police Department, Peking [京师警察厅公共卫生事务所]. In 1928 as the city's name was changed to Beiping and city districts were re-organized, the station's name was changed to Health Station of the First Health Area, Special Municipality of Beiping [北平特别市第一卫生区事务所]. In 1930, the Municipal Department of Public Health was merged with the Police Department to reduce municipal expenditure and the station became Health Station, First Health Area, Department of Public Safety, Beiping [北平市公安局第一区卫生事务所]. (Ting-an Li, Director, "The Health Station of the First Health Area, Beiping,"1930, 2–5, folder 366, box 44, series 601, RG1, RF, RAC.)

104 Letter of W. S. Carter to R. F. Johnston of British Legation, June 9, 1926, p. 2, folder 465. Box 66. RG IV 2B9, CMB Inc., RAC.

105 Grant, November 2, 1928, 1, attached to his third annual report on the Health Station, folder 2736, box 219, series 3, RG5, RF, RAC.

106 Ting-an Li, "The 6th Annual Report of the Health Station" submitted to John B. Grant, August 15, 1931, 5, folder 2739, box 219, series 3, RG5, RF, RAC.

107 Memo, from H. Barchet to M. K. Eggleston, April 18, 1925, folder 525, box 75, RG IV 2B9, CMB Inc., RAC. The station was often referred to as the health center or unit in the early stage of its existence.

108 Grant to Dr. Dunlap, re Public Health Nursing, April 10, 1926, folder 465, box 66, RG IV 2B9, CMB Inc., RAC.

109 Grant, "Department of Public Health and Preventive Medicine, PUMC," January 18, 1929, p. 18, folder 533, box 75, series 2B9, RG IV, CMB Inc., RAC.

110 A classification of causes of death in China was created by the staff of the station based on the model of the International Classification, and it was adopted for national use by the China Medical Association in 1927. The classification offered a uniform standard that Western and Chinese doctors could use in death reports. Major causes of death according to the station's 1927–28 report were tuberculosis, respiratory diseases, gastro-intestinal diseases, and cardiac and renal diseases. ("Report of Peking Health Station, 1927–1928," Third Annual Report, p. 6, folder 469, box 66, RGIV 2B9, CMB Inc., RAC.)

111 "Health Station Report," September 1925 (Chinese version), p. 2, folder 465, box 66, RG IV 2B9, CMB Inc., RAC.

112 "Health Station Report," September 1925 (English version), p. 5, folder 465, box 66, RG IV 2B9, CMB Inc., RAC.

113 "Health Station Report," November 1925 (Chinese version).

114 Grant, "Health Station—First Quarterly Review," December 24, 1925, pp. 5–6, folder 465, box 66, RG IV 2B9, CMB Inc., RAC.

115 "Health Station Report," November 1925, p. 1 (Chinese version).

116 Grant, "Second Annual Report—Health Station, July 1, 1926–June 30, 1927," folder 2735. box 219, Series 3 IHB/D, RG5, RF, RAC.

117 Yang Nianqun, " 'Lan Ansheng moshi' yu minguo chuqi Beijing shengsi kongzhi kongjian di zhuanhuan"['Grant Model' and the Spatial Transitions of Life/Birth and Death Control in Early-Republic Beijing], *Shehuixue yanjiu* [Sociological Studies], no. 4 (1999), 98–113.

118 Grant, "Second Annual Report—Health Station, July 1, 1926–June 30, 1927," pp. 7–8.

119 Grant, "Health Station—First Quarterly Review," December 24, 1925, p. 8.

120 Ibid., 2–3.

121 Grant, "Second Annual Report—Health Station, July 1, 1926–June 30, 1927," p. 7.
122 Ibid., 6.
123 Ibid.
124 "The First Report of Flies Survey and Preliminary Recommendations for Eradicating Flies," Public Health Experimental Station, Beijing Metropolitan Police Department, August 1925. J181-18-18179, pp. 18–27, Beijing Municipal Archives.
125 "Monthly Report for October 1925, Public Health Demonstration Station, Metropolitan Police Department," pp. 1–2, folder 465, box 66, RG IV 2B9, CMB Inc., RAC.
126 Grant, "Second Annual Report—Health Station, July 1, 1926–June 30, 1927," p. 9.
127 "Monthly Report for October 1925, Public Health Demonstration Station, Metropolitan Police Department," pp. 4–5.
128 Grant, "Second Annual Report—Health Station, July 1, 1926–June 30, 1927," p. 9.
129 Ting-an Li, "The Health Station of the First Health Area, Beiping,"1930, p. 8, folder 366, box 44, Series 601, RG1, RF.
130 "Fifth Annual Report of the Health Station," September 30, 1930, p. i, folder 2738, box 219, Series 3, RG5, RF.
131 Ting-an Li, "The Health Station of the First Health Area, Beiping,"1930, p. 9.
132 "Report of Peking Health Station, 1927–1928," p. 16, folder 469, box 66, RGIV 2B9, CMB Inc., RAC. J.B. Grant and P.Z. King, "Tentative Appraisal Form for Health Work in Large Cities in China," *National Medical Journal of China* 14 (1928), 81–104.
133 Grant to R. S. Greene, "8th Annual Report—Health Station," September 1933, p. ix, folder 2741, box 220, Series 3, RG5, RF, RAC.
134 Letter, Grant to Heiser, "Proposal for Midwifery School," September 20, 1926, pp. 1–2, folder 669, box 94, RG IV 2B9, CMB Inc., RAC.
135 Ibid., 2. This sounded a recipe for what the PRC did decades later in training barefoot doctors.
136 Ibid.
137 Tina P. Johnson, *Childbirth in Republican China: Delivering Modernity* (Lanham, MD: Lexington Books, 2011).
138 Grant to Heiser, "Proposal for Midwifery School."
139 Letter, Roger Greene to John D. Rockefeller, Jr., October 17, 1933, folder 250, box 35, RG IV 2B9, CMB Inc., RAC.
140 Chen Chih-ch'ien, "The Development of Systematic Training in Rural Public Health Work in China," *Milbank Memorial Fund Quarterly Bulletin*, vol. 14 (1936), 370–387, on midwifery, 381–84.
141 C. C. Chen, "China-Health, Training of Personnel: First Semi-Annual Report for 1945," box 218, Series 3, IHB/D, RG 5, RAC.
142 Shanghai Medical College was founded in 1927 and began classes in October that year. Yan Fuqing was president of the college and also served as chair of the Department of Public Health.
143 Zhang Daqing, *A Social History of Diseases in Modern China, 1912–1937* (Shandong jiaoyu chubanshe, 2006), 183–84.
144 C. C. Chen, *Medicine in Rural China: A Personal Account* (Berkeley, CA: University of California Press, 1989), 70.
145 Wen Tsing Tao to Dean J. E. Russell, February 16, 1916, folder 755D "Livingston Scholars, 1915–1916," series 10, RG 6, James Earl Russell Papers, Teachers College Special Collections. Tao changed his name to Xingzhi in 1934 after he published his article "Practice to knowledge to Practice" (行知行) to promote the idea that practice is the beginning to know and the end of knowledge is practice. Xingzhi means practice to know. Tao was very much influenced by the American educator John Dewey's theory on practice in education. Tao's education thought contributed significantly to China's modern education, particularly elementary education.
146 C. C. Chen, *The Binying Weekly* 4 (Beijing, 1926), 21–23. *The Binying Weekly* was initially published in *Peking World Daily* and then in *Dagongbao* by a group of first-year students at PUMC who organized a Binying Society (丙寅医学社). The *Weekly*

promoted awareness of public health and the role medicine in national strength, and the responsibility of the state for the healthcare of people.

147 Chen, *Medicine in Rural China*, 68.

148 Ibid., 69.

149 Chen, *Medicine in Rural China*, 67–69; and Ka-che Yip, *Health and National Reconstruction in Nationalist China: The Development of Modern Health Services, 1928–1937* (Ann Arbor, Association for Asian Studies, Inc., 1995), 76–77.

150 Guy S. Alitto, *The Last Confucian: Liang Shu-ming and the Chinese Dilemma of Modernity* (Berkeley: University of California Press, 1979).

151 The MEM chose Dingxian as its base after its successful operation in Changsha of Hunan province in 1922 because Dingxian had all the known statistics useful for MEM experiment. Ginling University (merged with Nanjng University in 1952) had been conducting socioeconomic surveys of Dingxian since 1923, with information on population, income, and traditional medical practice. Ginling University was quite a pioneer in rural health study. It started an agricultural experimental area in Wujiang (乌江) of Hexian County of Anhui in 1923. It built a Wujiang Peasant Hospital with the help of Gulou missionary hospital to improve peasants' health, although the medical services were limited. See Chen Haifeng, *Zhongguo weisheng boajian shi* [*History of Health Care in China*] (Shanghai kexue jishu chubanshe, 1992), 16; and C. C. Chen, *Medicine in Rural China*, 73–74.

152 Grant, "A Proposal for a Department of Hygiene for Peking Union Medical College," 30.

153 Sidney D. Gamble, *Ting Hsien: A North China Rural Community* (Stanford: Stanford University Press, 1968); Charles W. Hayford, *To the People: James Yen and Village China* (NY: Columbia University Press, 1990); Mary Bullock, *An American Transplant*, chapter 7; and C. C. Chen, *Medicine in Rural China*.

154 On October 18, 1928, the Executive Committee of the RF passed a resolution on the budgets for two Shanghai health units: (1) rural demonstration unit with $21,580 for first year (1928–1929) and $9,790 for second year (1929–30), and (2) school demonstration unit with $16,296 for first year and $7,140 for second year. ("Resolutions on Shanghai health units," folder 368, box 45, series 601, RG 1, RF.) Shanghai municipal government was to provide the rural demonstration area with $4,500 for first year (1928–29) and $14,290 for second year (1929–30). (Grant to Heiser, September 3, 1928, folder 368, box 45, series 601, RG 1, RF., RAC.)

155 In the 1920s, individual behavior was a prominent topic of public health discussion, especially the training of school children. Newsholme was a strong advocate of incorporating hygiene into elementary school curriculum. (John M. Elyer, *Sir Arthur Newsholme and State Medicine, 1889–1936*, Cambridge: Cambridge University Press, 1997.) Newsholme, "On the Study of Hygiene in Elementary Schools," *Public Health*, vol. 3 (1890–1), 134–6. Grant was also a believer in changing people's health behavior through education, particularly via school health education and preventive medicine.

156 Memo from R.S. Greene to M. K. Eggleston, on Dr. Li Ting-an, November 24, 1928, folder 535, box 76, CMB Inc., RAC (David L. Edsall was Dean of School of Public Health, Harvard University.)

157 Grant, February 1929, folder 368, box45, series 601, RG 1, RF, RAC.

158 Letter of Li Ting-an to Richard M. Pearce, March 6, 1930, folder 535, box 76, RG IV 2B9, CMB Inc., RAC.

159 "First Quarterly Report Ending September 30, 1929, Rural Health Demonstration, Kao-Chiao, The Municipality of Greater Shanghai, China," 1–3, folder 2742, box 220, Series 3, RG 5, RF, RAC.

160 Ibid., 7–19.

161 Liping Bu, "From Public Health to State Medicine: John B. Grant and China's Health Profession," *Harvard Asia Quarterly*, vol. 14, no. 4 (December 2012), 8–15.

162 "Traveling Clinic of Kao-Chiao," folder 2742, box 220, series, 601J, RG 5.3, RF, with pictures attached.

163 "Traveling Clinic of Kao-Chiao," folder 2742, box 220, Series 601J, RG 5, RF, RAC, with pictures attached.

164 "Sixth Quarterly Report Ending Dec. 31, 1930, Kao Chiao Rural Health Demonstration Station, Bureau of Public Health, City Government of Greater Shanghai," folder 2743, box 220, series 3, RG 5, RF, RAC.

165 Except Dingxian, little detailed studies have been conducted of these rural health stations. Their importance in Chinese rural health development calls for more scholarly investigation of rural health in the 1920s–1930s.

166 Li Ting-an, "Report of Rural Public Health Survey in China," *National Medical Journal of China*, vol. 20, no. 9 (1934) [Chinese version, 李廷安, "中国乡村卫生调查报告, 中华医学杂志, 20卷，9期 (1934)], 1113–1201; and T. A. Li, "Summary Report on Rural Public Health Practice in China," *The Chinese Medical Journal*, vol. 48 (October 1934), 1086–1090.

167 T. A. Li, "Summary Report on Rural Public Health Practice in China," 1090.

168 J. B. Grant and T. M. Peng, "Survey of Urban Public Health Practice in China," *The Chinese Medical Journal*, vol. 48 (October 1934), 1074–1079.

169 Grant and Peng, "Survey of Urban Public Health Practice in China," 1075–78.

170 Ibid., 1078.

171 "Excerpts from J.B. Grant's Notes of October 1929," folder 368, box 45, series 601, RG 1, RF, RAC.

172 Grant, correspondence, 1925, folder 3006, box 235, series 1.2, RG5 IHB/D, RAC.

173 Letter from C. C. Williamson [director of information service of RF] to Grant, March 20, 1923, folder 1805, box 78, Series 1, RG 4, RF, RAC.

174 Grant, "Plans for Public Health Work in China, 1925," folder 532, box76, RG IV 2B9, CMB Inc. RAC.

175 The English version of the pamphlet had 6 pages with single space, titled "Public Health in Peking." It gave a brief history and the organizational divisions of public health, and defined public health as "that branch of government undertaking the prevention of disease in the community. . . . the business of health protection is being undertaken." (Attachment to Grant, "Plans for Public Health Work in China," 1925.)

176 Grant to Hsueh Tu-pi, February 13, 1925, folder 532, box 76, RG IV 2B9, CMB Inc. The story was when Grant contemplated a rural health station near Beijing, he had to walk a delicate line not to upset Chinese nationalist sentiment; so he made sure the appeal for public health assistance came from the local county, San Ho Hsien [Sanhe xian, 三河县]. Grant wrote: "Although, as a private organization, we are not desirous of undertaking anything in the Public Health line, we feel it incumbent upon us to answer the appeal for help from San Ho Hsien." The project of San Ho Hsien did not work out, which led Grant to seek the opportunity to partner with James Yen on a public health program in Dingxian.

177 Grant to Greene, December 13, 1926, folder 465, and Inter-office memo, Greene to Houghton, March 23, 1927, folder 466, box 66, RG IV 2B9, CMB Inc. On the Chinese competition for the use of British Boxer Indemnity, refer to chapter 4 of See Heng Teow's book, *Japan's Cultural Policy toward China, 1918–1931: A Comparative Perspective* (MA: Harvard University Asia Center, 1999), 130–132.

178 Memo to Greene, July 27, 1927, folder 466, box 66, RG IV 2B9, CMB Inc.

179 G. Douglas Gray to Huang (Zifang), 22 August 1927, folder 366, box 44, series 601, RG1, RF, RAC.

180 China had been ravaged by wars between warlords since the end of the Qing dynasty. In 1924, a revolutionary government of the United Front between the Guomindang (the Nationalist Party, 国民党) and the Chinese Communist Party was established in Guangzhou under the leadership of Sun Yat-sen to challenge the warlord-controlled central government in Beijing. The revolutionaries launched the Northern Expedition against warlords in 1926–27 with much popular support and success. Jiang Jieshi, leader of the Northern Expedition and Guomindang after Sun Yat-sen's death in 1925,

turned the guns around to kill the communists and purge them just before the new national government was established in Nanjing.

181 John B. Grant, "State Medicine –A Logical Policy for China," *National Medical Journal of China*, vol. 14 (February 1928), 65–80.
182 Ibid., 75.
183 Ibid.
184 "Public Health in Peking," p. 2, attachment in Grant, "Plans for Public Health Work in China 1925." Chinese medical scientists such as Jin Baoshan and Huang Zifang frequently cited this allegedly Gladstone's statement in their advocacy of state responsibility for public health.
185 "Rural Public Health," p. 1, attachment in Grant, "Plans for Public Health Work in China 1925."
186 John B. Grant, "State Medicine – A Logical Policy for China."
187 Ibid., 76–77.
188 Ibid., 78.
189 Ibid., 79.
190 Gao Xi, "Between the State and the Private Sphere: Chinese State Medicine Movement, 1930–1949," in *Science, Public Health and the State in Modern Asia*, 144–160.
191 Iris Borowy, "Thinking Big—League of Nations Efforts towards a Reformed National Health System in China," in *Uneasy Encounters,*205–228; and AnElissa Lucas, "Changing Medical Models in China: Organizational Options or Obstacles?" *The China Quarterly*, vol. 83 (Sept. 1980), 461–489.
192 Iris Borowy, *Coming to Terms with World Health* (Germany: Peter Lang GmbH, 2009), chapter III.
193 For general history of China, see Immanuel Hsu, *The Rise of Modern China* (New York: Oxford University Press, 1983); and Jonathan Spence, *The Search of Modern China* (New York: Norton and Company, 1990).
194 Gyan Prakash, *Another Reason*, 12.
195 S. P. Chen, "Greetings on Behalf of the Ministry of the Interior," in *Addresses & Papers, Dedication Ceremonies and Medical Conference, Peking Union Medical College, September 15–22, 1921*, 48.
196 His Excellence, President Hsu Shih-Ch'ang, "Address at the Reception at the President's Palace," in *Addresses & Papers, Dedication Ceremonies and Medical Conference,* 67.
197 Mary E. Ferguson, *China Medical Board and Peking Union Medical College,* Appendix C, 245–253.
198 For their careers up to 1937, see Mary Bullock, *An American Transplant*, Appendix A, 233–237.
199 Grant, "State Medicine," 65–66.
200 Chen, *Medicine in Rural China*, 38.
201 Chen Zhiqian thought that Grant emphasized academic research but not enough attention to the value of clinical training of public health specialists, which limited their capability in dealing with diseases in real life. (Chen, *Medicine in Rural China*, 39.)
202 Minutes of the Peiping Union Medical College, Committee on the Health Station, May 19, 1932. PUMC archives, #391.
203 Ting-an Li, "A Critical Study of the Work of the Health Station, First Health Area, Department of Public Safety, Peiping, for the Years 1925–1931 with Suggestions for Improvement, January 1932." PUMC archives, #387, p. 12; and Grant's response to Li Ting-an's study, February 9, 1932. PUMC archives, #388, Beijing.

3 Building a modern health system

GMD's state medicine and CCP's people's health, 1920s–40s

Introduction

China was divided and devastated by wars in the 1920s–1940s. Guomindang (GMD, the Nationalist Party) and the Chinese Communist Party (CCP) formed a United Front to fight against the warlords in 1924. After they won great victories in the Northern Expedition, Jiang Jieshi (Chiang Kai-shek) turned the guns on the Communists in a political betrayal, just before he formed the Nationalist government in Nanjing to replace the warlord-supported government in Beijing (Beiyang government) in 1927. The CCP, after surviving the bloody setback, re-grouped in the rural mountains in southeast China of Jiangxi and Fujian to start all over again. The Nationalist government, however, faced both domestic and foreign challenges in the effort to create a unified modern sovereign state of China. On one hand, it continued the negotiations with foreign powers that had been carried on by the Beiyang government to recover the sovereign rights that China had lost through the unequal treaties. Those rights included sovereignty over customs and quarantine services, tariffs, medical regulations, and education. On the other hand, the Nationalist government attempted to eliminate the CCP, its political rival, by launching major military campaigns against the Communist bases in the Jiangxi and Fujian border regions. The Communists, against all odds, survived the attacks and completed the Long March in 1934–1935 to resettle in Yanan (Yan'an, Yenan, 延安) in north central China, where they continued the revolution. When the Nationalists were fighting the Communists, Japanese military forces in northeast China (Manchuria) orchestrated the aggressions in 1931 to expand their territory in China, and then launched the full-scale invasion in 1937, starting World War II. In this national crisis, patriotic Chinese called to unite against the Japanese invaders, leading to the formation of a Second United Front of the GMD and the CCP in 1937. China's war against Japanese invasion, which became part of World War II, did not end until the Allies' victory over Japan. Against this background of wars and political upheavals, health modernizers of the Nationalist government made substantial efforts in creating an institutional system of modern national health, with significant assistance of the League of Nations and the Rockefeller Foundation. The Communists, in the meantime, managed to create health programs in rural areas with limited resources but relied on local people and used both Chinese and Western medicines. International medical aid from the anti-fascist movement helped improve the standards of the CCP's medical services and influenced the health development in CCP regions.

This chapter examines the ambitious creation of a national health system by the health modernizers of the Nationalist government, and their collaboration with the League of Nations Health Organization (LNHO) and the Rockefeller Foundation (RF). It also investigates the creative efforts of the Communists in establishing medical services and healthcare programs, with the mobilization of local population and the help of international aid, for military soldiers and civilian peasants in their regions. The different approaches to health construction by the Nationalists and the Communists illuminated the contrasting priorities of their health programs and medical policies. The Nationalist health programs constituted an important part of institutional-building of a new modern state. Health modernization programs functioned as social transformative agents to change society from a traditional to modern mode of operation. In this process of modernization, Chinese medicine faced the threat of being abolished by the state. The crisis triggered new efforts of self-rejuvenation by Chinese medicine men through political as well as medical activism. In contrast, the CCP's health programs emphasized the usefulness of both Western and Chinese medicines and integrated health activities in social and land reforms. The GMD's health construction reflected a different set of medical and health concerns of the Western-oriented medical elite who focused their attention on building a centralized health administrative system.

Part I: GMD's state building and health modernization

State medicine (公医): construction of a centralized national health system

Health modernizers of the Nationalist government considered public health a major component of state-building that would contribute to national prosperity and modernity. The Nationalist government claimed, at the inauguration of the Ministry of Health in October 1928, that the quality of health administration not only concerned the health of the people but also the prosperity of the Chinese nation.[1] The political thinking of Nationalist leaders in the matter of national health continued to echo the intellectual discourse that the late Qing reformers had articulated. To the Nationalist modernizers, China was still in a state of "medieval society" and national health would play an important role in modernizing the society in the overall socioeconomic reconstruction.[2] They believed that scientific application of Western medicine would transform China from a traditional society into a modern nation, and that health improvement would be conducive to national strength and economic prosperity. In his study of the Nationalist health construction in the 1930s, Ka-che Yip pointed out: "Nationalist leaders perceived health to be part of the nation-building process. . . . Individual health concerns therefore should be subordinated to the national priorities of state-building, military might, and economic development."[3]

The Chinese medical elite who led the health construction accepted state medicine as the model of national health system. State medicine, a concept first introduced by John B. Grant at the 1928 conference of Chinese medical professionals, meant state responsibility for national health. Chinese medical leaders had different interpretations of the concept when they tried to deliver state medicine under the Nationalist government. Grant's advocacy of state medicine emphasized a national health system that would provide health services to *all* people. Chinese health modernizers, particularly those of the Ministry of Health such as Liu Ruiheng (刘瑞恒, 1890–1961) and Jin Baoshan (金宝善, 1893–1984) concentrated on building a centralized health administrative system as the priority. They reasoned that an adequate institutional system of health administration was the first step of implementing state medicine in China. In other words, health service could not be delivered without an administrative system established in the first place. The debate on the meanings of state medicine continued throughout the 1920s–1940s among Chinese medical professionals, with the Health Ministry officials emphasizing centralization of health administration and medical educators and practitioners argued for a national health service to the people.[4] At the Symposium on State Medicine in 1937, Wu Liande mentioned three different forms of state medicine:

> The panel system in Great Britain is solely devoted to curative purposes, whilst the State medical organization built up in Soviet Russia is characterized by ample provision of hospitals, clinics and *crèches* as well as by public health and socio-medical institutions. The State Health Insurance system sponsored by the League of Nations, though at present opposed by many organized medical associations in several countries, will undoubtedly be a feature of the medicine of the future.[5]

These discussions and debates indicated that Chinese medical professionals took a broad view of all the possible models of health system practiced by other nations. They sincerely sought to find a suitable and practical model for China. Perhaps tired of the endless debate and few solutions adopted for the urgent need of China, Wu Liande told his colleagues: "instead of indulging in theoretical considerations we should concentrate attention upon the practical possibilities of introducing a State medical system into China."[6] The real difficulty in doing so, he acknowledged, "lay in finding sufficient and adequate workers for this purpose."[7] Health officials' concentration on building a centralized health administration may have been driven by a combination of factors, such as bureaucratic convenience, shortage of financial and human resources, and lack of political will of the government to deliver health service.

Politics of medicine in the Nationalist government complicated the creation of a modern health system and the implementation of state medicine. Jiang Jieshi, leader of the Nationalist government, showed more interest in eliminating the

Chinese communists than health construction for the people. In the autumn of 1931 when Yan Yangchu urged the Nationalist government to coordinate the various rural improvement activities of literacy and public health to develop a blueprint of national programs with government financial support, the Nationalist government ignored his ideas.[8] Jiang Jieshi told Yan Yangchu: "Calm down, Jimmy. First we'll defeat the Communists and then we'll implement your program."[9] In April 1931, the Nationalist government abolished the Ministry of Health and established, instead, a National Health Administration (NHA, 卫生署) within the Ministry of Interior. One third of the staff and two departments of the Ministry of Health were eliminated as a result, though Liu Ruiheng kept his leadership position as the Director of NHA.[10] Health modernizers worried about the government commitment and used personal connection and persuasion to extract support of Jiang Jieshi. Liu Ruiheng and Ludwik Rajchman, the LNHO representative in China, used all the "flattery and arguments at their command" to obtain Jiang Jieshi's agreement to continue the health modernization scheme.[11] The Nationalists did not restore the Ministry of Health until 1947; but by then the end of the Nationalist power was in sight as the CCP moved on to win the civil war in 1949.

Delivering a health service to the people was difficult to achieve without the full commitment of the state. For the health bureaucrats, it was a manageable and pragmatic task to build an institutional structure of health administration as long as the government continued modern state-building with health as a component. In all practical terms, a nationwide health service would not be possible without a national health administration and adequate medical facilities and personnel. Wu Liande found China terribly inadequate in both the numbers of modern-trained health professionals and the ability of people to pay for a health service. He pointed out that in comparison with Great Britain and the United States where the ratio of medical practitioners with inhabitants was 1:800 and 1:1000 respectively, China's ratio was 1:30,000.[12] Wu counted only doctors of Western medicine, as he and his colleagues already dismissed Chinese medicine as unscientific and unreliable. Wu Liande's articulation on the shortage of medical doctors echoed the view of John Grant and other medical elite who urged that China needed first and foremost to train competent technical personnel to staff a national health administration.[13] Statistics on modern medical doctors in the 1930s showed that the number of medical doctors registered with the NHA during 1929–1932 was 2919 with 2646 male and 273 female. 2567 of them were domestic graduates (88 percent) and 352 graduated from abroad (12 percent, including 194 from Japan, 74 from USA, 42 from Germany, 15 from Britain, 13 from France, 6 from Korea, 4 from Austria, 4 from others).[14] A 1935 survey indicated that the total had increased to 5390 doctors, with 4638 of Chinese nationality (87 percent) and 752 of foreign nationalities (13 percent).[15]

China had about 450 million people in the 1930s with 85 percent living in poverty in rural villages. Eleven epidemic diseases, namely, smallpox, meningitis, diphtheria, scarlet fever, cholera, dysentery, typhoid fever, plague, typhus fever, relapsing fever and malaria, were defined notifiable infectious diseases and monitored by the government. Surveys of 19 provinces with limited statistical data indicated that cholera, dysentery, malaria, typhoid fever, and smallpox were the major causes of death.[16] The national average death rate was estimated at 30 per thousand for China.[17] Sample surveys conducted in the 1920s–1930s offered statistical glimpses of rural and urban China. The Ginlin University (Nanjing) study of 101 rural districts across 17 provinces in 1920–1931 indicated the birth rate at 39 per thousand, death rate 28 per thousand, and infant mortality 156 per thousand among the rural population. A survey of Jiangying county of Jiangsu province in 1931–1934 indicated that the birth rate was 44 per thousand, death rate 43 per thousand, and infant mortality 278 per thousand. The 1934–1935 surveys of Nanjing showed that the birth rate was 23 per thousand, death rate 18 per thousand, and infant mortality 123 per thousand. In Beijing in 1936 the birth rate was 26 per thousand, death rate 17 per thousand, and infant mortality 149 per thousand. Life expectancy in China was about 35 in the 1930s.[18]

Most of modern doctors stayed in urban centers to secure lucrative practices. Shanghai, Guangzhou and Nanjing were the three most popular cities for them, with the two provinces of Jiangsu and Guangdong having the largest concentration. In the mid-1930s, Shanghai alone had 22 percent of China's doctors of Western medicine.[19] Despite the severe shortage of medical personnel, Nationalist health modernizers excluded physicians of Chinese medicine and healers of various Chinese traditions from the construction of modern health. They even attempted to eliminate Chinese medicine once and for all in 1929. In drawing the blueprint of a modern health system of China, the Chinese medical elite relied on Western models with complete faith in Western bio-medicine.

Sun Yat-sen had framed a three-phase process for China's modernization—the military campaigns, the tutelage, and the constitutional governance. Nationalist leaders followed this theoretical framework by defining 1928 as the beginning of the tutelage phase after the military expeditions against warlords and the unification of China. In the tutelage phase of nation-building, the government would enact laws and send qualified people to every county to educate people on how to use the rights and responsibilities of citizens in the construction of local self-governance.[20] Following this outline of national construction, the medical elite envisioned that the creation of a national health system would go through stages from urban centers down to rural villages. They seemed to ignore the fact that modern rural health programs had been carried out for some time by various groups and individuals, such as the MEM, universities, missionaries and Chinese local elite. The rural reforms proved that the process of health modernization did not have to take the top-down approach from urban to rural areas. But the medical elite stressed that health institutions ought to be first built in major municipalities such as Shanghai, Beijing, Tianjin, Nanjing, and Guangzhou, and then extend to provincial capitals and the lower administrative level of *xian* (县, the county). Basically, the health modernizers tried to construct a health structure using the existing bureaucratic administrative system. But they outlined a rural health system with *xiancheng* (县城, the county town) as the center to extend health service into rural villages.

Ideas of building urban health institutions and connecting them into a national network had been circulated, as discussed in chapter 2, among Chinese medical leaders and American and British medical officers in China before the establishment of the Nationalist government. These ideas were formally expressed in 1926 when the Association for the Advancement of Public Health in China, an organization formed by prominent Western-trained Chinese medical doctors including Liu Ruiheng and Wu Liande, sent a proposal to the British Boxer Indemnity Commission in an attempt to obtain portions of the British Boxer Indemnity funds to turn these ideas into reality.[21] Although there was no evidence that any money was obtained from the British Boxer Indemnity for public health work, the proposal showed concepts of a national health system already in circulation before the organization of the Ministry of Health in 1928. Once the medical elite gained leading positions in the Health Ministry, they lost no time in implementing their ideas. The result was the creation of a modern national health system with two major segments: one was the central health institutions, and the other was the local health institutions from provincial to county/*xian* levels. The feature of two segments reflected the political relation between the central and the local. The Nationalist government, which encouraged local self-governance (地方自治), did not have effective control over the provinces. The Health Ministry, later the NHA, delegated the work of local health construction to provincial and county governments with technical assistance and some funds. Consequently, provincial health institutions developed without a uniform standard and the health institutions built in different locales varied significantly, depending on local conditions.[22] Although county health centers, which were called hospitals, were established gradually with some health service, modern health construction in the villages basically remained on paper. (**Table 3.1 local health institutions, 1937–1947.**) This proved a contrast to the CCP rural health development, which is discussed later in this chapter.

Embracing international standards: formation of the Ministry of Health

The Ministry of Health was inaugurated in October 1928 with the promulgation of the "Organizational Laws of the Ministry of Health." The legal procedure of organizing a health ministry followed the international standard of institutionalizing a modern health agency. Xue Dubi (薛笃弼, 1890–1973), formerly Minister of Interior, was appointed Minister of Health. This appointment was Jiang Jieshi's political maneuver to balance the power of different factions within his government. During the process of organizing the Ministry of Health, Chinese medical elite of different factions—the Anglo-American, the Japanese, and the German—vied for the leading positions of health administration. Candidates for the position of health minister included prominent medical leaders of different factions such as Liu Ruiheng and Yan Fuqing (American-trained), Wu Liande (British-trained), Hu Ding-an (German-trained) and Tang Erhe (Japanese and German trained).[23] Political forces of different warlords (Yan Xishan and Feng

Table 3.1 Local medical and health institutions, 1937–1947

	1937			*1945*			*1947*		
	P	*M*	*C*	*P*	*M*	*C*	*P*	*M*	*C*
Hospitals	15	11		53	10		110	56	
Infectious disease hospitals	3	6		7			6	19	
Health field station	3	2		10	14		12	7	
Other health agencies	31	63							
Maternal hospitals							11	13	
TB hospitals							4	4	
Mental hospitals							2	2	
Leprosy hospitals							3	1	
Anti-smoking centers								3	
County health centers			162			1013			1440
District/village sub-station									353/783

Notes: P = province, M = municipal, C = county. The 1947 statistics included those of Taiwan and Taibei city.

Sources: compiled from data from Jin Baoshan, "Brief History of Health Development since the Founding of the Republic," *Zhonghua yishi zazhi* [Chinese Journal of Medical History] vol. 2, no. 1 (1948), 18–25; Jin Baoshan and Xu Shijin, "Pubic Health Facilities in the Provinces," *Zhonghua yixue zazhi* [Chinese Medical Journal], vol. 23, no. 11 (1937), 1235–1248; and Gong Chun, "Medical and Health Institutions of the Republic of China, 1912–1949," *Chinese Journal of Medical History*, vol. 19, no. 2 (1989): 80–85. See also Qian Xingzhong, *Encyclopedia of Chinese Medicine, Social Medicine and Health Administration* (Shanghai keji chubanshe, 1984).

Yuxiang, for instance) and the Nationalists also juggled for the position to award their protégés. The RF and the LNHO, with offers of technical and financial assistance, quietly worked behind the scene to make sure the leading position was to be held and sustained by professional expertise to neutralize factional in-fighting politically and professionally.

John B. Grant and his associates at PUMC made sure that persons of the best standard of expertise, meaning the American standard, were to take the leadership of the new ministry. Grant and Yan Fuqing had been in contact with the Nationalist leaders in Hankou including Mme Sun Yat-sen—Song Qinglin, sister of Mme. Jiang Jieshi—Song Meilin, for the creation of a ministry of health. The political coup of Jiang Jieshi in attacking the Communists and breaking up the United Front of the Nationalists and the Communists in 1927 to establish his own government in Nanjing, however, upset this plan. But Grant and his Chinese colleagues did not give up their pursuit of a health ministry. They seized the opportunity in Nanjing to work on Jiang's government for the cause of public health. Xue Dubi, a protégé of the warlord Feng Yuxiang and a friend of Grant and those at PUMC when he was mayor of Beijing, was awarded the position of the Minister of Interior after Feng Yuxiang pledged loyalty to Jiang. Grant and Fang Shishan presented Xue a proposal for a health ministry, but Xue thought the time was not ripe for it yet. Liu Ruiheng almost lost heart, thinking the government lacked interest in public health.[24] Never giving up, Grant and his associates approached Li Dequan, Feng Yuxiang's wife, for help with the creation of a health ministry, even providing her with a list of candidates. Li Dequan, who was active with YWCA social reform services in Beijing before her marriage to Feng in 1924, was well known among the PUMC circle. In the attempt to shape up the leadership of the new health ministry, Grant recalled that Li Dequan "asked us to draft the wire, which we did. She sent the wire to her husband, and each of the men named in the wire was appointed to the position that was indicated."[25] As Special Advisor to Chinese government on all health matters, Grant had personal access to almost all the cabinet members of the Nationalist government. At one point, when he heard the rumor that Tang Erhe was offered the position of minister of health, he asked Yan Fuqing to look into it.[26] In the end, Liu Ruiheng, the Harvard-trained physician and Director of PUMC, was appointed Vice Minister of Health, the technical and real leader of the health administration. Jin Baoshan, Liu's colleague at PUMC who was serving as Health Commissioner of Hangzhou at the time, was appointed as Liu's assistant at the Health Ministry. In August 1929, less than a year in the position of Health Minister, Xue Dubi resigned and Liu became the Minister of Health. The PUMC circle dominated the leadership of national and municipal health administrations, significantly shaping the policies and programs of a national health system. Table 3.2 shows the leadership of the Health Ministry and NHA during 1928–1949, held by people of American training and of the PUMC circle. Following Liu Ruiheng (Harvard graduate), Yan Fuqing (Yale graduate) and Jin Baoshan (Public Health at Johns Hopkins), Zhou Yichun (周贻春, a Harvard graduate and a PUMC trustee) served as Health Minister; and Zhu Zhanggen (朱章赓, a PUMC graduate with a PhD in Public Health from Yale Univeristy) served as Acting Minister before the Nationalist government retreated to Taiwan in 1949.

The Health Ministry had five departments: general affairs, medical administration, health and sanitation, epidemiology, and vital statistics. It supervised medical practice, medical education, studies and prevention of epidemic diseases, sanitary inspection, and quarantine. Two advisory boards assisted the ministry in planning and organizing a national health system. One was the Central Board of Health (中央卫生委员会), which comprised the most prominent medical doctors such as Wu Liande, Yan Fuqing, Lin Kesheng, Niu Huisheng and Hu Xuanming. They made recommendations on health policies. The other was the International Advisory Council made up of three international health leaders: Ludwik Rajchman (1881–1965) of the League of Nation's Health Organization,

Table 3.2 Heads of Ministry of Health/National Health Administration, 1928–1949

1928–1929	Ministry of Health	Xue Dubi
1929–1930	Ministry of Health	Liu Ruiheng
1931–1947	National Health Administration, Liu Ruiheng (1931–1937), Yan Fuqing (1938–1939), Jin Baoshan (1940–1947)	
1947–1949	Ministry of Health, Zhou Yichun (1947–48), Zhu Zhanggen (1948–1949)	

Victor Heiser (1873–1972) of the Rockefeller Foundation's International Health Division, and Arthur Newsholme (1857–1943) of the British Ministry of Health (he declined because of advanced age).[27] John Grant had been working with Liu Ruiheng and the Chinese medical elite to make the Health Ministry a reality. The international significance of the Nationalist construction of a modern health system was not merely shown in the existence of an international advisory council but the deep collaboration with the League of Nations and the Rockefeller Foundation. From surveys of port quarantine service in the 1920s, the League's technical assistance expanded in 1931, at the request of the Nationalist government, into broader areas of economic reconstruction such as water conservation, transportation, and agriculture.[28] Only the eruption of World War II ended this bold, ambitious, and to a great extent, successful assistance of the LNHO in China.

National Quarantine Service: initial success of collaboration with the LNHO

In 1924, Norman White of the League of Nations did a survey of health administration at Chinese port cities and wrote a critical report of the bad situation. White found the health administration so inadequate that Shanghai, the largest and supposedly the best managed port in China, had the possibility of being "classified as a third class port."[29] Grant seized the opportunity to suggest that the RF's International Health Board should use White's report as a point of action to reform health administration at Chinese ports. Due to the unequal treaties, health officers at China's treaty ports were foreigners and quarantine administration was controlled by the authorities of foreign settlements and concessions in the port cities. Problems of quarantine service were concerns of both the IHB and the League of Nations because they mattered in international prevention of epidemic diseases. Grant urged Heiser:

> to start steps leading to pressure from The League of Nations to the British and French Governments and through the latter to their legations in Peking, bringing about a situation permitting of the establishment of a Chinese Quarantine Service in place of the inadequate customs service now in force.[30]

The Chinese government and health modernizers were anxious to take back the sovereign right over customs and quarantine services through diplomatic negotiation and international cooperation. To the LNHO, competent quarantine service was vital in the gathering and exchanging of epidemiological data for preventing epidemic diseases globally. Chinese ports were of important interest and concern to the LNHO, and Chinese control over quarantine would effectively facilitate the LNHO's work. The intricate situation of foreign control and Chinese eagerness to restore their sovereignty over customs and quarantine services made the health matter quite a delicate political and diplomatic maneuver. Grant, being the representative of the IHB in China, worked to network

Chinese officials with the League's health leaders in the restoration of Chinese sovereignty over the quarantine service.

In 1925, at the invitation of Chinese government (Beiyang government), Ludwik Rajchman, Medical Director of the League of Nations Health Organization, came to visit China while on a tour in Asia. The LNHO had just opened a Far Eastern Bureau in Singapore to collect epidemiological data in the region for international prevention of epidemics. Rajchman was shocked to find no systemic quarantine service at China's port cities along its 5000 miles long coast.[31] Chinese health modernizers and government officials requested that the League take a comprehensive survey of Chinese ports. They understood that working with the League would secure China the League's technical expertise in the creation of a national quarantine service. The plan was delayed by domestic political upheavals in 1926–1927 when the coalition government of the Nationalists and the Communists in Guangzhou started the Northern Expedition against warlords to unite China. The Nationalist government continued cooperation with the League of Nations after it replaced the government in Beijing. It went further to request the League's assistance in its national health modernization. Health leaders of the Nationalist government were the same group of people who had influenced the previous government in working with the League of Nations. They invited Rajchman to join the International Advisory Council of the Health Ministry, and Rajchman came in November 1928 and made a comprehensive survey of port health and quarantine service as well as medical and sanitary institutions.[32] He stayed on for several weeks, gaining a better understanding of the Chinese situation and developing close relations with Liu Ruiheng and Song Ziwen (T. V. Soong), China's Finance Minister and brother-in-law of Jiang Jieshi. The factional fight within the Chinese medical elite made Grant and Rajchman aware that the involvement of the League might exert a neutralizing influence with emphasis on technical expertise and professional competence. In 1929, the Ministry of Health sent proposals to the LNHO, requesting specific assistance of a broad range, including the re-organization of quarantine service, the creation of a central field station as the nucleus of national health service, the establishment of a national hospital for undergraduate and graduate training, the organization of a provincial health administration as a model [Zhejiang was intended as such] for other provinces, the creation of a medical education system, and joint studies on epidemics of smallpox and cholera.[33] Most of these were suggested originally by Grant in his talks and correspondence with Liu Ruiheng.[34] The League's Health Committee approved the proposals and committed considerable professional expertise as well as financial support to assist China.

Wu Liande had led Chinese health modernizers working on restoring Chinese control of port quarantine service. They had urged the Beiyang government to negotiate with foreign powers on a series of sovereignty issues including tariff and quarantine service. The negotiations continued under the Nationalist government. In 1929 the government successfully won tariff autonomy from foreign powers and began the re-organization of the Customs Service. The diplomatic achievement over Customs Service was intertwined with the restoration of the quarantine service to Chinese authority. The LNHO experts, such as Rajchman, Frank Boudreau and C. L. Park, together with Chinese medical scientists Wu Liande, Jin Baoshan and Cai Hong (蔡鸿) conducted surveys of port conditions in 1929 and proposed the creation of a central administration of a quarantine service with local organizations at individual ports. To accomplish the task, the League created a commission, comprising "Chinese medical officers, representatives of the Office international d'Hygiene publique, and of health services of all the important maritime Powers" and League's experts, to discuss and approve a plan for the organization of a new National Quarantine Service of China.[35] With the help of the League, the Nationalist government skillfully negotiated a diplomatic victory in restoring sovereignty over the quarantine service. In July 1930, the National Quarantine Service was established with headquarters in Shanghai, and Wu Liande was appointed the director. In keeping up with international standards, the National Quarantine Service promulgated new quarantine regulations based on the1926 International Sanitary Convention. The National Quarantine Service maintained close relations with the League's Far Eastern Bureau in Singapore as well as offices in Europe. Chinese health officers updated their technical expertise by taking study tours to Europe and North America. The Shanghai headquarters was equipped with laboratories and hospitals. Quarantine administration gradually extended to all the coastal ports north from Dandong and south to Guangzhou as well as all the river ports of international concerns. The National Quarantine Service collected statistics on epidemics and communicated the information to the LNHO while it carried out sanitary control, detection, and inspection of epidemics of international traffic of ships, animals and humans in China. Most European countries accepted Chinese authority and the health certificates issued by the National Quarantine Service. Interestingly, the United States government discouraged and actively opposed Chinese management of the quarantine service. As late as 1934, American ships still refused to accept the authority of the Chinese quarantine officers.[36]

The National Quarantine Service played an active role in domestic public health activities as well. Wu Liande and his colleagues regularly gave public lectures on infectious diseases and methods of prevention. Collaborating with municipal and local authorities, the Service launched public health campaigns and vaccinations against cholera and smallpox. When a cholera epidemic broke out in 1930–1932, the Service carried out vigorous campaigns, providing hundreds of thousands of free vaccinations. It acted as the Central Cholera Bureau in 1932 to coordinate anti-cholera campaigns in coastal cities. Vaccinations and inspection of water supplies kept cholera under control. From 1930 to 1934, "over four million inoculations against cholera were carried out with vaccines prepared in the Shanghai municipal laboratories."[37] Moreover, the Service conducted studies of plague in eastern port cities and took measures of prevention.[38]

Education of the masses about epidemic diseases such as cholera and plague were of deep concern among health modernizers. The 1930s cholera epidemic prompted Wu Liande and his colleagues to publish a handbook on fighting the disease, which devoted an entire section, titled "Education and Propaganda," to anti-cholera health education campaigns.[39] They believed: "Public health progress in China is in the main dependent upon the awakening of sanitary consciousness among the masses." When laws were enacted before people were mentally, politically, and economically prepared for them, they "were just *paper tigers* (纸老虎), incapable of producing more than a ripple in the tide of the nation's destiny."

> It is only through systematic early training and education and the application of intensive scientific methods of propaganda that our law-makers and our public health workers can count on the intelligent participation of the common man, without which their labours would be but a delusion and a snare.[40]

These remarks echoed the sentiment of many public health advocates at the time. Jin Baoshan, for instance, criticized that China in the past often blindly copied methods from other countries without knowing whether they fit the socioeconomic conditions within China. He recommended not using health laws to coerce people in health matters but to educate people without limiting their freedom. "If the people believe the good of health, they will follow without the coercion of laws."[41] Health modernizers emphasized a comprehensive program in dealing with public health problems, namely, educating people about public health, training health professionals of technicians, managers and law enforcement, establishing health stations, enacting laws suitable for Chinese situation, and developing a complete public health system.

Building the national health system with international assistance: the central institutions

The Health Ministry issued the "Guideline for the National Health Administration System" (全国卫生行政系统大纲) in December 1928 as the blueprint for a centralized system of national health administration. According to the guideline, each province was to establish a health department and each municipality a health bureau. The government put lots of effort and resources into Zhejiang province, designated to develop a model health administration for other provinces to emulate. Central medical and research institutions were to be built under the jurisdiction of the Health Ministry to train technical personnel in medical research, disease prevention, health administration, midwifery, and health education. The trained personnel were to staff the institutions of a centralized system of national health. In 1929, the Central Hygienic Laboratory (中央卫生试验所) was established in Shanghai for chemical and pharmaceutical research and analysis; the Central Epidemic Prevention Bureau in Beijing was moved to Nanjing and placed directly under the Health Ministry; and the National Midwifery Board was formed to promote modern midwifery training with the creation of the First National Midwifery School in Beijing and the Central Midwifery School in Nanjing.

To the Health Ministry officials, the most immediate tasks:

> were to organize training facilities for health officers, midwives, nurses, sanitary inspectors and the other health staff of which China stood in such urgent need, and to work out a national health programme which meant an intensive study of the problems to be solved and of the methods to apply.[42]

China had only a handful of modern-trained medical and health professionals. Few of them had the experience of preparing and organizing a national health system. The LNHO's assistance and the medical enterprise of the RF in China filled the gap by providing technical and financial support. Training technical personnel became a priority in China's collaboration with the League. The Health Ministry proposed to the LNHO in 1929 establishing a Central Field Health Station (CFHS, 中央卫生实验处) in Nanjing as the center of national medical and public health research and training. A central hospital was to be established for the CFHS for undergraduate instruction and postgraduate training. Nine Chinese medical officers of the Ministry of Health and three foreign experts formed the original group working on the organization of the CFHS under the direction of Jin Baoshan. The foreign experts were Dr. Berislav Borčić (1891–1977), Dr. Brian R. Dyer, and Dr. W. W. Peter (1882–1959). Berislav Borčić was the Director of Zagreb Health Institute of Yugoslavia and a specialist in medicine and veterinary studies. He was sent to China by the LNHO to specifically assist the organization of the Central Field Health Station. Brian R. Dyer was a specialist in sanitary engineering of the Rockefeller Foundation. W. W. Peter, who had led the popular health campaigns in China in the 1910s, was now of the Cleanliness Institute in New York.[43] Borčić and Dyer stayed in China and worked with the CFHS till the outbreak of World War II, whereas Peter returned to the US shortly afterwards. Borčić came to Nanjing in May 1930 with the plan to stay for two years, but he was so much needed and appreciated by the Chinese government that he ended up working in China for nine years till 1938 when Japanese invasion disrupted the functions of CFHS and forced it to move to the southwest with the Nationalist government. As an employee of the Rockefeller Foundation, Dyer worked with CFHS and later the North China Program of the RF till Japanese invasion derailed the program and his service in China.

Rajchman and Borčić provided an organizational chart of the CFHS based on the experience of Yugoslavia and other European countries, but they insisted that the Chinese should take charge of the CFHS with financial commitment when it was obvious that the RF intended to shape the station's development with financial support. In a meeting with Rajchman, Roger Greene mentioned the RF's intention to provide both financial support for the organization of the station and the technical training of Chinese personnel of public health abroad. Rajchman accepted the offer of technical training of personnel but resisted the financial contribution of the RF, despite Greene's argument that "the accomplishment of the project" might be delayed without RF's financial support.[44] The RF representatives in China had PUMC in mind as the model for the CFHS, while the League's experts had little interest in building another PUMC. Rajchman and Borčić were deeply interested in helping China create an institution that would adequately address the general public health needs, not an elite medical research institution like PUMC. Their negotiations with the RF over the organization and operation of the CFHS demonstrated different approaches to the solutions of national health needs, with the League promoting state medicine and the RF elite medical research.

The LNHO and the RF had been in cooperation and collaboration on many fronts of international health affairs.[45] The RF provided the LNHO with considerable financial funds and worked with the LNHO on a wide range of health projects. Their close collaboration led Martin Dublin to claim that the "LNHO and the RF enjoyed a symbiotic relationship in which the former acted in important respects as a surrogate for the latter."[46] The China case demonstrated that the LNHO's relation with the RF was not a symbiotic but negotiated collaboration. Rajchman and the League's professionals resisted the RF's attempt to set the agenda and impose standards on the LNHO's work with the Chinese government. Both the League and the RF wielded influence on China's development. Rajchman worried about possible open conflict with the RF. He suggested that the RF concentrate on the work of PUMC and efforts in North China while the League concentrate on the government's health construction.[47] Chinese officials and health modernizers understood the limits of the PUMC model in serving the health needs of the people and the challenge of delivering state medicine when they sought to work out a feasible system of modern health administration in China.

The Central Field Health Station began operation in 1931 with Jin Baoshan as the director.[48] It had nine departments: Bacteriology and Epidemic Disease Control, Chemistry and Pharmacology, Parasitology, Sanitary Engineering, Medical Relief and Social Medicine, Maternal and Child Health, Industrial Health, Epidemiology and Vital Statistics, and Health Education and School Health. The CFHS engaged in the investigation and research of the treatment of epidemic diseases such as malaria, schistosomiasis, kala-azar and plague but also helped create health laboratories at municipal and provincial levels. It conducted a wide range of public health projects, such as sanitary engineering in cities, collecting vital statistics, training maternal and child hygiene specialists, and promoting health education, school health and nutrition studies.[49] The ambitious work of CFHS was made possible by several newly created institutions, including the Central Hospital, the Central Hygienic Laboratory, the Central Midwifery School and the Central School of Nursing. Undergraduate and graduate courses were taught through partnership with these new institutions. Its graduates became key medical, hygienic, maternal and child health specialists occupying leading positions at municipal and provincial health institutions that were being developed. The CFHS, working with the Central Hospital in Nanjing, used internships to train doctors and nurses for public hospitals that were being built in major cities. Important to the development of a national structure of medical research and health administration, CFHS established 35 local laboratories and branch stations in the capitals of eight provinces by 1934.[50] The newly created central and local institutions together with the National Quarantine Service were the first concrete steps of national health construction.

In the meantime, Chinese professionals were being sent abroad for advanced training in special areas of health administration and disease control. Both the League of Nations and the Rockefeller Foundation provided fellowships for Chinese health specialists to have advanced training in Europe and the United States. By 1935, the LNHO had granted 28 members of the CFHS and its affiliated institutions fellowships to study for three to six months in Europe on subjects of public health organization, fumigation of ships, organization of quarantine stations, malariology and parasitology, maternal and child welfare, industrial hygiene, and hospital administration. The RF had provided 32 members with fellowships for training in the United States on topics of bacteriology, entomology, hospital administration, public health, and midwifery. [51] The League also sent experts to China to help with specific projects on short and long visits. Dr. Andrija Stampar (1888–1958), the health expert of social medicine from Yugoslavia and a colleague of Borčić, was sent to China in 1933 by the League to help develop a rural health service. He traveled across China investigating the socioeconomic and health conditions before making recommendations to the Nationalist government. He worked in China till 1936 and published his studies with critical assessment of the Nationalist rule not only in reports to the League but also in academic periodicals.[52]

The Central Field Health Station was the technical nerve center of China's health modernization construction. Its work constituted an important component of the League's broader assistance to China's modern reconstruction that was being directed by the National Economic Council (全国经济委员会) personally chaired by Jiang Jieshi. The League's assistance furthered China's integration in the international community. Major international health figures, such as Berislav Borčić, Andrija Stampar and Ludwick Rajchman, spent years working in China, and their contributions left the imprints of state medicine on China's modern health system. China, in turn, offered the LNHO a unique opportunity to practice the visions of a modern health service. The LNHO leaders had adopted a comprehensive scope of health that integrated medical, political and social responsibilities. Iris Borowy called these three corner-stones of the LNHO's operating principles.[53] The China project was one of the most ambitious international engagements of the League, "a once-in-a life opportunity for the LNHO" to put into reality the interlocking ideas of health.[54] The LNHO leaders aspired to have a system of international standards adopted by individual countries. They believed that the LNHO had the responsibility to supply, upon the request from any country, a blueprint for a national health system and the practical support to build it in the endeavor of developing international health, which would contribute to world peace and justice. The work of the CFHS bore significant input from the LNHO. The CFHS suffered when the Japanese invasion forced it to retreat with the government to western China in 1937.

By the time of the Japanese invasion in 1937, the National Health Administration had established the Northwest Epidemic Prevention Bureau and the Mongolia Suiyuan Epidemic Prevention Bureau.[55] Branches of the Central Hospital were built in Guiyang, Lanzhou, Guangzhou, and Tianjin as centers of clinical research and training for advanced medical personnel. Before the outbreak of the war, there were 52 health institutions of various types established at the provincial level and 82 at the municipal level, totaling 134 health institutions. By 1947, the peak time of health construction of the Nationalist government, the growth of health institutions was seen across local levels, with 148 provincial health institutions, 105 municipal health institutions, and 1440 county health centers, even though many county centers had limited functions.[56] (See Table 3.1.)

Constructing local health institutions: the xian*-centered rural health*

Nationalist health modernizers fully understood the difficulty in building rural health due to the large population (88 percent of national population) and poor socioeconomic conditions. Nonetheless, at the 1932 NHA meeting on rural health work, Jin Baoshan reiterated the government plan of using *xian* (县, county) as the center to create a health administration system in rural China. Jin Baoshan cited two reasons for the need to pay attention to rural health: (1) devastating effect of epidemic and endemic diseases on rural population and farming, and (2) winning rural support for the government.[57] In 1931–1932, floods and Japanese military attacks on China caused epidemic crises in large parts of China. The government was frustrated at not being able to provide medical relief to the disaster areas because of the absence of health administration. Responding to the dire situation, the Nationalist cabinet approved, in December 1932, the proposal that each county, according to local circumstances, should establish a health administration agency as the center of health affairs and medical relief.[58] The proposal was presented with political persuasion that the medical service would help win the hearts of the people for the Nationalist government in competition with the Chinese Communist movement. The Nationalist rural health plan basically mapped a system upon the existing administrative structure with *xiancheng*, the county town, as the center to extend health administration into villages. Nationalist leaders expected that the *xian*-centered rural health system would be able to perform simple health work such as epidemic prevention, basic medical service, midwifery, health education and anti-opium smoking.[59]

Rural health received serious attention of studies at the time, with proposals from various organizations.[60] The National Medical Association of China formed a Rural Health Survey Committee in October 1932 and appointed Li Ting-an as chairman of the committee to investigate rural health work. The task was to find out the number of rural health institutions, their organization and work so as to inform national rural health construction. With the assistance of Yao Xunyuan, Li gathered data of 17 rural health stations and districts in 6 provinces and two municipalities. They were Qinghe Health Demonstration Area of Wanping County of Hebei, Dingxian Village Health of Hebei, Xishan Village Health of Beiping, Longshan Demonstration Area of Shangdong, Wujiang Peasant Hospital of Hexian County of Anhui, Xiaoxian County Hospital of

Jiangsu, Yancheng County Hospital of Jiangsu, Taixian County Hospital of Jiangsu, Jurongxian County Hospital of Jiangsu, Tangshan Health Station of Jiangning County of Jiangsu, Jiangning Town Health Station of Jiangningxian of Jiangsu, Wusong Health Station of Shanghai, Gaoqiao Health Station of Shanghai, Jiangwan Health Station of Shanghai, Wuxingxian County Hospital of Zhejiang, Wukangxian County Hospital of Zhejinag, and Guangzhou Family Health Promotion Association of Guangdong.[61] Out of the 17 stations and centers, only one, the Tangshan Health Station in Jiangsu, was administered by the central government, i.e. the National Health Administration; two by city government; and the rest by a combination of local government, universities and private organizations and individuals. The health stations were established to conduct preventive medicine, dissemination of health information, school hygiene, midwifery and maternal and child healthcare, industrial health, collection of vital statistics, training of health workers, and anti-opium smoking. The actual work of each station, however, varied a great deal, as well as the staff and facilities. All the stations had been established in economically favorable locations; and except for Dingxian and Tangshan stations, they were confined mostly to curative medicine—the only thing locals showed some interest in.

Li's rural health survey provided an overview of the methods and programs of rural health development for the National Health Administration when it drafted a "Plan for County Health Administration" (县卫生行政方案) based on the 1932 cabinet-approved proposal. The NHA promulgated the plan in 1934, whereby each county was to establish a health center hospital (卫生院), each rural district a health station, and each village town a sub-station and each village a health worker. The *xian* health center was to be staffed with doctors, nurses, midwives and assistants. The NHA named the *xian* health center "county hospital" (县立医院) mainly for the convenience of popularizing this new term of modern institution to rural people. The organizational structure of a three-tiered rural health administration from *county* (*xian*, 县) center to rural *district* (*qu*, 区) to individual *village* (*xiang*, 乡) clearly indicated the influence of the operational formula of Dingxian and Tangshan model. The NHA considered making health facilities available to the populace a necessary step in the implementation of state medicine.[62] Therefore, it was important to create the *xian*-centered rural health system. To facilitate the organization of rural health, the NHA issued the "Guideline for the Implementation of County Health Administration" (县卫生行政实施办法纲要) in March 1937, just a few months before the Japanese invasion disrupted the whole program. The NHA delegated the task of establishing *xian* (county) hospitals to provincial government, with the promise of technical assistance. County administration, hence, relied on the direction and support of provincial health institutions in the creation of county hospital. Consequently, rural health construction developed sporadically and unevenly across the country. Most of the county hospitals and rural health centers were short of staff and equipment, as modern-trained doctors were scarce and unwilling to work in rural towns.

Institutionally, there was a lack of uniformity for the newly established health administration at both provincial and county levels. Across the different provinces, the name of the county hospital varied in as many as eight different types.[63] Some were called hospitals, and others health centers or stations. The confusion had much to do with the chaotic development of provincial health institutions that helped organize county hospitals/centers. Provinces developed their health administration within their bureaucratic structure with local characteristics. The name of provincial health departments differed from one to the other, some calling it *weisheng chu* (卫生处, health department), others *weisheng shiyan chu* (卫生实验处, health demonstration station), or *weisheng yuan* (卫生院, health institute/hospital).[64] In an effort to standardize provincial health institutions, the National Health Administration issued the "Organizational Guideline for Provincial Health Department" (省卫生处组织大纲) in 1940, which made it clear that provincial hospitals, health field stations, junior-level health training centers, and factories of health materials should be established under the health department of each province. The guideline, which intended to bring uniformity to provincial health administration across the nation, imitated the organizational structure of the NHA and its affiliated institutions.

Nine provinces (Jiangxi, Hunan, Gansu, Qinghai, Ningxia, Shanxi, Zhejiang, Yunan, and Aihui) had set up a provincial health department by 1937. The number of health administrators and technical persons of each province was relatively small—on average fewer than 10 administrators and 20 technical staff. Jiangxi province was an exception, which claimed to have 52 health administrators and 53 technical persons.[65] Jiangxi was unusual because the Nationalist government put lots of resources and energy in the province with military and political campaigns against the Chinese Communists who had created several rural soviet bases there with more than 10 million people. In the attempt to drive out the Communists and win the support of local people, the Nationalists started mass mobilization campaigns to revive Jiangxi with broad reform programs of literacy, public health, and agricultural improvement. Jiang Jieshi flew to Nanchang, the capital of Jiangxi, in February 1934 to provide an ideological guidance for the New Life Movement. Personal hygiene was a prominent element of Jiang's ideological instruction for a new life that was promoted as the pathway for modern China. In Jiangxi, there was great fanfare about rural reforms through the New Life Movement. The government conducted campaigns mainly by relying on Christian organizations and semi-governmental organizations, such as the YMCA, the service corps (*fuwutuan*, 服务团), clubs, civic associations and societies, and schools.[66] The fundamental need of tackling poverty, however, was conspicuously left out in the New Life Movement. To get things started, the central government provided Jiangxi local governments the entire operational budget of the programs in 1934. The propaganda campaigns of rural reforms were well coordinated with the GMD's military campaigns against the Communists. Jiangxi rural health stations were built along GMD's military routes against the Communists. The Nationalist army handed out free medicine and smallpox vaccines to local people in the campaigns against the Communists.[67] In the end when the CCP was driven out of Jiangxi, the GMD's reform programs of rural education, health, cooperatives, and social services largely stayed in cities and county centers, barely reaching the lives of villagers.

Just before the Japanese invasion in 1937, a total of 162 county health centers or hospitals were established in several provinces, including 35 in Jiangsu, 14 in Zhejiang, 83 in Jiangxi, 2 in Shandong, 1 in Hebei, 9 in Shanxi (陕西), and 18 in Fujian, in addition to 12 health districts in Guangxi.[68] The services of county health centers, rural district health stations and village town health substations were clearly defined in the Nationalist plan of rural health construction. Specifically, the county health center was to have the functions of a clinic and hospital, maternal and child care, laboratory, drug and supplies, health education and health administration; and the rural district health station a clinic, preventive medicine, sanitation, school health and health education.[69] In reality, few performed these responsibilities. Some of the health centers/hospitals conducted preventive service of vaccination and medical reliefs while others did little because they were simply converted from anti-opium smoking offices with few personnel and facilities. Nationalist health leaders were aware that most of the county health centers were poorly equipped and ineffective. Jin Baoshan admitted that few had adequate facilities and personnel. The few counties that had functioning health centers and health stations in rural districts were those operated by private groups, such as the stations in Jiangning, Dingxian, Zouping, and Lanxu.[70]

Andrija Stampar of the League observed the attitude and working style of the medical staff at local level, which defined the success and failure of the county (*xian*) health centers. Stampar contrasted two health centers with similar financial support and facilities to illustrate the problems of *xian* health centers. One *xian* health center concentrated its work in *xiancheng*, the county town, without paying attention to farmers in adjacent rural villages. The service was almost entirely curative and for commercial purposes, where preventive measures of public health were totally neglected. In the course of one entire year, the nurses attended only 20 deliveries, all for the families of merchants and officials, not one for farmers. The center was designed as a free service facility with financial support from the provincial government, but it charged fees and drove away many needed patients who could not pay. As a result, it accumulated a considerable budget surplus. The other *xian* health center studied the health and social conditions in adjacent villages, conducted vigorous health propaganda and education among farmers, and followed the example of Dingxian by training selected villagers as assistants to work with the health program. The midwife, instead of waiting for patients to come to her, went to visit pregnant women in their rural homes. Her distribution of sterilized navel dressings considerably reduced infant mortality from tetanus. Vaccination and preventive measures led to a decrease in the death rate among farmers. Lessons learned: the first county center failed because it paid too much attention to *xian* city and too little to farmers in villages; whereas the second succeeded because it directed its work towards farmers with the greater part of its service free.[71]

The Nationalist government made little effort to tackle poverty problems in the old land and tenancy system. The League experts made specific recommendations on land reform to reduce poverty and ameliorate rural conditions, but their ideas were ignored. During his three years of visiting and observing different Chinese rural regions, Stampar witnessed the terrible social conditions and the landlord system in rural villages. The Council on Rural health Reform concluded after studying the tenancy system and rural taxation: "The abuses of the tenancy system have been . . . the main cause of the present social unrest in China . . . the landlord system is one of the chief obstacles to the technical improvement of agriculture."[72] In Stampar's view, health was integral to the general improvement of social and economic conditions. "Successful health work is not possible where the standard of living falls below the level of tolerable existence. Public health policy must be intimately connected with a programme for general social improvement."[73] The League's recommendation on land and tenancy reforms, however, proved too radical for the Nationalist leaders, who took no action of land reform for rural improvement. Instead, taxes and levies of various kinds increased continuously when the government squeezed the peasantry for revenues, labor, and conscription.

Shortage of medical personnel and proposed medical education reform

The shortage of medical personnel was a main challenge to building modern health in China. Wu Liande pointed out that the current medical service was not available to the majority of people even in big cities like Nanjing where one third of the population received no medical treatment at all. Even in the most developed rural districts "old-style practitioners still attend over 65 percent of all patients, while about 26 percent die without receiving any treatment at all."[74] Nationwide, doctors of Western medicine were of a small number who were concentrated in large cities of Shanghai and Nanjing.[75] Situations were much worse in the rural villages where doctors and healers of any type were scarce and poverty was prevalent. Old-style physicians of Chinese medicine also preferred to practice in cities and county towns (*xiancheng*) rather than in villages. Financially, it was impossible for rural towns to support modern doctors of private practice. Wu Liande calculated that it would take 10,000 people to support a physician in the minimum manner according to the 12 cents contribution per capita for the annual income of $600 and basic equipment costs of $400 of a physician.[76] The poor socioeconomic conditions of China made modern medical service inaccessible to the majority of people unless the state took over the financial responsibility and trained more medical professionals.

To produce more medical personnel with faster speed, medical education had to be reformed in terms of training time and curriculum. The Ministry of Education and the National Health Administration formed the Commission on Medical Education to tackle the problem. The Commission, with financial support from the RF, carried out studies and issued a report in 1935 that outlined a new approach to the training of medical personnel in response to the needs of China.[77] The key recommendation was a shift from research-oriented elite education to the training of a quantity of medical professionals. Since the early 1930s, different proposals on medical education reform had been presented to the government. One proposal recommended a two-tiered approach that would continue the training of "fully qualified physicians for central institutions" while setting up "subsidiary schools of lower standard to train a kind of second-class doctors for service in rural districts."[78] The two-tiered proposal, which gained favorable reception among policy-makers of the Nationalist government, was supported by the recommendation of Knud Faber of the University of Copenhagen, a League expert who came to China in 1930 to investigate the state of medical education and assist Chinese policy-makers on the reform.[79] The other proposal, which was presented by Robert Lim and C. C. Chen, aimed to combine a senior middle school science curriculum with college courses to reduce the cost and time of medical training at medical colleges. They recommended a broad education in natural science at middle schools so as to reduce the length of medical science courses at colleges. Stampar, who came to China in 1933, did not think the two-tiered approach plausible because it would create new problems associated with hierarchical classes of doctors. He favored Lim and Chen's proposal, considering it worth serious consideration. The Ministry of Education eventually decided to adopt Lim and Chen's proposal and contemplated testing a pilot curriculum at selected middle schools in 1936.[80] But Japan's invasion of China derailed the plan.

Reforms also aimed at midwifery and nursing schools. Dozens of midwifery schools and over one hundred nursing schools—most of them were affiliated with missionary hospitals and clinics—were in operation when the Nationalist government was established.[81] The quality of nurse training varied significantly and the curriculum lacked uniformity and quality control, which posed a challenge to health modernization. Yang Chongrui, who had worked with John Grant in the modernization of midwifery training in Beijing in the late 1920s, was now appointed to chair the National Board of Maternal and Child Health. She worked hard to create a new profession of midwifery, separate from the nursing profession, by promoting midwifery schools across China. The First National Midwifery School in Beijing and the Central Midwifery School in Nanjing produced leading modern midwives who filled responsible positions in urban hospitals and the teaching positions at midwifery schools in major cities of the provinces. They were the face of new women—modern, educated, confident, and chic in fashion—in the Nationalist construction of modern health.[82] The vast majority of Chinese women, however, did not have access to the service of modern midwifery, nor did they trust, in delivering babies, those young modern professionals who had no personal experience in childbirth. Professionally, Yang's insistence on separating midwifery from nursing profession, and giving it a higher standard of training, met resistance from the Nurses' Association of China over the control of childbirth. The League's experts did not favor the separation, either. The common understanding was "a good midwife needs a good general education in nursing, as a good nurse should be capable of practicing midwifery."[83] Yang's advocacy for a new midwife profession led some medical leaders to question the wisdom of separating midwifery from nursing because specialization meant more training time and costs, which China could not afford. Suggestions were made to examine the value of separating midwifery and nursing schools. But the war disrupted this effort as well.

The famous Peking Union Medical College was also contemplating reorganizing itself to better serve the needs of China. The PUMC had focused on research and the elite medical education of a small number of students, without maximizing its utility for the needs of Chinese population. In the spirit of educational reform, PUMC—the best equipped medical college with world-class medical education and research—was considered an ideal place to train future teachers for Chinese medical schools without giving up its high standard of research. Public health training was to be expanded with increased staff, training time, and courses in the curriculum. The Chinese language was to be used broadly in the training.[84] The change of language from English to Chinese had profound implications that the education now was to be for the Chinese and by the Chinese.

The re-organization of the PUMC's work constituted a re-orientation of the RF's enterprise in China. A new generation of leadership emerged in the Rockefeller Foundation after its re-organization in late 1920s. They were eager to generate better social returns of the foundation's financial and human investments. Selskar Gunn, Vice President of the RF, came to visit China in early 1930s. He was deeply impressed with the Dingxian rural health programs and felt that a shift to rural development was urgently needed for the RF's policy in China. With John Grant and Ludwik Rajchman as his close associates in China, Gunn submitted to the RF a 61-page proposal, outlining a rural development program that integrated public health in the general improvement of agriculture and education of rural communities. The RF board approved the proposal and the China Program of rural development was officially launched in July 1935.[85] The China Program recruited major Chinese universities to train rural development specialists: agriculture at the University of Nanjing, sanitary engineering at Qinghua University, economics at Nankai University, social administration at Yanjing University, and public health and social medicine at PUMC. Dingxian became the training ground for public health fieldwork. As of February 1937, the China Program had made 429 fellowships for professional training within China, including 103 in public health, 62 in nursing, 56 in public health nursing, 54 in agriculture, 44 in education, 35 in social science, 21 in rural economy and sociology, 14 in midwifery, 12 in sanitary engineering, 12 in maternal and child welfare, 10 for technicians, and 6 in natural sciences. Additionally, the China Program made 177 fellowships to the Nanjing Public Health and Medicine Program run by the Commission of Medical Education for training in public health, nursing, midwifery and sanitation inspection.[86] The RF's China Program collaborated with the National Health Administration and the Ministry of Education to influence medical education reform and rural health construction.

Grant and Gunn wanted to coordinate the different groups of Rural Reform and Mass Education Movement and the reformers at Chinese universities into one united force under the China Program to train a corps of professionals to tackle the problems of rural China. However, the collaboration of different institutions and leaders of rural reform movement turned out to be quite challenging. It was not the local and national politics that got into the way but the institutional walls and individuals' egos. To better coordinate projects and different players, the China Program established a North China Council for Rural Reconstruction in 1936 with Grant, the only Westerner on the Council, in charge of cooperation.[87] Sadly, the China Program, like other GMD reform programs, was disrupted and derailed by the Japanese invasion in July 1937. In the war years, the China Program lingered on, managing to develop a few rural programs in inland and southwest China where the Nationalists were in control, but these small local programs exerted little meaningful influence on national rural reconstruction.

Exclusion of Chinese medicine from health construction

Doctors of Chinese medicine and healers of all types of indigenous medicine were excluded from the Nationalist construction of a modern health system. The Western-trained medical elite were eager to replicate what the West had. They considered Chinese medicine, commonly referred to as old-style medicine, an obstacle to health modernization. Since the turn of the twentieth century, Chinese medicine as a system of knowledge and practice was increasingly dismissed as a useless superstition by modernizers. The health modernizers of the Nationalist government continued this bias with intensified attack on Chinese medicine. However, Chinese herbal drugs (*materia medica*), due to their effectiveness in treating illnesses, could not have their valuable qualities flatly denied. Therefore, the modern medical elite took a more receptive approach to Chinese herbal medicine. Scientific research on herbal medicine also substantiated the value of Chinese medicine. Medical scientists conducted research on the pharmaceutical nature of the Chinese herb *mahuang* at PUMC in the 1920s. Their scientific discovery that ephedrine from *mahuang* could effectively treat asthma made world news in the medical field.[88]

The scientifically proved quality of herbal medicine, however, did not change the attitude of modern medical elite toward Chinese medicine. Officials of the RF and the LNHO held similar attitude toward Chinese medicine. They played an encouraging role in denying Chinese medicine the opportunity to contribute to national health modernization. The RF, in introducing medical science to change China, advocated Western scientific medicine, furthering the divide of Western and Chinese medicines. The PUMC, however, offered old-style midwives short-training courses in hygienic knowledge of midwifery in the effort to reform old-style midwifery. When it was suggested that doctors of Chinese medicine be trained in basic scientific practices, the League's expert Knud Faber dismissed such training as doing "more harm than good" because it would be taken as "an official authorization of native doctors."[89] The RF and the LNHO worked with the Nationalist government to exclude Chinese medicine from China's health modernization process.

In February 23–25, 1929, the Ministry of Health held a Health Administration Conference, at which "heads of municipal health bureaus were expected to report their work and offer proposals to formulate a national plan of health administration."[90] More than 50 Chinese medical leaders attended the conference presided by Liu Ruiheng, Minister of Health. They offered a wide range of proposals, including those on eliminating Chinese medicine. Yu Yunxiu (余云岫, also Yu Yan, 余岩, 1879–1954), head of the Shanghai branch of the Pharmaceutical Association of China, submitted a proposal titled "Abolition of Old Medicine to Remove the Obstacle of Medical Health" (废止旧医以扫除医事卫生之障碍案).[91] Hu Ding-An (胡定安, also Hu Ping, 胡平), head of Nanjing Health Bureau, presented eight proposals, including the ban on dissemination of unscientific medical information, which targeted Chinese medicine.[92] The National Board of Health combined those different proposals into one proposition and approved it under the heading "Abolition of Old Medicine to Remove the Obstacle of Medical Health." According to the proposition, Chinese medicine would be eliminated in six steps: (1) registering old medical doctors within a certain time limit, (2) training old medical doctors in Western medicine, (3) setting a timetable to limit the use of an old medical doctor's license, (4) banning information on old medicine in newspapers and magazines, (5) prohibiting the dissemination of unscientific medicine, and (6) prohibiting the establishment of schools of old medicine.[93]

The Health Ministry's attempt to abolish Chinese medicine led to all-out opposition by practitioners of Chinese medicine across the country. They held a national meeting of Chinese medical and pharmaceutical delegations in Shanghai on March 17, 1929, and rallied popular support with the slogan that Chinese medicine was national medicine (国医). They empowered the protest with the statement that Chinese medicine was the essence of Chinese culture concerned with the health of every individual and that Western medicine was part of foreign imperialist invasion. They called for the "promotion of Chinese medicine to guard against cultural invasion" and "promotion of Chinese drugs to guard against economic invasion."[94] These statements and slogans demonstrated that practitioners of Chinese medicine had become politically savvy in the struggle against the state-sponsored hegemony of Western medicine and the oppression of Chinese medicine. They organized a National Federation of Medical and Pharmaceutical Associations (全国医药团体总联合会), whereby the National Medicine Movement was born. March 17 was designated National Medicine Day and was celebrated in China and overseas Chinese communities until the People's Republic of China was established and Chinese medicine was promoted by state health policy. Supporters of Chinese medicine across Asia and North America lent their voices to the National Medicine Movement. Practitioners of Chinese medicine became united as never before in face of the government attempt of abolition. More than 130 groups formed a petition delegation to put pressure on the Nationalist government. Imagine the political implication for the Nationalist Party to abolish national medicine! Faced with widespread protests and petitions at various government departments, the Nationalist government sensed the medical dispute was spinning into a political crisis. Jiang Jieshi became personally involved by ordering the repeal of the abolition resolution to calm down the situation. The government subsequently forced the National Federation of Chinese Medical and Pharmaceutical Associations to break up but permitted the establishment of the Institute of National Medicine with branches in local places. The compromise of the government in recognizing Chinese medicine as National Medicine resulted in the formation of a Commission on Chinese Medical Studies.

The victory of Chinese medical practitioners in the fight for Chinese medicine did not mean that Chinese medicine had gained an equal footing with Western medicine. The Nationalist government continued to discriminate against Chinese medicine.[95] Schools of Chinese medicine, which had been established by Chinese medical specialists and intellectuals in resistance to the hegemony of Western medicine, were not allowed to be part of the national education system under the Nationalist government.[96] These schools were regarded as offering medical apprenticeships, not a real education. Moreover, Chinese medical practitioners were banned from using modern devices such as stethoscopes and syringes. The Legislative Yuan of the Nationalist government approved the "Regulations of Chinese Medicine" in 1933 but did not promulgate it until 1936 after the NHA and the Ministry of Education formed the Commission on Chinese Medical Studies. Within the Nationalist government were different views of Chinese medicine. While the NHA bureaucrats were all trained in Western medicine and had deep bias against Chinese medicine, some Nationalist political leaders like Chen Guofu (陈果夫, 1892–1951) and Chen Lifu (陈立夫, 1900–2001) supported Chinese medicine.[97] The Nationalist Party was divided on the issue, with supporters of Chinese medicine mostly found in the party higher echelons and the Legislative Yuan, whereas supporters of Western medicine were found in the Executive Yuan, particularly in the ministries of health and education.[98] Zhang Zanchen (张赞臣, 1904–1993), a renowned physician of Chinese medicine, pointed out that the main reason the National Health Board decided to abolish Chinese medicine was because:

> the old-style medicine does not understand germ theory to treat the legally notifiable contagious diseases (法定传染病) and therefore it becomes an obstacle of disinfection and prevention, which is the first task of health administration. A look at the reality of disinfection and prevention reveals nothing but propaganda hyperbole of the government.[99]

Biomedicine, in short, dominated the NHA's health modernization policy at the expense of Chinese medicine.

Popular health movement: propaganda and education

Institutional construction of a modern health system was accompanied by a national health movement to educate people on the importance of health to national revival and people's livelihood. The government and educational and social organizations produced materials of health propaganda and education.[100] The Propaganda Department of the GMD Central Executive Committee published a booklet, titled "Guideline for the Propaganda of Health Movement" [卫生运动宣传纲要], which explained in plain colloquial language:

> National competition for existence . . . has entered the most urgent moment. There are six key elements of competition: physique, intelligence, bravery, vigilance, tenacity, and unity. . . . The label of "sick man of East Asia" indicates to us that you are physically weak, deficient in knowledge, lacking bravery, having little will to improve, having no tenacity, not solid in unity, and having no ability to compete but be bullied and dismembered.

It concluded: "If you are physically strong, then you will be mentally healthy; if you are mentally healthy, then you will have a strong will; if you have a strong will, then you will be united as a nation."[101] The guideline had three chapters and specific slogans for health campaigns. The first chapter defined the meanings of health movement in relation to national revival and people's livelihood, using Sun-Yat-sen's Three People's Principles as the guidance.[102] Chapter 2, titled "Common Knowledge for Health Movement," defined diseases (疾病) and pests (害虫) as the enemies of health movement, and provided information on personal hygiene and public health. Chapter 3 was about the endeavor of the health movement, such as what facilities the government should have and to what people should pay attention. The slogans in the booklet emphasized that health movement would increase population, strengthen the body, prolong life, uplift people, promote unity, relieve national sufferings, and create happiness of life. It promoted the health movement as the movement to improve conditions of national independence, the movement of national salvation, and the movement of liberation. Therefore, the health movement must be popularized among the masses and conducted scientifically.[103]

Health movements were carried out most actively in big cities, though county towns also conducted sporadic health campaigns of general cleanliness against flies and pests, displayed public health notices on bulletin boards, and promoted anti-opium movement.[104] Nanjing, Beiping (北平, name of Beijing during 1928–1949), and Shanghai regularly conducted campaigns of health propaganda and education that consisted of parades, exhibitions, radio talks, lectures and distribution of health leaflets in addition to week-long summer and fall health campaigns of general cleanliness. Shanghai carried out 16 city-wide health campaigns in 1927–1937 that were led by the municipal government with the cooperation of civic organizations. The campaigns mainly conducted health propaganda and activities of sanitation and general cleanliness.[105] Nanjing, as the capital of the Nationalist government, built new health facilities and created health programs to catch up with Beijing and Shanghai, the two pioneering centers of modern health movement. The following discussion focuses on Nanjing, Beijing, and Hangzhou to illustrate the diverse efforts of health propaganda and education.

The Health Bureau of Nanjing was formed in October 1928, with Hu Ding-an (胡定安) as the Health Commissioner. Previously, Nanjing municipal government had only a police unit in charge of health matters. Hu complained: "Nanjing has no basic hygiene facilities such as running water, sewage system, toilets and street garbage collections, and residents did not have training in health matters."[106] Hu faced an urgent need to build up the city's modern health infrastructure, but he was short of human and financial resources. In 1930, Nanjing municipal government made a request of half a million from the Dutch Boxer Indemnity to build a running water system and a sewage system in the city, which the Executive Yuan of the Nationalist government approved in April 1932.[107] Nanjing also built an infectious disease hospital in 1933–34. For health education and propaganda, Nanjing municipal government published a journal called *Shoudu Weisheng* (首都卫生, *Hygiene of the Capital*). The first volume appeared in 1929 with Jiang Jieshi's inscription as public endorsement. The journal claimed that the state had the moral responsibilities to protect the health of people in four basic areas of needs—food, clothing, shelter, and transportation (衣食住行). It called for a medical revolution in China where national medicine, i.e. Chinese medicine, was to be transformed according to hygiene and science (卫生化科学化). The journal discussed drinking water and disease, mosquitoes and flies, and the criteria of municipal health construction, laws and regulations, statistics, planning, and an overview of health conditions.[108]

In preparing the public for health campaigns, the Nanjing city government expounded:

> The foundation of health depends on people's understanding that health was intertwined with the weal and woe of our nation and race. Only when people are thoroughly awakened can health work make achievements. Health education is for the long-term effect.[109]

Following the instruction of the central government, Nanjing city government emphasized the three strategies of propaganda (宣传), training (训练), and awakening (唤醒) to meet the needs "of lower general ordinary people" in obtaining common health knowledge. They expected people to use health knowledge in daily life after they gained the knowledge.[110] Both written and oral methods were used in propaganda work. Written material included health leaflets, booklets, posters, slogans and charts of vital statistics. Posters and charts were posted at major traffic junctures, and common health knowledge was published in newspaper supplements. Nanjing municipal government compiled pamphlets on such topics as daily personal hygiene, hygiene for women and children, the danger of carbon monoxide poisoning, venereal diseases, school health, running water and hygiene of the capital, smallpox vaccination, factory hygiene, and why refuse must be cleaned up. Oral dissemination of health information featured indoor lectures by celebrities, outdoor lectures by traveling teams of government officials and professionals, and the use of slang and songs for women and children.

In the work of training, Nanjing Health Bureau designed short courses to train people of different vocations about health rules, particularly those whose work had direct impact on public health, namely, workers of restaurants, teahouses, bathhouses, barber shops, theaters and hotels. The bureau worked to improve the transportation methods of garbage and waste, and organized self-governing district committees on street cleaning. The city promoted physical education—martial spirits among people, built public cemeteries, banned exposed coffins, and buried dead animals. The bureau supervised medicine through licensing, promoted health and disease prevention by setting up health stations and conducting vaccinations, and paid attention to women and children's hygiene by advocating new delivery methods and training midwives to reduce death rate. Health stations distributed information leaflets on pregnancy and infant health, and produced and sold soy milk for infants who did not have mother's milk.[111] These efforts reminded people of what American city health stations and laboratories did at the turn of the twentieth century.

In the work of awakening, Nanjing Health Bureau held health campaigns with meetings, parades, and slogans; it carried out disinfections, anti-pest movements against mosquitoes, flies, fleas and rats; launched city-wide general cleaning campaigns (required by the Health Ministry) twice annually to remove street refuse and dirt and to give vaccinations against smallpox. Health exhibits were displayed with pictures, posters, slogans, images of microbes, charts of diseases and vital statistics, and model devices of pathology.[112] The government used health propaganda campaigns to promote vaccinations to fight against epidemic diseases, such as smallpox and cholera. Vaccination against smallpox, an epidemic disease that was prevalent in China, was carried out in cities under the Nationalist government. Although China produced its own vaccines, there was a shortage of technical persons to carry out the vaccination. To solve the problem, the Health Ministry established Smallpox Vaccination Training Centers (种豆传习所) in 1929 at provincial and municipal health departments, to offer training classes at public and private hospitals. Each class had 20 students for 3 weeks. Men and women of 20–45 years old were recruited, who were expected to be healthy and literate and of good moral character. The training was free but students or their sponsoring units had to pay for food and lodging. Training lectures included overviews of smallpox, its transmission, comparison of old methods of inoculation and new methods of cowpox vaccine, history and rules of vaccination, vaccination principles and an overview of immunology, choosing and preserving the living viruses of cowpox, an overview of disinfection, methods of vaccination, normal experience of the vaccine and treatment of abnormal situation, and time and age and frequency for vaccinations. After their studies, students practiced vaccinations on each other, at least one on ten people.[113]

The importance of health was interpreted beyond the physical well-being of individuals. "Health is a matter that concerns the international status of a country and the nation's spirit, hence national health is a very important matter."[114] In a radio health lecture titled "The Medical Question for the Reviving Nation," Zhu Xiangyao (诸相尧) of Beijing interpreted national revival and racial health in explicit eugenic terms.[115] He asked his audience: "When we shout the slogans of reviving the nation and saving the country and working hard for the national struggle, do we ask ourselves what is the power to revive the nation? And with what to overcome the enemy?" He continued;

> The answer is clear: first is the supreme quality of the race; and second is a healthy body. . . . for a nation to survive properly it needs a race of superior quality and healthy individuals before it can talk about working hard for progress and national revival.[116]

To join the chorus of national revival and healthy body, merchants advertised their products, such as the Ovomaltine (麦乳精), with the slogan, "To Strengthen the Nation and the Race, We Must First Strengthen the Body (强国强种必先强身)."[117]

Beijing had been holding regular health campaigns since the 1920s. Every year on May 15 and December 15, the city would organize private organizations and government agencies to carry out a thorough cleaning campaign. The cleaning campaign of December 1928 demonstrated the official propaganda and the participation of the public. First, a general meeting was held at Tiananmen Square to mobilize people before the attendants set out in three routes—south, east, and west—to do the cleaning. Shouting health slogans, the procession of the cleaning parade started with an opening team, water-spraying vehicles, a military band, and leaders of various government departments sweeping the streets with brooms (to promote the cleaning campaign). Participants of the cleaning procession included police, schools, boy scouts, private organizations, government employees, and street-cleaners.[118] To make the campaign felt everywhere in the city, public health lectures, radio talks and exhibitions were carried out simultaneously with the cleaning parade.

Doctors at different hospitals in Beiping, such as the Outer City Hospital (外城医院), the Inner City Hospital (内城医院), the East Suburb Hospital (东郊医院), and the Infectious Disease Hospital (传染病医院), were organized to give health lectures every day at their hospitals where patients and their relatives were supposed to have genuine interests in health matters. Table 3.3 shows the topics of health lectures and the numbers of attendance in 1930. Starting in 1935, Beiping Municipal Health Bureau collaborated with the city's Radio Station to create a health lecture program on the radio every Friday afternoon from 4 to 4:30.[119] Departments of the Beiping Health Bureau took turns to give the weekly radio lecture, which covered a wide range of social and health issues. For example, the radio lectures talked about why the city's cleanliness relied on the cooperation of the people, what disease was, what health examination was, why people needed to register births and deaths, smallpox prevention and vaccination, the need to promote family hygiene, symptoms of meningitis and its treatment, medicine and the nation, opium and China, clothes for babies, venereal disease and marriage problems. The talks were supposed to be delivered in a colloquial style and easy for people to understand.[120]

Table 3.3 Health lectures at inner city hospital of Beiping, 1930–1931

Lecturer	*Topic*	*Number of audience*
An Shiyuan, head of the hospital	Clinical diagnosis of typhoid	168
He Qiaoquan President of Inner City Hospital	Incidence and prevention of trachoma	173
He Qiaoquan	Public health	142
An Shiyuan	Hygiene of spitting	112
Dong zhihe	Introduction to public health	148
Zhang Hualong	Information on public health	115
Zhang Yanhe	Three benefits of public health	142
Zhang Han	Foundation of public health	141
Jiang Baohe	An ounce of prevention is better than a pound of treatment	125
Jing Zecheng	Personal hygiene makes public health	144
He Qiaoquan	Introduction to infectious diseases	148
Dong Zhihe	Public health and infectious diseases	137
Zhang Hualong	Hygiene of digestive system	125
Zhang Yanhe	Prevention of infectious diseases	135
Zhang Han	Good and bad of public health	167
Jing Zaixiang/Yang Fangyi	Prevention of cholera and dysentery	126
Jiang Baohe	Hygienic methods in the summer	130
He Qiaoquan	Clean food and drinks	168
Fan Zangqing	Mosquitoes and malaria	170
Dong Zhihe	Prevention of plague	180
Zhang Hualong	How to prevent hookworm	175
Yang Fangyi	Trachoma and its prevention	274
Jing Zecheng	Catch and eliminate flies for public health	304
He Qiaoquan	Causes of TB	240
Fan Cangshu	Common treatment of typhoid	239
Fan Cangshu	Preventive methods of intestinal parasites	300
Zhang Hualong	Hygiene for pregnant women	300
Jiang Baohe	Cause and treatment of TB	340
Dong Zhihe	Common knowledge for bathers	328
Zhang Hualong	Hygiene of nervous system	338
Zhang Anhe	The cause of indigestion	104

Sources: Public health lectures, 1930–1931, the 4th municipal hospital of Beiping, Beijing Police order, #419. Beijing Municipal Archives, J182-1-680, Beijing.

Exhibition, a popular method of displaying science and health in the West, was eagerly copied by Chinese health modernizers. Exhibitions were held in Beiping, Shanghai, Nanjing, and other big cities. They often made requests of each other about items for display and circulated them among different cities, as none of the cities had a good stockpile of materials for exhibitions alone. For instance, the Health Bureau of Beiping requested exhibition materials from Shanghai to be displayed at the first and fourth mass education institutes and in Zhongshan Park during the 4th Health Campaign on May 15–29, 1928. Requested material included specimens, pictures, posters and charts, medical instruments, health and hygiene tools, and food and drink hygiene. These materials would be categorized into biology, pathology, pregnancy and babies, nutrition, environmental sanitation, school and factory hygiene, personal hygiene, common knowledge on medicine, vital statistics, and emergency treatment and instruments.[121] Beiping Health Bureau also created a permanent Health Exhibition Hall (*weisheng chenglie guan*, 卫生陈列馆) in Zhongshan Park, free to the public and open on all national holidays and Sundays. The bureau assigned people to take care of the exhibit items, write explanations and make pictures and charts. Health police kept order and safeguarded the exhibition rooms, keeping a record of visitors.[122] Even the Social Bureau of Beiping caught on the passion to create a Health Exhibition Institute (*weisheng chenglie suo*, 卫生陈列所) to explain diseases and social problems to the public in plain and simple language with new and refreshing images and pictures.[123]

The enthusiasm for exhibitions seemed contagious as many cities vied for the best show of exhibitions. The Health Exhibit Hall at West Lake of Hangzhou during the 1929 World Fair was probably the largest with 16 exhibition rooms of different departments. They displayed current ideas on hygiene and health with a wide spectrum of topics. The pharmacy department showed products by students from Zhejiang pharmaceutical schools and Chinese medical drugs and formula/recipe. The cosmetics department showed the full range of poisonous elements in cosmetics that caused facial complexion to become yellowish and sickly after long-time use due to lead poison. Perfumes were revealed as made of alcohol and irritant agents. The health protection department showed posters and images of new and old methods of midwifery and interpretation of the human body, whereas the prevention department featured posters and films of parasitic diseases, images of the spread of diseases and methods to prevent infectious diseases. The exhibit on babies showed a deformed fetus, the death rate of mothers and children, an animal fetus, dystocia, and charts of the age of pregnant women. The school health department promoted physical examination, sports meets and physical education charts, dental and eye health, and postures of sitting and standing. The Ministry of Health had a room of its own to display calls on people to change their unhygienic habits and learn health knowledge. The health education department showed posters, charts and books on the lack of health education in the past four thousand years in China and why China was labelled as the "sick man of Asia."[124] The exhibition was carefully organized to achieve health propaganda and education of the public. The health message basically followed the decades-long argument of the modernizers that a strong body was important for national revival but added scientific persuasion this time.

Government promotion of public health encouraged civic-minded people to form health organizations of their own. Organizations such as the Society of Health Education in China (中国卫生教育社) created in Zhenjiang (镇江) in 1935, aimed to promote national health (民族健康) by individual actions. The society held health education exhibits and meetings and published weekly on health education to awaken the masses to hygiene and to promote a physical health movement of the nation. The society advocated ten principles of health: sunshine, fresh air, healthy food and drinks, being tidy and clean, diligence, good rest, good sanitation, positive thinking, balanced emotions and moderate drinking. Its four major missions were to disseminate reasonable and effective health knowledge, correct unreasonable and harmful habits, create a tidy and clean environment, and promote a healthy and orderly new life.[125] The society was obviously a product of the New Life Movement.

School hygiene and health programs

School hygiene and health were important components of national health modernization. Programs of school hygiene started in Beijing in the 1910s. The Education Department of Beijing municipal government issued ten regulations regarding school hygiene in 1917 and for the first time, assigned a government official in charge of school hygiene. The regulations only stayed on paper, however, due to budget limitations. In 1918, clinics for students in each section of the city (south, north, east, and west) were planned, and again the government did not follow through due to budget problems. By 1925, a physical examination committee and a smallpox vaccination committee were established, despite the fact that they were of temporary nature and convened only when condition of budget favored. In 1927, recommendations were made to set up a health affairs' office to take care of school hygiene. An administrative organizational chart showed that under the School Hygiene Office of Beijing Education Department were units of medical clinics, prevention, health, general affairs, nurses, and hospitals to take care of ear/nose/throat (otolaryngology), interior health and eye, exterior health and skin, and dental care.[126] Little evidence indicated the plan was put into practice. After the Nationalist government was formed, the Health and Education Ministries organized a School Hygiene Committee in Nanjing to promote school hygiene education and health services. The health and education bureaus of Beijing, now designated as the Beiping Special Municipality, also formed a School Hygiene Committee to take charge of school hygiene and health. Following the central government policy, the Beiping municipal government created a pilot hygiene program in the spring and summer of 1930 at all municipal elementary schools, to which the Beiping Health Bureau assigned doctors and health instructors with provisions of smallpox vaccination and treatment of trachoma. The health and education bureaus collaborated in offering a course on school hygiene for elementary school teachers, with each school sending two teachers, or at least one teacher, to attend. Schools were expected to use the funds provided by the Education Bureau to buy the health posters designated by the Health Bureau. The training course started in the spring term, with two hours a day for theory and practice, and lasted for four weeks. Those attending the course would become responsible for the creation of a hygiene program at their schools. The Health Bureau's doctors and health instructors would visit the schools regularly to assist the teachers with school hygiene.[127]

In February 1931, the Beiping city government started a comprehensive health demonstration program at No. 2 School with a doctor, a nurse and a health inspector to instruct students about healthy habits, examine and improve school hygiene, prevent epidemics, treat diseases, correct students' and teachers' posture, and conduct physical examination. The nurse went to the school every day, and the doctor every Tuesday and Friday for treatment of diseases. The school health office opened every afternoon from 3:30 to 4:30 and carried out weekly school hygiene and sanitation inspection. Students received a physical examination once every month.[128] The demonstrative program at No. 2 School was later expanded to other schools in the city. The Hygiene Education Commission of Beiping Education Bureau reported that in 1931 schools had conducted physical examinations, hygiene education training classes, hygiene discussion meetings for school principals and teaching staff, sanitary inspection of schools, epidemic disease inspections, and medical treatment for school students. Statistics on students indicated that 26.6 percent had trachoma, 8.8 percent had vision problems, 18.5 percent had tonsillitis, 1.1 percent had lung problems, 15.8 percent had hearing problems, 36.6 percent had dental problems, 0.5 percent had heart problems, and 20.4 percent had malnutrition. These data came from 2015 students of all the 67 municipal schools that included nine middle schools, 57 elementary schools, and one kindergarten.[129]

Health programs at schools in 1933 included health education, preventive work, correction of defects, and environmental sanitation. Health education trained elementary and middle school teachers who were in charge of school hygiene, which led to the formation of a Health Education Research Society by those interested in school hygiene. Preventive work included health examination, inspection of possible epidemic diseases, smallpox vaccination, and preventive injections against typhoid, diphtheria and scarlet fever. Correction of defects focused on trachoma, teeth, and vision. Environmental sanitation targeted the cleaning of campus and the toilets. Schools kept health records of students, such as medical treatment records, statistics of physical defects of students in every grade, height and weight of students, and certificates of students' medical treatment transfers.[130]

In 1934, the Beiping city government designed an elaborate institutional structure of school hygiene (**Figures 3.1 and 3.2**) for inner city schools.[131] Figure 3.1 "School Hygiene Organization and Administration System" shows that the health and social affairs bureaus together with the Beiping School Hygiene Committee led school health. Figure 3.2 "Tasks and Contents of Health Classes" shows that under the category of health classes (*weishengke*, 卫生课) are three sub-categories

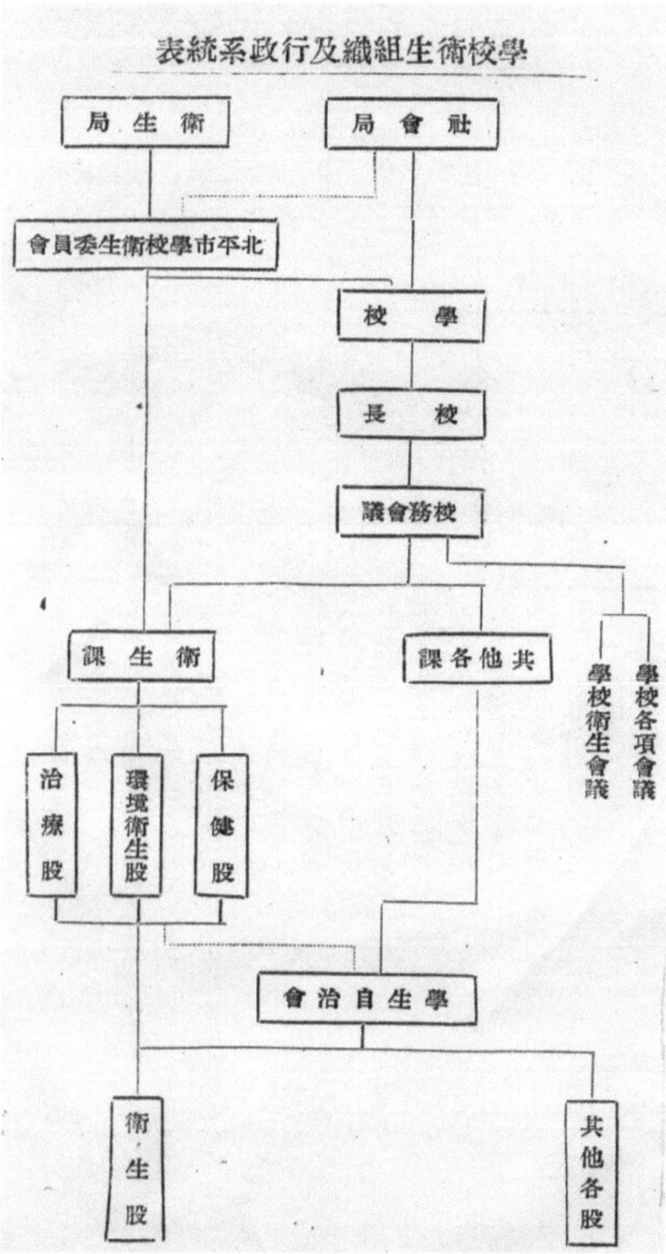

Figure 3.1 School hygiene organization and administration system

Sources: "Beiping shili xuexiao weisheng shishi fangan 北平市立学校卫生实施方案, 1934", p. 3 [Health implementation plan for municipal schools in Beiping], J2-3-232-171, Beijing Municipal Archives. Title: "Chart of School Hygiene Organization and Administration System."

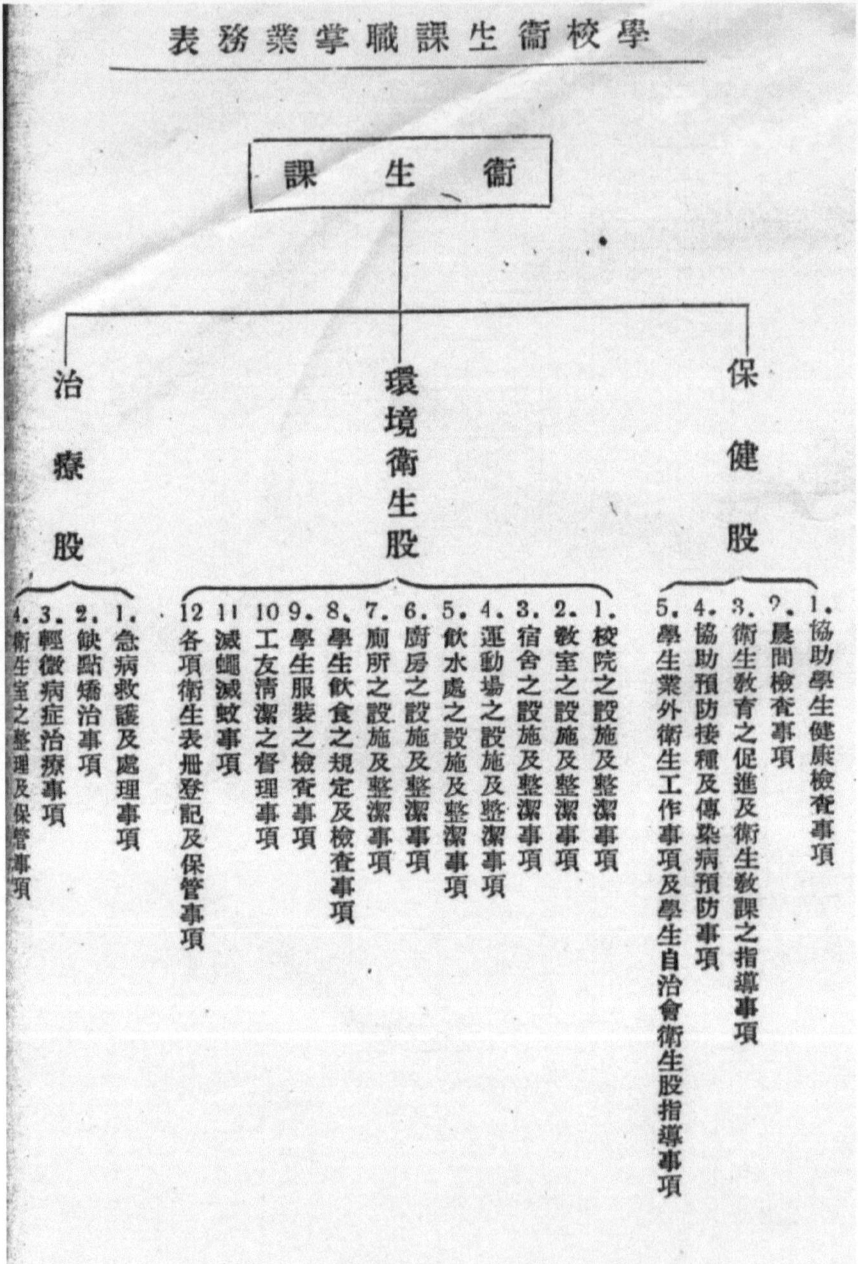

Figure 3.2 Tasks and contents of health classes

Sources: "Beiping shili xuexiao weisheng shishi fangan, 1934," p. 4, J2-3-232-172, Beijing Municipal Archives. Title: "Tasks and Contents of Health Classes."

of health protection (*baojian*, 保健), environmental sanitation (*huanjin weisheng*, 环境卫生) and treatment (*zhiliao*, 治疗). Each category included several tasks with sanitation having a dozen. There was little information on whether the detailed plan was put into practice. Archival data indicate that health programs at individual schools were less consistent, due to factors of shortage of funds, lack of technical personnel, and a mechanism to enforce health plans. Nonetheless, the charts of Beiping school hygiene show the sophisticated understanding and high expectations of school health programs in a modern society.

In Nanjing, school hygiene and health programs started in 1930 at only five schools. After the city government organized the Health Education Committee in 1933, school health extended to 136 schools in 1935, covering a total of 40,000 students. School health service included physical examination, defect correction, vaccination, health education, improvement of sanitation, and visits to student homes. Additionally, Nanjing had 304 private academies [*sishu*, 私塾] with over 8000 students, mostly children from poor families, who needed to know hygiene and health urgently. The municipal government decided in 1936 that the health station at Fengfu Road (丰富路) took charge of the health education at 53 private academies in the 5th police district. When the work proved successful, the city government decided to expand it to all private academies. Nanjing Health Bureau, in collaboration with Social Affairs Bureau, held advanced health training sessions for teachers of private academies at health stations and municipal hospitals in February 1937 with courses on 10 subjects: vaccination, disinfection, emergency aid, trachoma, skin disease, infectious disease, sanitation, school hygiene, and women and children's health. In order to encourage attendance, anyone who did not miss a session would be awarded a certificate of merit.[132] Nanjing also organized activities of children's health on June 1, Children's Day, in 1935–37.[133]

Training for elementary school health was conducted in cooperation with Nanjing Education Bureau, which used posters and charts to show population and death rates of different countries, infectious diseases in Nanjing, channels of tuberculosis transmission, horror of smallpox, and children's life and habits and improvements. Health lectures for elementary and middle school teachers were held in the summer, where government health leaders, such as Liu Ruiheng, Jin Baoshan, and Hu Ding-an, came to give talks on various topics, including methods of disinfection, emergency aid, infectious diseases and their prevention at schools, overviews of school hygiene, responsibilities of school doctors, physical examination, personal hygiene, hygiene of sex, and the meaning of immunity.[134] Subsequently, schools added courses on hygiene and biology to the curriculum. Posters on children's hygiene, scientific explanation of the human body, and public health became useful tools in school health education.[135]

In the movement for school health, the National Beiping University Medical School reformed its curriculum of health education by offering one year of public health theories and one year of practice of public health. Physical examination and correction of defects were conducted on all students, faculty and staff with special attention to plague and venereal diseases. Anyone with plague or venereal disease would be banned from school. Categories of examination included malnutrition and anemia, skin diseases, deformity, tonsillitis, lymphnoditis, goiter, eye disease, ear disease, nose disease, dental disease, heart disease, lung disease, spleen disease, intestinal disease, reproductive organ disease, nerve and mental diseases. Physical examination started at the beginning of the academic year with recommendation for treatment if one was found having any of the diseases. The school encouraged physical exercises with a football field, basketball courts and tennis courts in addition to martial arts and military drills. For prevention, the school's vaccination office carried out smallpox and cholera vaccinations once a year, typhoid vaccinations every the other year, and plague vaccinations when plague broke out. The school also experimented on the prevention of diphtheria, using the Schick test, and the prevention of scarlet fever, using the Dick test. Faculty and staff received free medical services at the school's hospital. Environmental sanitation was taken seriously with attention to light, air circulation, temperature at dorms, clean chairs and desks, clean kitchen utensils, clean toilets and bathrooms, and sanitation of ditches and play grounds. Sanitation was inspected monthly by the department of hygiene and public health along with relevant persons from the school's secretary office and hospital. Kitchen staff had weekly meetings with public health faculty and nurses. Kitchen utensils were boiled three times a day for disinfection, and kitchen sanitation was inspected by the head nurse. Drinking water was tested daily by the bacteria department, toilets were disinfected with sodium cyanate (氰酸纳) to kill flies, and cleaners took care of the garbage at school.[136] There were, however, little data to indicate that all these health programs were effectively implemented. Nonetheless, they demonstrated the school administration's response to the central government's call for school hygiene and health modernization. Interestingly, some wanted to take advantage of the health movement for personal benefits. The *Beijing Daily* publisher sent a letter to municipal hospitals and asked if they would give its staff a special treatment, i.e. to reduce and waive the costs of treatment, because they reported on their health work.[137] The incident showed that state medicine in the sense of free medical service was not yet available even to urban professionals in the mid-1930s.

Wartime health efforts

As mentioned before, Japan's invasion of China in 1937 disrupted the Nationalist state-building and modernization programs. The Nationalist government was forced to move west, settling in Chongqing as the wartime capital, but the health modernization efforts continued with the wartime rally to "strengthen the race and build the nation" and to "increase the power of Anti-Japanese War."[138] The National Health Administration was relocated with the government in Chongqing with half of its employees dismissed due to wartime hardships. Key institutions such as the Central Field Health Station and the Central Hospital had to be relocated in Guiyang, 330 kilometers away, because Chongqing was not able to house all the government agencies. As an indication of medical importance during wartime, the NHA was made to report directly to the Executive Yuan; and practitioners of Chinese medicine were increasingly given license of practice. The presence of the central government brought new energy of health construction to western China. Health stations, hospitals, and health training and research institutions were being created in local areas, benefiting from the expertise and facilities of NHA. Local health bureaus were established to direct health campaigns and develop rural health and sanitation units in the Sichuan and Yunnan region. In cooperation with the Allied military campaigns during World War II, Nationalist health workers built more than 70 health stations along the China–Burma road, with every 50 miles a station, contributing to military disease prevention and anti-malaria work.[139] These stations were turned into county hospitals and health institutes after 1949, forming part of the institutional infrastructure of post-1949 health reconstruction.

More importantly, the National Health Administration, under the leadership of Jin Baoshan (1940–47), continued the commitment of state medicine in the sense of building local health administrative institutions with a medical service. In 1940 the Nationalist government adopted the state medicine system (公医制) as the fundamental health policy of China. By that, the government meant a state controlled central system of health administration, which was not different from what the NHA had been doing before the war. Nonetheless, the announcement of the state medicine system as the health policy had profound political implications for the Nationalist regime in competition with the CCP for popular support. The legislation of a state medicine system projected the government commitment to the promotion and protection of the nation's health as its ultimate objective. During the war against the Japanese invasion, the CCP had gained increasing popular support with rural reforms, while the GMD had suffered corruption and demoralization. Public commitment of state medicine might help gain popular support for the GMD.

The NHA promulgated the "Resolution on Implementing State Medicine" in 1941, with the ambition to create health institutions at every level of the administration, from province to municipality to county and to village town, as preparation for the delivery of state medicine.[140] A health administrative system was considered imperative for the delivery of medical service. The government allocated funds for state medicine and sent people to provinces to promote and plan state medicine. As a result, the number of health institutions and centers increased in the following years at all local levels except rural villages. The numbers of county health centers increased to 1013 by 1945 when the war against Japan ended. In the next two years when the civil war was going on between the Nationalists and the Communists, county health centers continued to grow and rural district sub-stations began to be established. By 1947 the peak time of Nationalist health work, there were 1440 county health centers, 353 district health stations and 783 village town health sub-stations (see Table 3.1). With these numbers, about half of the counties (*xian*) in China had established some sort of health center by then. The number of rural health stations and sub-stations, however, was only a small fraction of the hundreds of thousands of villages in

China. The *xian* health centers, however, found it difficult to obtain funds and competent administrative and technical staff. The efforts little changed the poor landscape of rural health. Health activists were constantly frustrated in their promotion of public health in local communities. C. C. Chen complained that to the Nationalist government leaders public health was only a matter of "theoretical and remote importance."[141] Regarding the position of public health in national priorities, Nationalist political leaders did not change their attitude even in wartime, despite the constant push of health modernizers.

When the government returned to Nanjing at the end of World War II, the NHA shifted its focus to building public hospitals. It issued the "Rules of Establishing Public Hospitals" in 1945 to standardize the operation of public hospitals. By 1947, 40 public hospitals were established in 11 provinces. Health institutions at provincial level increased to 148, including 110 provincial hospitals, 11 maternal and child health hospitals, 4 tuberculosis hospitals, 6 hospitals for infectious diseases, 2 hospitals for mental diseases, and 3 leprosaria.[142] Additionally, the Southeast Plague Prevention Office in Fuzhou and the Kala-Azar Prevention Office in Huaiyin of Jiangsu hired specialists to conduct field investigations, prevention, and laboratory research on epidemic diseases.[143] The Nationalist government also established a military medical administration system, and medical departments of different ministries such as the industrial and the railway ministries. All of these health facilities and institutions, though incomplete and accessible only to a small portion of the 500 million Chinese people, laid the groundwork for the post-1949 development under the PRC.

Part II: Health development at CCP revolutionary bases

Jiangxi Soviet bases, 1927–1934

While the Nationalist government concentrated on the institutional construction of a modern health administration system, the Chinese Communist Party (CCP), after its terrible setback in 1927, regrouped to establish themselves in the Jinggang mountain (井冈山) region in the southeast of China, on the borders of Jiangxi and Fujian provinces.[144] They created revolutionary bases, which they called "the soviet bases," by working with local people and winning their support. They took as their revolutionary missions to solve people's problems of food, shelter, sickness, hygiene, and marriage. They formed a new government, the Soviet Republic of China (中华苏维埃共和国), on November 7, 1931 with Ruijin (瑞金) as the capital, and started land reforms by confiscating land from big landlords and redistributing it among poor peasants. A new marriage law was promulgated to forbid arranged marriage and the sale of marriage contracts. Marriage was defined as based on the free choice of spouses, and divorce was allowed at the request of either of the spouses. These reforms, which were carried out by the peasant associations in the villages, fundamentally improved the status of poor peasants and women in general. Women's rights and liberation, instead of a separate agenda and movement, were integrated in the overall social reforms of the CCP revolution. With these reforms, the CCP created a new social order that gave hope and opportunity to the poor and the oppressed in the struggle against the oppressors of the rich and powerful.

Mao Zedong, the CCP leader, made it clear at the 1934 Workers and Peasants' Congress at Ruijin that:

> all the practical problems in the masses' daily life should claim our attention. If we attend to these problems, solve them and satisfy the needs of the masses, we shall really become organizers of the well-being of the masses, and they will truly rally around us and give us their warm support.[145]

The Communist health work in the soviet bases began and remained as an integral part of fundamental social reforms of institutions, traditional habits and norms, and old behavior and attitudes of people. The health policy aimed to serve both the revolutionary Red Army and local civilians in the effort to strengthen the CCP's fighting ability and popular support for the revolution. Facing extreme material shortages of modern medicine and health personnel, the Communists were innovative and resourceful in fully exploiting the use of herbal medicine and utilizing all types of healing practices of traditional Chinese medicine, in addition to modern Western medicine. When no saline solutions were available, they made liquids from coptis roots (*huanglian*, 黄连, Chinese goldthread, an anti-inflammatory drug) and honeysuckle flowers (*jinyinhua*, 金银花, an antibacterial drug) to cleanse the wounds. They used pig lard as Vaseline and opium as an anesthetic.[146] It was during those difficult years that they mastered the functions and the use of hundreds of herbs to offset the lack of Western medicine. Mao Zedong's instruction to use both the Chinese and the Western methods of healing and treatment encouraged the support of Chinese medicine practitioners for the CCP. After the Red Army settled in the Jinggang mountains, they turned an old site of Panlong Academy (攀龙书院) in Maoping of Ninggang county into a hospital, called Maoping Red Army Hospital (茅坪红军医院). Although treatment of wounded soldiers was the task of the hospital, local civilians received free medical service as well.

The early CCP health professionals of Western medicine came from a diverse background. Some were Communists trained in modern medicine, others were from missionary medical schools and hospitals, and others were captured medical officers of the Nationalist forces who decided to join the Communists. The first hospital that treated the CCP wounded soldiers in 1927 was a missionary hospital in Tingzhou (汀州) in northeast Fujian where Dr. Fu Lianzhang (傅连暲, 1894–1968) was the director. Fu had saved many CCP lives, including Chen Geng (陈赓, 1903–1961), later a famous military general, and Xu Teli (徐特立), Mao Zedong's teacher. Fu graduated from a missionary medical school and worked in a missionary hospital, but he decided to join the CCP revolution. He moved his hospital from Tingzhou to Ruijin in 1930, and expanded it into the Central Red Army Hospital (中央红色医院). Fu was one of the founders of the CCP health profession, serving as a leader of the Red Army's hospitals and medical schools; and after 1949, he was Vice Minister of Health of the PRC and president of Chinese Medical Association. He died a victim of the Cultural Revolution in 1968.[147] In 1930, He Fusheng (何复生， 1902–1934), an underground CCP member, convinced his colleagues at the British Methodist Hospital (普爱医院) to join the CCP's Third Army Corps, which significantly strengthened the health force. He organized and headed the general hospital of the Third Army Corps, but he was killed during the Nationalist fifth anti-CCP military campaign in 1934.

Mao Zedong considered health work a key component of the revolutionary movement, just as important as the construction of defense works and the food supplies in the consolidation of revolutionary bases.[148] At one time, he heard about a well-known physician named Dai Jimin (戴济民, 1888–1978), and decided to personally invite him to help the Red Army with revolutionary humanism (革命的人道主义). Dai had studied medicine at a missionary hospital in Wuhu of Anhui province in his youth, and served with the Red Cross in the 1911 revolution. Dai had long determined to dedicate himself to the needs of people, and that was why he adopted *Jimin*, meaning helping people, as his own name. Dai agreed to help the CCP's revolution and converted his entire clinic, together with equipment and a dozen doctors of Western and Chinese medicines, nurses and aides, into the Workers' and Peasants' Revolutionary Red Hospital (工农革命红色医院). Winning Dai to the revolutionary cause was an example of the CCP's determination to gain health support. Dai later headed the New Fourth Army Rear Hospital and served as Duty Health Minister of the New Fourth Army. He was Director of the Supervision Bureau of the Health Ministry (卫生部监察局局长) of the PRC after 1949.[149]

The arrival of He Cheng (贺诚, 1901–1992) and two other Communist physicians from Shanghai to Jiangxi in 1931 injected new blood in the health work and leadership of public health work. The three men were all trained in Western medicine and became key health leaders in the Red Army. Educated at National Peking University Medical College, He Cheng participated in the Northern Expedition, but opened a hospital in Shanghai to practice medicine as a disguise for his underground revolutionary activities after Jiang Jieshi's attack and suppression of Communists in 1927. At the Jiangxi soviet base, He Cheng organized a Military Medical Office in Longgang (龙岗), which became the Health Department of the Red Army in 1932. He also served as the first president of the Red Army Medical School. After 1949, he was Vice Minister of Health of PRC and Vice Minister of Health of the Central Military Commission. The CCP soviet government had established a Bureau of Health Affairs under the Interior Ministry that oversaw the units of medicine and health. Public clinics and drug/herbs cooperatives were developed, and doctors and drugstores registered. Additionally, households were formed into health teams with four, seven, or twelve in each team, where a team leader was put in charge of promoting sanitation, food hygiene and personal hygiene, and enforcing health regulations.

As the CCP developed more soviet bases, new hospitals were established for the military and civilians. From 1932 to 1934 before the Long March, the Red Army had established ten rear hospitals, with each having five to six stations, where 300 wounded soldiers could be accepted at each station. Additionally, there were six mobile military hospitals, two hospitals for the disabled and one for recuperation. Each soviet base had its hospitals, such as Huanggang Hospital in the Hunan-Hubei border area, Cidu Hospital in Fujian, and Luokounan Hospital in Jiangxi.[150] These medical hospitals and facilities demonstrated the fast growth of the Red Army's health institutions, when the revolutionary bases were expanding.

The first CCP medical school was called the Chinese Workers and Peasants Red Army Medical School (中国工农红军军医学校, renamed as the Red Army Health School, 红军卫生学校, in 1932). It was created in November 1931and opened for classes in January 1932 with He Cheng as president. It merged with Fu Lianzhang's Red Army Medical Affairs School in October 1934 at Ruijin and used the Central Red Army Hospital as the field-training hospital. Medical training followed Mao Zedong's instruction "to train red doctors with firm political belief and superior skills."[151] Students were recruited from the 18 to 23-year-old men and women, healthy and literate with some experience of health work. With limited resources, they studied medicine for one year, plus five-month clinical training and two-month residency. Their curriculum included anatomy, physiology, histology, materia medica, diagnosis, bacteriology, foreign languages (Japanese, German), pathology, internal medicine, surgery, hygiene services, skin and venereal diseases, basic otolaryngology (ear, nose, and throat), basic ophthalmology, military medicine, prevention of poisonous gas, and forensic medicine. Students took exams to graduate with credentials and were assigned to work in medical and health units. The hospital of the Red Army Health School was equipped with an X-ray machine and a laboratory. Up to October 1934 before the Long March, the school had graduated 181 medical doctors, 75 pharmacists, 300 nurses, 7 researchers, and 123 hygiene workers, totaling 686 graduates to supply the military and civilian hospitals. The CCP also established nursing schools, medical administration schools, and paramedics training classes to meet the urgent needs of health staff.[152] The first major health publication of the CCP was *Health Newspaper* (健康报), which started in 1931 but was published irregularly due to wars. Contents of the publication included health administration, political affairs of hospitals, and information on medical knowledge and techniques. *Health Newspaper* resumed regular publication in August 1946 first in the northeast and then in Beijing under the auspices of the Health Ministry.

The difficult conditions and shortage of modern medicine made the CCP adapt to local resources of herb medicine and traditional healing practices. Different from the Nationalist government, the CCP advocated that Chinese medicine and drugs be combined with Western medicine in medical and pharmaceutical work. At the Red Army's hospitals, Western medicine took care of surgery and Chinese medicine took care of internal diseases. Organized teams went to collect herbs in the mountains to deal with a shortage of medical supplies. Physicians of Chinese medicine were recruited to work in the CCP hospitals, which had a department of Chinese medicine and a department of herbs. The CCP relied on herbs to treat various kinds of illnesses including those of internal medicine, surgery, and obstetrics and gynecology. Some Chinese medical doctors used acupuncture to treat soldiers and peasants. Relying on herbal plants, the Red Army produced medical supplies at workshops under the direction of Tang Yizhen (唐一珍，唐义贞, 1909–1934), a young woman of 23 years old who had grown up in a family of Chinese pharmacists and studied medicine in Moscow.[153] The use of Chinese medicine during the difficult wartime years laid the foundation of CCP's appreciation of Chinese medicine as an important component of healthcare. Doctors of Western biomedicine and physicians of Chinese medicine worked together and learned from each other. Those trained in biomedicine learned the use of Chinese herbal medicine and those in traditional Chinese medicine learned anatomy and surgery.[154]

Prevention of disease was carried out in a health movement via the mobilization of peasants and soldiers in 1932. The CCP's newspaper, *Red China* (红色中华报), published an editorial on January 13, 1932, which explained that disease prevention aimed to ensure the health of workers and peasants and the Red Army, and the consolidation of the revolutionary forces. CCP authorities defined eight rules of the anti-disease movement, integrating health movement into the overall work of class struggle and revolution. The Red Army adopted a "prevention first" policy at the third health meeting in 1932 and encouraged the use of all possible means to educate and mobilize the soldiers and the masses to get rid of four major epidemic diseases—malaria, dysentery, scabies, and leg ulcers. Soldiers did "legs up" exercises to prevent varix and ulcers. The Red Army also carried out hygiene week with local residents to do general cleaning. It became a regular activity for the Red Army to disseminate health information wherever they went. They encouraged the masses to dig wells, open windows and do weekly cleaning of the house. Well water improved the sanitary conditions of water supplies, which was an important source of disease prevention. The hygiene work cost people little but accomplished much; and more importantly, it significantly changed their health attitude and behavior to safeguard their own well-being.

The CCP government issued the "Guideline of the Health Movement" in March 1933 to promulgate that the workers and peasants' government sought to solve the problems of people's sufferings and that filth and disease were part of the problems. It called on local governments and mass organizations to lead the people to fight against filth, disease, and old ideas and habits of superstition. The guideline spelled out methods and requirements for the masses to follow in the health movement. After Mao Zedong conducted an investigation at Changgang village of Xingguo county, he concluded in December 1933 that disease was a serious enemy of the soviet base because it weakened the revolutionary force and plagued the people. Mao wrote that it was the responsibility of the CCP soviet government to mobilize the masses in a health movement to reduce and eliminate diseases. Hygiene was expected of soldiers in the rules of "Three Disciplines and Six Attentions" (三大纪律、六项注意) of the Red Army. Moreover, the CCP established a Central Disease Prevention Committee in March 1934 to promulgate regulations on communicable diseases. The Committee developed methods of disease-reporting and isolation and disinfection, created health education plans, carried out training classes for health administration, and held health contests among the masses.[155]

All of these health efforts were destroyed by the Nationalist fifth suppression campaign against the CCP in 1934. The military setback forced the CCP Red Army to abandon the soviet bases and start the Long March in October 1934. The medical and health infrastructure that the CCP had built was completely wiped out along with those left behind to defend the bases—soldiers, health workers, and communist supporters, including Tang Yizhen, leader of the medical supplies production workshops. She was pregnant with a second child and decided to stay behind at the base, but she was captured by the Nationalist forces and murdered. Those who went on the Long March endured extreme hardship and constant battles with the Nationalist military forces. More than 1200 medical workers at the beginning of the Long March were reduced to about 200 when the Red Army reached Yanan in October 1935.[156] The CCP literally had to start all over again by re-building their revolutionary bases in north China, including medical institutions and staff, and led the people there for a new society.

Health development of the Yanan era, 1936–1948

Yanan (Yan'an, Yenan, 延安) was located in Shanxi (陕西) province of north China, a region, at the time, plagued with extreme poverty, disease, and human suffering where people sheltered, if they had any, in caves on the plateau of yellow earth. Terrible communicable diseases such as plague, cholera, smallpox and tuberculosis, coupled with high maternal and child mortality, were rampant during years of famines.[157] More than three million people died in the famine of 1928–1930 in the northwest of China. The population of Shanxi alone was reduced from 11.8 million to 8.9 million.[158] In 1932, the region was hit by bubonic plague, followed by cholera.[159] The crisis prompted the Nationalist government to establish the Northwest Epidemic Prevention Bureau in 1934. Other diseases, such as typhoid, dysentery, typhus, relapsing fever, tuberculosis, Kaschin-Beck disease, and neonatal tetanus, were widespread in the region. The infant mortality rate was as high as 60 percent, almost three times the national average.[160] Selling of women and children was widespread, and poverty-stricken people migrated in search for food and survival. It was in such circumstances that the CCP Red Army settled in the region in late 1935. Surprisingly, they successfully rebuilt their bases and expanded their governance over a region of 180 thousand square kilometers (the size of North Dakota of US) by 1937, with 1.5 million people that covered northern Shanxi, eastern Gansu and southeastern Ningxia.

The Xi'an Incident (西安事变) occurred in December 1936, when Jiang Jieshi, who went to rally his troops to fight the Communists, was kidnapped by his own soldiers in their attempt to force him to change his policy from fighting the CCP to fighting the Japanese.[161] The peaceful solution to the Xi'an Incident led to the formation of the United Front of the CCP and GMD for the second time, the first being in 1924–1927 to fight against the warlords.

The Second United Front was a new turning point in the GMD–CCP history of competition and collaboration while they carried the war against Japanese invaders. In accordance with the terms of the United Front, the CCP changed the name of their soviet government to ShanGanNing Border Region Government (陕甘宁边区政府) in September 1937 and adopted a series of moderate social and political reforms, such as rent reduction instead of land confiscation and redistribution, and democratic representation of all social classes in the region's political assembly. The Red Army was re-organized into the Eighth Route Army of the Nationalist military forces but remained under the CCP leadership and control. The Second United Front (1937–1945) lasted till Japan's defeat at the end of World War II. This period, despite tensions and distrust between the CCP and the GMD, saw CCP's expansion and growth of popular support. The CCP also built bases in the JinChaJi Border Region (晋察冀边区), areas bordering Hebei and Shanxi (山西) and Inner Mongolia, and pocket areas in central, eastern and southern China during the war.[162]

The CCP-controlled regions developed into a unique society in north China during 1937–1949, where extensive state-building and rural reforms took place.[163] Public health, along with the promotion of literacy and women's liberation and equality, was an important part of the social reforms in the border-region society and the growth of a popular political system. As in Jiangxi soviets, the CCP had severe shortages of medical personnel, facilities and resources in north China, but the health work persevered in the overall revolutionary movement. The CCP leaders called on the Communist revolutionaries to continue the spirit of the Jinggang era in undertaking active prevention and treatment of diseases and developing a people's medical and health enterprise in the pursuit of revolution and social transformation of China. Early in 1938 the border-region government created a Health Commission to guide and oversee medical and health affairs of local health agencies. The Commission emphasized the priorities of health work in increasing people's health knowledge, improving public health and maternal and child health, establishing pharmacies, training health workers, attacking superstitions and campaigning against witch doctors and sorcerers.[164] Health policies continued the tradition of the Jiangxi era by emphasizing the combination of Chinese and Western medicines, prevention as the first priority, and mass health movement. The guidance was self-reliance but actively seeking outside aid as well.

The border-region government delegated responsibilities to local administrations and encouraged them to take initiatives in providing services and organizing production. Every county organized medical and health co-operatives to deal with health and sanitation problems, and mobilized people to take their own responsibility in hygiene and disease prevention. The effect of mass mobilization in health campaigns was noted by various Western journalists like Edgar Snow, Agnes Smedley, Robert Payne, Gunther Stein, and members of the Dixie Mission.[165] They were impressed with the hospital work in Yanan, even though the hospital was a "rows of caves in a steep, yellow hillside."[166] In contrast to the Nationalist military medical facilities, Smedley found the CCP's hospital orderly and clean, with doctors of modern medicine and modern-trained women nurses.

She saw records of patients, operations and examinations being kept in a Chinese hospital, for the first time.[167] The reports of Western journalists made known to the world their observations of the efficiency and confidence as well as the apparent lack of squalor and disease in CCP's Yanan, which formed a sharp contrast to the bureaucracy and the squalor in wartime GMD's Chongqing.

The anti-fascist movement and international medical aid

The Yanan era witnessed diverse international support for CCP's fight against Japanese invasion, as the Anti-Japanese War was part of the international anti-fascist movement of World War II. Medical support came from doctors of many different countries, such as George Hatem (Ma Haide, 马海德, 1910–1988) from the United States, Norman Bethune (白求恩, 1890–1939) from Canada, and Dwarkanath Shantaram Kotnis (柯棣华, 1910–1942) from India. International medical doctors made significant contributions to CCP's revolution and China's medical and public health development.[168] Some of them, such as Bethune and Kotnis, sacrificed their lives in the fight against Japanese aggression and fascism in China during World War II.

George Hatem came to Yanan in 1937 after he had spent some time investigating tropical diseases in China. Upon his arrival, he saw primitive conditions in the CCP controlled area—no electricity, no running water, no plumbing, and no sink in the hospital. The Japanese blockade and GMD's restrictions meant a lack of supplies of modern medicine and equipment in CCP areas. Hospitals were established in caves, old temples, and even peasant houses, but the health workers were innovative in making creative use of what was available.

> I saw instrument sterilizers made of old gasoline cans, catgut containers used as test tubes, cuticle scissors serving the ophthalmologists for eye operations, and strange contraptions of old dye cans and cardboard for eye testing. I heard of doctors who for days carried test tubes with bacterial cultures on their bodies to secure the even temperature which is needed for their growth.[169]

In an attempt to fully understand the situation, Hatem conducted a detailed survey of the health and medical units in the region and made suggestions for improvement. Mao Zedong was impressed with his work and appointed him health advisor to the CCP military.[170] Hatem even joined the CCP in 1937, becoming the first foreign member. Hatem, called Ma Haide in Chinese, was a precious addition to the CCP's international outreach. He was instrumental in getting the news of CCP's fight against Japanese fascism to the outside world and obtaining international medical aid to the CCP. He worked with Song Qinglin (宋庆龄, Soong Ching-ling, Mme. Sun Yat-sen, 1893–1981), Agnes Smedley and other notable progressives to recruit foreign medical personnel for the CCP soldiers who were wounded in the fighting against Japanese in China.

Dr. Norman Bethune was one of those international medical specialists who came to help the CCP in the international anti-fascist movement. He arrived in

Yanan in March 1938 and brought the CCP the badly needed military medical expertise. More importantly, his total dedication to medical work with high standards injected new professional ethics to CCP's medical service. Having served in both World War I and the Spanish Civil War against fascism, Bethune had the unrivaled knowledge of battlefield medical work and the skills of battlefield blood transfusion, which he applied immediately to saving the lives of the Eighth Route Army soldiers. Bethune stressed the importance of frontline mobile medical units in saving soldiers' lives, which meant that medical staff followed battlefield actions and sought the wounded instead of waiting for the wounded to come to the rear hospitals. Surgery and blood transfusion were crucial in battlefield medical operations and they became the new weapon in reducing military casualties. Bethune demonstrated the operation of blood transfusion to Chinese medical staff and villagers and persuaded them to organize a blood transfusion corps for medial needs. He often spent long hours operating on patients without a break, sometimes up to 72 hours. Bethune was made the medical advisor to the JinChaJi military administration, in charge of developing a medical system. He helped create medical supplies workshops to solve the problems of medical shortage. He wrote training manuals on surgery and medicine and taught medical staff battlefield rescue skills. He worked on improving hospital organization and cleanliness, and the standards of medical work of his staff. He was anxious to train a whole generation of skilled doctors, but his life was cut short when he contracted septicemia during an emergency operation. He died in the village of Huangshigou (黄石口) in Tang county (唐县), Hebei province on November 12, 1939. Bethune's contributions went beyond his unique medical skills and his training of medical cadres and improving medical work. His total dedication and selfless service to patients impressed all who had worked with him. His death was a major loss to the CCP and its medical work. In his essay, "In Memory of Norman Bethune," which immortalized Bethune in China, Mao Zedong defined "selfless service to the people" the medical ethics and expectations of every Chinese communist. Chinese medical workers and Communist members were instructed to work like Bethune with dedication and selfless service. The motto was "to serve the people whole-heartedly."

In celebrating Bethune's dedication to international peace, the JinChaJi Model Hospital was renamed as Bethune's International Peace Hospital. Dwarkanath Shantaram Kotnis, an Indian-born doctor, was appointed the first Director of Bethune's International Peace Hospital. Dr. Kotnis had been working as a battlefield doctor with the Eighth Route Army in JinChaJi border region. Like Bethune, Kotnis spent long hours operating on wounded soldiers. He trained Chinese medical staff on surgery at the Bethune Health School and drafted a curriculum on nursing. He originally came as a member of the Indian Medical Mission Team of five doctors (Drs. M. Atal, leader of the team, M. Cholkar, D. Kotnis, B. K. Basu and Debesh Mukherjee) dispatched to Yanan by the Indian National Congress in 1938. They were personally welcomed by Mao Zedong and Zhu De (朱德, 1886–1976), the top leaders of the CCP. The team, like other international aid groups, brought much appreciated medical equipment like an X-ray machine to

Yanan. The Indian doctors worked in frontline mobile clinics to treat wounded soldiers for almost five years before they, except Kotnis, returned to India. Long hours of stressful work in difficult conditions severely affected Kotnis' health. He suffered a series of epileptic seizures and passed away on December 9, 1942. When the sad news reached Yanan, Mao Zedong observed that the Eighth Route Army had lost a great fighter and the Chinese nation had lost a great friend. Mao and Zhu De wrote to the Indian National Congress in praise of Dr. Kotnis' international spirit and dedication to fighting against fascism. They believed:

> the two great nations of India and China will be more closely united than ever before, so as to fight alongside other anti-fascist countries to smash fascism and liberate all the people who are under fascist yoke, and at the same time liberate India and China and win independence for these two great nations.[171]

Development of health institutions

Health institutions of the CCP were created along these three lines: the central, the military, and the border-region local. The central system was under the leadership of the Central Health Commission, including the Yanan Central Hospital and the Central Outpatient Department. The military system was led by the Health Department of the Military Commission, including the Bethune International Peace Hospital, United Military Hospital, and Chinese Medical University. The border-region government developed a health system with a Department of Health at the top, followed by a health station at each county, a health worker at a rural district, and a health committee in a village. This rural institutional system was similar to that of the Nationalist government, but the CCP supported private-run Chinese health and medical clinics (保健药社) and health cooperatives (卫生合作社) for medical and pharmaceutical services, in addition to having a health committee to take charge of health activities in village communities. Mao Zedong encouraged the promotion of health and the establishment of a village clinic in every one of the thousand more villages of the border region when he gave the commencement speech at Yanan University in May 1944. Moreover, under the jurisdiction of the border-region government were hospitals, the Society of National Medicine Studies, and the Association of Chinese and Western Medical Research. Every hospital of the central and the military systems had an outpatient department and clinics with service available to local civilians and villagers. The Chinese medical clinics and the health cooperatives had their headquarters in Yanan but branches in counties and rural towns. These different institutions and organizations formed a system of healthcare network that penetrated rural communities with Chinese and Western medical and pharmaceutical workers.[172]

A brief look at the different institutions of the three systems provides a sense of CCP health work during the wartime.[173] The Yanan Central Hospital was the best hospital in the region. It was established in April 1939 with He Mu (何穆, 1905–1990) as director. He Mu was trained as a pulmonary physician in France.

He was highly appreciated in Yanan and north China where tuberculosis was a terrible epidemic. The hospital had 170–180 beds and two small X-ray machines, one of which was brought to Yanan by He Mu. After 1949, the hospital moved to Beijing and acquired some staff from the Bethune International Peace Hospital, becoming the Beijing Hospital. The Bethune International Peace Hospital, originally the JinChaJi Model Hospital of the Eighth Route Army, became a major hospital in Shijiazhuang (石家庄) of Hebei province. The Border-Region Hospital was established in 1938 for the health service of government officials, but more than a quarter of the patients were ordinary people from local areas. The hospital had 150 beds by 1946. In collaboration with other medical groups, the hospital sent medical teams to different counties to provide healthcare services, set up health stations, train new midwives, hold health exhibits and talks, and promote model hygiene households. The China Red Cross donated medicine and equipment when its medical teams visited the ShanGanNing border region. When the Nationalist forces occupied Yanan in 1947 during the civil war, the hospital was changed to the First Rear Hospital of the Northwest Field Army.

Private health organizations such as the Chinese health and medical clinics were organized by Li Changchun in 1938, who headed the Yanan Municipal Organization Department but was a physician of Chinese medicine by training. The clinics, which were very popular with local people, were of Chinese medicine and pharmacy where Chinese physicians treated patents and dispensed herbal medicine. More than 20 counties established the clinics with branches in village towns. They lasted till 1955 when they were merged with the Chinese medicine department of Yanan prefecture hospital. The health cooperatives were established as a result of response to the epidemic outbreaks of typhoid fever and relapsing fever in 1944. They used both Chinese and Western medicines to treat people and live stocks. They were sponsored and operated by people's cooperatives (大众合作社)—a type of commercial stores of private enterprise, and the Chinese health and medical clinics. The government provided them assistance and donated medical supplies. The health cooperatives, which continued till 1952, were private health organizations financed by citizens and supported by the government for the public good.

Different from the Nationalist-controlled area, practitioners of Chinese medicine were respected and appreciated by the CCP, even though the CCP attacked witch doctors and superstitions and tried to modernize people's health behavior and attitude. Chinese medical doctors, using the network of the Chinese medical clinics, formed the Society of National Medicine Studies in 1941 to update their medical knowledge and skills. They met weekly and had speakers of prominent doctors of Chinese medicine, such as Li Dingming (李鼎铭, 1881–1947) and Bi Guangdou (毕光斗, 1879–1970). The Society had a library, a research room, and an outpatient department, in addition to training classes in Chinese medicine to produce more Chinese medical and pharmaceutical professionals.

The formation of the Chinese and Western Medical Research Association (中西医药研究会) in March 1945 aimed to carry out the policy of combining Chinese and Western medicines for the advancement of medical knowledge and skills. The Association congregated all persons of Chinese medicine, Western medicine, veterinary medicine, and pharmacy in the Yanan area for mutual learning and improvement and the promotion of people's health. It organized teams of Chinese and Western medicines to go to villages to offer medical services and disseminate health information. The Association's activities were the precursor of the post-1949 nationwide implementation of the policy to combine Chinese and Western medicines. Members of the Association also investigated Chinese and Western pharmacology with the Guanghua Pharmaceutical Production Factory and the Chinese Medical University. Shortage of medical materials was a serious challenge to the CCP, which sought donations of medical supplies and equipment from groups at home and abroad. When underground CCP groups obtained medicines, they often had to smuggle through the Japanese blockade to get the medicine to Yanan. During World War II, Song Qinglin was particularly helpful in sending medicine and equipment to the CCP. When she received a large X-ray machine donated from abroad in 1941, she asked General Stilwell to use an American plane to carry it together with other surgery equipment and medicine to Yanan.

Medical education and training

Medical education and training were expanded and strengthened as more professionally trained medical graduates from well-known schools in China and abroad came to Yanan to join the CCP to fight against the Japanese. The Chinese Workers and Peasants Red Army Medical School (founded in 1931 in Jiangxi) was re-organized with expansion into the China Medical University in 1940.[174] The formation of China Medical University was a turning point in the CCP's health education and professionalism, which advocated "firm political belief and superior skills" (政治坚定，技术优良). The teachers were mostly trained in Western medicine at major universities and medical colleges in China and abroad. They taught regular medical courses on anatomy, physiology, pharmacology, pathology, bacteriology, internal medicine and surgery. They purchased equipment, books, and teaching devices from Chongqing and Hong Kong, and created a library. Wang Bin (王斌, 1909–1992), a renowned surgeon who had led the Workers and Peasants Red Army Medical School, became the first president, and Zhu Lian (朱琏, 1909–1978), a female doctor, served as the deputy president. Zhu Lian was trained in Western medicine but she learned and researched Chinese medicine. She made impressive new discoveries by applying Western medical theories to Chinese acupuncture and published her explanation of the therapeutic functions of acupuncture in her book *The New Acupuncture* (新针灸学) in 1951. Her career was a good example of the benefit of combining Chinese and Western medicines.[175] Nicknamed as the cradle of red doctors, the university received encouragement from Mao Zedong, who wrote the graduates of 1940 an inscription: "Recue the dying and heal the wounded; practice revolutionary humanism" (救死扶伤，实行革命的人道主义).

Nursing schools as well as medical and pharmaceutical training schools were also established by the military and the border-region government.

Training classes for doctors, physician assistants, pharmacists, nurses and health assistants were offered on a rotation manner, where people could get training while working on the job. The short training courses usually lasted for a few months or up to half a year depending on the needs. There was also training in health administration for those who were health team leaders of regiments, recuperating station heads, and hospital department heads. The purpose was to combine the needs of actual work with the training in order to solve immediate problems.

The CCP government made health education and disease prevention the primary task of health work for the populace. High death rates and high maternal and child mortality rates were manifestations of many underlying conditions of the region. Mao Zedong pointed out: "the human and animal mortality rates are both very high, and at the same time many people still believe in witchcraft. In such circumstances, to rely solely on modern doctors is no solution."[176] Thousands of young peasant men and women were trained as health workers and midwives via short-term courses in the basics of diagnosis and treatment. Many of them returned to set up health co-ops in their counties and offer training of others. In the health movement, every village strived to have a health worker or a midwife (they were called doctors) who coordinated public health activities and popular health education with both the military and civilian hospitals. The medical staff at hospitals participated in the health work by offering lectures and classes on sanitation and public health as well as medical services.

Scientific theories of modern medicine, such as of bacteriology and cytology, were introduced in medical studies and explanation of diseases, as were Marxist theories of socialism and communism propagated as the guidance of revolution. Health workers disseminated medical science and revolutionary ideas simultaneously to help soldiers and peasants understand modern hygiene and public health and to attack the folly of old superstition and feudal thought. Traditional doctors of Chinese medicine were recruited to participate in the revolution and become an important group of health force in the CCP-led revolution.[177] There was, however, bias among modern doctors against Chinese doctors even in the CCP controlled region. Mao Zedong made it clear that the task of modern doctors and old-style Chinese doctors was nothing but serving the people.

> Of course, modern doctors have an advantage over doctors of the old type, but if they do not concern themselves with the sufferings of the people, do not train doctors for the people, do not unite with the thousand and more doctors and veterinarians of the old type in the Border Region and do not help them to make progress, then they will actually be helping the witch doctors and showing indifference to the high human and animal mortality rates. . . . Our task is to unite with all intellectuals, artists and doctors of the old type who can be useful, to help them, convert them and transform them. In order to transform them, we must first unite with them. If we do it properly, they will welcome our help.[178]

Mao had more than once stressed the role of Chinese medicine in the expansion of the health work in the border region but emphasized re-education "so that they can acquire a new outlook and new methods to serve the people."[179]

Health and social reforms

As poverty, unhygienic conditions and sanitary problems, illiteracy, superstitious attitude and feudal thinking characterized the socio-economic landscape of the Border Region, the CCP-led health movement was a social reform movement that addressed these problems together to change the old mentality and social norms. Public health education activities for the people were integrated in the programs of literacy, women's equality, nutrition and farming production with the aim of disseminating hygienic and health information, advocating new hygienic and sanitary practice, propagating revolutionary ideas to liberate people from feudal traditions and poverty, and changing people from superstitious to scientific outlook.[180]

The "Administration Guideline of ShanGanNing Regions," issued on May 1, 1941, contained the statement of clause 15 that health administration was to be expanded to enhance the medical and pharmaceutical construction and to recruit more medical personnel for the purpose of reducing people's suffering from diseases. The border-region government was to carry out regular inspection of hygiene and public health, strengthen the research of Chinese medicine and drugs, and expand health education and propaganda. The government sent medical teams to local counties for preventive and curative work and expanded hospitals, published popular readings and pictorials on maternal and infant health, rural health and prevention of infectious diseases, held training classes of midwifery and nursing to produce more health workers and to transform the old ones. The medical teams, who worked with the masses on health matters, were political activists eager to mobilize people for social reforms and the revolution. They emphasized the improvement of sanitation and disease prevention by paying special attention to better managing human excrement and animal dung. People were encouraged to build latrines away from home and to keep animals away from their living quarters. Soldiers and peasants were called upon to dig wells and boil water, as clean water was important to safeguard hygiene and the health of people.

> We try to teach the peasants not to live with their animals and to dig their latrines far from their houses. Ultimately of course the problem is economic. The tempo is slow. We try to educate the primary school children and the soldiers—especially the soldiers, because they are usually in close contact with the villagers, but we wish sometimes were going faster.[181]

The CCP Red Army worked with peasants in producing crops and food supplies with the spirit of self-reliance and self-sustainment. Public health and hygiene work was carried out in the army and villages simultaneously.

A major commitment of the CCP health work was to reduce infant mortality by training midwives in aseptic-procedures of delivery and encouraging pregnant women to go to the trained midwives. Consequently, the risk of neonatal tetanus and septicemia to mothers were reduced, leading to a significant drop in the death rate of women and children. Women during pregnancy would receive better nutrition with extra meat, oil, vegetables and salt; and new babies were allotted locally produced cotton and cloth for clothes.[182] In order to ensure food production and the increase of nutrition, the border-region government curbed opium addiction and provided special care for mothers and children. Women and children were mobilized to report on opium smokers and smugglers who would be reformed into productive workers through education and thought reform programs. These programs and health services for mothers and babies drastically reduced infant mortality and improved the health of mothers. By 1943, the infant mortality rate dropped to 2.8 percent in the border region, compared with the national infant mortality rate of 20 percent.[183]

To change people's old attitude and behavior, health workers and Communist cadres used familiar folk entertainment to convey messages against superstition and witch doctors. The favorite peasant dance "yang-ge" (秧歌) and short skits became popular propaganda tools to disseminate revolutionary ideas and health information and to expose the lies of witch doctors and superstitious ideas. People, watching the shows, would laugh at the witch doctors and silly superstitions, and even their own ignorant behavior. Witch doctors were banned and reformed while traditional Chinese doctors were recruited and updated with modern medical ideas. Ma Haide informed visitors:

> we got them [witch doctors] better jobs—gave them farms—anything as long as they would stop harming the people. The herb doctors, the acupuncturists and the midwives we kept but we gave them training in the essentials of Western medicine. Chinese herb doctors have done an enormous lot of good.[184]

Health cooperatives in counties and towns were the major players in organizing and coordinating health propaganda activities with social reforms against superstition and witch doctors. They gave health talks on hygiene and disease prevention and put on shows of health exhibits with drawings and posters. Festivals and temple fairs were great opportunities for public education and propaganda on health and new ideas. Teams of health workers and cadres would gather large crowds of audience with talks about modern hygiene and sanitation, and they encouraged people to get rid of superstitious beliefs. Women medical workers would mix with the female audience and perform short plays on child rearing and home hygiene. Mobile exhibits on pregnancy, delivery and child rearing went to counties during the festival of International Women's Day on March 8.[185]

Each county had mobile medical teams to respond to emergencies and epidemics. They worked in cooperation with health cooperatives and district health workers in mobilizing peasants to do general cleaning and maintain hygienic conditions. "Walking the mass line" (走群众路线) was a principal method of the CCP-led social reforms, which meant going to the masses, listening to them and letting people take initiatives. Peasants were mobilized with new knowledge of hygiene and sanitation and made to understand that practicing hygiene would cost them little but time and effort. Villages would hold contests to challenge each other for the honor of being the "cleanest village in the district." Local governments, in collaboration with production cooperatives and schools, promoted community health through mass hygiene campaigns and public health education. People's health was of vital importance for the revolution, as it was expressed:

> The mass movements are of central importance to us; all our policies are carried out through them. To carry on a prolonged war and to achieve progress in every field, we have to rely on the masses of the people. We could not rely on bureaucratic methods or a dictatorship if we did not want to fail as the KMT did. We had to mobilize the masses, to awaken, educate and guide them to the goal of self help.[186]

Even with active education and guidance, habits of self-help took time to develop among the common people. Old habits and attitudes were deeply entrenched in superstition and traditional ways of life, which were not easily transformed, especially among the adults. In many cases, when peasants had been taught methods of personal hygiene and prevention of disease, they would, out of habit, continue their old ways of doing things. In contrast, children were eager to practice what they learned about hygiene and health. They received health education and became activists in pushing the practice of hygiene and sanitation at home and in the community. To change the deep-rooted social habits and attitude, the Communist Youth Corps (共青团), in particular, played an active role in promoting hygiene and public health among soldiers and villagers. They carried out propaganda work to encourage soldiers to do the "Three Oughts and Three Noughts—to "obey discipline, be clean, and be polite; and don't drink alcohol, don't smoke, and don't drink cold unboiled water." They even gave lectures on disease prevention and simple remedies, administered first aid, and supervised the construction of latrines.[187] When Norman Bethune arrived in Yanan in 1938 he was impressed that the city was clean and had more latrines than cities ten times its size.[188]

Primary school pupils in Yanan were trained to have the routine of getting up in the morning to clean their teeth, wash their faces, do physical exercises, clean their rooms and hunt down fleas.[189] Children brought home public health knowledge to their families and villagers. In north China, people had the old habit of keeping long fingernails, which often were an unhygienic source. Young students would sing the songs they learned at school to tell people the bad things of keeping long fingernails: "In long fingernails is stored up filth. Put in your mouth and your stomach will hurt; scratch itches and you will get boils. Quickly cut the long nails; don't leave them to store up filth."[190] Children learned the ideas of hygiene and public health along with social reforms and revolution when their textbooks taught hygiene, cooperation and courteousness as much as the glorification of labor and the abolition of feudal practices. The schools were dedicated to making the rural youth fully engaged in the revolutionary cause and the health movement as modern healthy and self-supporting citizens.

Conclusion

The GMD's state medicine and the CCP's people's health demonstrated different emphases in constructing a modern health system that was guided by their different visions of a modern China and shaped by different immediate needs and circumstances. The Nationalist government made significant achievements in building an institutional structure of a centralized health administration system. Institutions of health administration, hospitals and research laboratories were created with the assistance of the LNHO and the RF. National Quarantine Service and regional epidemic prevention bureaus were established to produce vaccines and to tackle outbreaks of epidemic diseases. Despite the continued endeavor of state medicine during the wartime, the GMD's health modernization barely reached the vast rural population in villages, which constituted 85 percent of Chinese society. Modern medical and health services were accessible in urban centers mostly to the educated and commercial classes who could afford to pay for it, leaving the poor to their own wits. The medical service was mainly in the hands of private practitioners, despite the government policy of state medicine. Public hospitals did not provide free medical care for the public, either. The majority of Chinese people still relied on, as they always had, traditional Chinese medicine and folk healings whenever available. In short, state medicine of the Nationalist government was the institutional construction of a central health administration system rather than a state-sponsored national healthcare service to the people. The Nationalist medical elite firmly believed that a national health administration system had to be established first before the delivery of medical service.

The Nationalist government tried to incorporate in the health modernization various rural health stations and projects that had been carried on by missionary organizations, the Rockefeller Foundation, the Rural Reform and Mass Education Movement, universities and local progressive individuals. However, it failed to set up an effective coordinating mechanism to connect these rural projects into a network of rural health modernization. The China Program of the RF tried to create a rural reform movement by using the same groups as the private force to stimulate and to supplement the government on rural health development, but the program was disrupted by the Japanese invasion and the outbreak of war in 1937. While the central health institutions were built with the financial assistance and professional expertise of the League and the RF, local health construction largely relied on provincial governments, as the central government delegated the responsibility to local officials. State medicine was officially adopted by the GMD as the national health policy in 1940 during the war with clear political motivations to gain popular support when the GMD had lost eastern China to Japanese occupation and the CCP was expanding its influence in rural China. The NHA focused its attention on increasing the numbers of county health centers in the implementation of state medicine with limited facilities and personnel. The number of county health centers grew from 162 in 1937 to 1013 in 1945 and to 1440 in 1947 (see Table 3.1). The increase of county health centers was not backed up by an expansion of medical training or increased health budget during the war. As a result, many of them did not have adequate staff or facilities for operation but stayed well on paper. Lower-level bureaucrats often played the number game by setting up a health center in response to the higher-level administration's demand. Some simply turned the anti-opium office into a health center, as Jin Baoshan noted.[191] They did not have the personnel, facilities and funds to operate the center as a health institution. Modernizers of the Nationalist government were good at designing and planning health institutions, but slow in getting things implemented on the ground. There was a bureaucratic indifference permeating the GMD officials, as witnessed by the League's professionals. When the Japanese aggression caused a national crisis in the fall of 1937, calling for most urgent action, the Nanjing officialdom seemed little affected. Dr. Berislav Borčić of the LNHO, who worked at the Central Field Health Station in Nanjing, wrote to Selskar Gunn of the RF:

> Nothing is there except the will of Chinese farmers to die. Nanking mandarins are just a little more mandarin-spirited than the Serbian pashas were [when World War I started]. There are about 120,000 wounded, and available accommodation for not more than half. On the Northern front even less. But we still find time to play mah-jong and enjoy dinner parties. For a whole week my mouth is bitter, very bitter.[192]

Western-educated medical elite occupied the Nationalist leadership of modern health administration. The minister of health and the head of the NHA were almost exclusively American educated PUMC men, who had a close association with the RF and John B. Grant. They were the products of Western medical education and relied on Western models for China's health modernization. With the deep involvement of the RF and the LNHO, the design of the GMD state medicine system was strongly influenced by a combination of the American research-centered and technical-focused model, the British state medicine model of a centralized health administration, and the League of Nation's state medicine model based primarily on continental European experience. The result, however, was a system that could not function in any similar manner of the models they emulated because of the huge gap between China's level of modern medical education and socio-economic conditions and that of the West. The Nationalist efforts at state medicine centered on building the institutional framework of a centralized health administration, whereby the central government delegated the development of local health administration to provincial government. In a sense, the Nationalist state medicine was not able to deliver what the LNHO emphasized, i.e. the state responsibility of providing healthcare to the national population. Stampar explained:

> The idea of State medicine is that the care of health should be a charge upon the people as a whole, not upon persons affected with disease. Sickness is chiefly a product of social conditions, and society as a whole should pay for its prevention.[193]

Referring to the health centers in China, he emphasized that "services of the centres should be free, or at a nominal charge."[194] Chinese health professionals continued the debate over the meaning of state medicine up to the end of the Nationalist rule on mainland China, as healthcare was still a paid service, not available to the majority of people.

Scholars have analyzed several factors that contributed to the Nationalist failure to build up a national healthcare service with a rural health infrastructure. Ka-che Yip argued that lack of funds and manpower, coupled with no land reform, were the reasons. Andrija Stampar seemed to concur with the argument with particular attention to land reform. During his investigation of China's social and health conditions in 1933–1935, Stampar noticed that the landlord system and poverty were the chief reasons for social unrest. Land taxes increased dramatically from the 1920s through the 1940s, with many other levies imposed by the government, putting tremendous pressure on the peasantry. The League's advisors recommended to the Nationalist government land reform as a top priority, but the government either did not agree or did not have the political will to carry it out.[195]

This study demonstrates that, in addition to the aforementioned factors, the GMD's exclusion of old-style Chinese doctors, inadequate communication of public health and work with ordinary people, and the lack of overall socio-economic reforms and improvement also contributed to its limitations in modern health construction. The central government's weak relations with local governments presented another challenge in the implantation of NHA's central plans and guidance. The Nationalist health leaders tried to abolish Chinese medicine even when the people relied on Chinese medical doctors and healers for their medical needs. A full utilization of practitioners of Chinese medicine would have significantly increased the manpower of health work, and helped mediate medical service and modern health institutions between the people and the Nationalist government. Chinese people trusted Chinese medical doctors culturally even when Western medicine gained the official support of the government and the medical elite. Moreover, the service of Chinese medicine doctors was generally much less expensive, an important factor for ordinary people.

To the majority of Chinese people, Western medicine was still an alien concept, much less a practice, due to a high illiteracy rate (over 90 percent in rural China) and traditional way of life. People in rural China were very much isolated from modern metropolis like Shanghai because of poor transportation, communication and poverty in general. The Nationalist health propaganda and education programs, such as lectures, exhibits, radio talks and parades, were geared towards the middle class in cities. Moreover, health propaganda was conducted without a reform of the medical service to the lower classes. One third of the city population did not have access to any medical service.[196] Health propaganda tended to lose effect among the ordinary people when they saw little improvement in the medical service. The gap between the educated upper class and the un-educated lower class presented a significant cultural divide and distrust, in addition to economic status, of different social classes. The health professionals faced a daunting task when they tried to institutionalize modern health in the society without having the illiteracy and poverty problems solved. Different from the CCP's health workers who lived and worked with peasants, the GMD's modern doctors and nurses were socially and culturally distanced from ordinary Chinese. They wore modern attire and white medical uniforms, and had to be carried to rural communities by the man-pushed wheelbarrow cart, rather than walking to peasant homes and being immersed in rural society. (See the image of the traveling clinic of Gaoqiao in chapter 2.) Among the small number of modern-trained doctors, there was the tendency that the better qualified sought to serve the government as health officials or took a private practice in big cities for social prestige and financial gains. The less qualified and inadequate ones would staff the *xian* health centers if they had no other options. Very few would choose to go and serve the people in the most needed areas. Consequently, the county-village modern health construction stayed well on paper, with few having the personnel and facilities to fully function.

The lack of commitment of the Nationalist political leaders to modern health construction posed a serious challenge for health modernizers. The Nationalist central government allocated large sums for the anti-communist suppression campaigns and limited funds for health programs when Jiang Jieshi focused his attention on eliminating the CCP. Only when health programs were used to win the hearts and minds of people in the Jiangxi campaigns against the CCP did the Nationalist government provide funds to mobilize local governments and private groups in an overall effort to improve agriculture, literacy and health in 1934. International assistance was significant for the GMD health modernization. The NHA and local health programs received significant financial support from the RF and the LNHO for research, training, and institution-building.

The Communists strove and sometimes throve in rural China where the Nationalists faltered. The CCP's health policy was guided by its revolutionary goals of changing the society and liberating the people from social, economic and health sufferings. The CCP leaders understood the fundamental importance of medical and health work in the overall revolutionary pursuit. The Communists relied on limited modern medical facilities and personnel and used traditional Chinese medical practices and herbs to tackle diseases and military wounds. They encouraged the education and practice of Western medicine but also actively recruited old-style medical doctors and creatively produced Chinese medical supplies at the same time. Mao Zedong and other CCP leaders recognized the usefulness of Chinese medicine and appreciated the contributions of old-style doctors in treating wounded soldiers and caring for the sick. Different from the Nationalists, the CCP promoted the unity of Chinese and Western medicines and encouraged them to learn from each other.

Health education and service work were incorporated in land reform, women's liberation, literacy movement, arts and entertainment, anti-superstition, and farming improvement. The party led movements against old shamanism and superstitions of spirits and gods and created model villages. Short-term training classes and training on the job were effectively used to produce health administrators, physician assistants, nurses, midwives, and health aids who could deal with basic medical and health needs in the military and rural villages. The CCP emphasized that it was the health professionals' responsibility to seek problems of the people and direct their research toward the problems to bring about social changes.

Situated in rural regions, the CCP health workers lived and worked with the peasants. As politically devoted communists, the health professionals carried out the task of educating, guiding and awakening the peasant masses with revolutionary ideas, hygiene and sanitation knowledge, and provision of medical services. They focused on the masses—peasants and soldiers—to motivate and guide them to take initiatives on hygiene and sanitation, instead of treating them as passive receivers of medical and health information. Private enterprises such as Chinese health and medical clinics, health cooperatives and production cooperatives were interconnected with local leaders playing the major role. Popular support for the CCP made "walking the mass line" productive, and in turn, the CCP gained people's trust via land and social reforms.

A comparative look at the GMD's and CCP's efforts at popular health education and propaganda indicates that they both emphasized disease prevention by disseminating knowledge of hygiene and sanitation. The difference was the methods of conducting the health propaganda. While the GMD directed the lectures and exhibits of propaganda, training and awakening at the people, the CCP mobilized the people to participate in health movements and do things themselves to achieve the awakening and education. The GMD's efforts often took the formality of parade and meetings, and general cleaning campaigns led by government officials in cities; whereas the CCP organized local health cooperatives and production cooperatives to work with villagers on hygiene contests and model village competitions. Without the luxury of indulging in the theoretical debate on health systems as the GMD medical elite did, the CCP health professionals of modern medicine and Chinese medicine had to solve many immediate problems with limited resources, often in very primitive conditions, despite international aid. The measure for a good doctor in CCP-controlled areas was whether the doctor would serve the people selflessly.

Notes

1 Ka-che Yip, *Health and National Reconstruction in Nationalist China: The Development of Modern Health Services, 1928–1937* (Ann Arbor, Association for Asian Studies, Inc., 1995), 26.

2 Lawrence M. Chen, *Public Health in National Reconstruction* (Nanjing, Council of International Affairs, 1937).

3 Yip, *Health and National Reconstruction*, 179.

4 Gao Xi, "Between the State and the Private Sphere: Chinese State Medicine Movement, 1930–1949," in *Science, Public Health and the State in Modern Asia*, 144–160.
5 Wu Lien-teh, "Fundamentals of State Medicine," *Chinese Medical Journal*, vol. 51, no. 6 (1937), 773–780, 778–9.
6 Ibid., 779.
7 Ibid.
8 Yip, *Health and National Reconstruction*, 93. Footnote 79. See James Yen to Dr. Stampar, May 18, 1932, folder 600.1, box 85, CMB, Inc. RAC.
9 Daniel Taylor-Ide and Carl Taylor, *Just and Lasting Change: When Communities Own Their Futures* (Baltimore: The Johns Hopkins University Press, 2002), 97–98.
10 Herbert Day Lamson, *Social Pathology in China: A Source Book for the Study of Problems of Livelihood, Health and the Family* (Shanghai, Commercial Press, 1935).
11 Dinner and Conference at the President's Residence, Nanking, January 7, 1930, Minutes drafted by Liu Ruiheng, and Rajchman to Liu, January 11, 1930. Quoted in Iris Borowy, *Uneasy Encounter*, 211–212 and footnote 34.
12 Wu, "Fundamentals of State Medicine," 777.
13 John B. Grant made the point clear in his article "State Medicine – A Logical Policy for China," *National Medical Journal of China*, vol. 14 (February 1928), 79; and then with T. M. Peng, he made the same argument in their publication, "Survey of Urban Public Health Practice in China," *The Chinese Medical Journal*, vol. 48 (October 1934), 1078.
14 Chen Haifeng, *Zhongguo weisheng baojian shi* [History of Health Care in China] (Shanghai: Shanghai kexue jishu chubanshe, 1992), 21.
15 Hsi-ju Chu and Daniel G. Lai, "Distribution of Modern-Trained Physicians in China," *Chinese Medical Journal*, vol. 49 (1935), 542–552; and Wu Liande, "Medical Renaissance in China," *Science*, vol. XX, no. 4 (April 1936), 256–266.
16 "Communicable Disease Report for 1942" in 19 provinces. The United Office of Plague Prevention during the War [zhanshi fangyi lianhe banshichu], chuan zong hao 372, juan hao708 (372–708), Second Historical Archives of China, Nanjing (Second Archives hereafter).
17 Huang Zifang, "Zhongguo weisheng chuyi [On Public Health in China]," *The National Medical Journal of China*, vol. 13 (1927), 338–354.
18 Chen, *Zhongguo weisheng baojian shi*, 15.
19 Wu, "Fundamentals of State Medicine," 777; and "Medical Renaissance," *Science*, 264.
20 *Health Policies during the Tutelage Phase* (Nanjing: Interior Ministry of the Republic of China, 1928), Nanjing Library. The Nationalist government announced that the tutelage phase of the Nationalist revolution started in 1928.
21 For the proposal, see Ka-che Yip, *Health and National Reconstruction*, 29–32. Different Chinese groups competed for the use of British Boxer Indemnity for industrial development and education. See Teow See Heng's book, *Japan's Cultural Policy toward China, 1918–1931: A Comparative Perspective* (MA: Harvard University Asia Center, 1999), chapter 4 on "The American and British Cultural Approaches" and chapter 5 on "The Issue of Cultural Imperialism."
22 An interesting study of Zhongshan county of Guangdong demonstrated the complex relations between the Nationalist government and local controls, and the policy negotiations between public and private interests. See Venus Viana, "Modernizing Zhongshan: The Implementation of Nation-Building Policies and Responses of the Local People, 1930–1949," PhD. Dissertation (School of Humanities and Social Science, Hong Kong University of Science and Technology, 2012.)
23 In 1929 when Liu Ruiheng was at the Ministry of Health, he wrote to Roger S. Greene at PUMC on the possible candidate for the directorship of the National Epidemic Prevention Bureau: "Dr. Grant agrees with me that Dr. Lim [C. E. Lim, Lin Zhongyang] would be a far more suitable person than Dr. Wu Lien-teh in this post." Liu Ruiheng to Greene, June 4, 1929, Liu Ruiheng papers, PUMC archives, #2144, Beijing. See also Grant's correspondence regarding Wu Liande and the Epidemic Prevention Bureau at RAC.

24 Yip, *Health and National Reconstruction*, 45–46.
25 "Grant Reminiscences," 271. For the politics of personal connections in this episode, see also Bullock, *An American Transplant*, 152–153.
26 Memo to Greene, July 27, 1927, folder 466, box 66, RG IV 2B9, CMB Inc., RAC.
27 Yip, *Health and National Reconstruction*, 47–48.
28 Margherita Zanasi, "Exporting Development: The League of Nations and Republican China," *Comparative Studies in Society and History* 49.1 (2007),143–169.
29 Letter from John Grant to Heiser, December 2, 1924, folder 601, box 202, series IHB/D, RG6, RAC.
30 Ibid.
31 "Mission of Dr. Rajchman in the Far East," Confidential Circular 1, 1926, February 5, 1926, League of Nations Archive, Directors' Meetings, p. 23, quoted in Iris Borowy, *Uneasy Encounters*, 206, footnote 5.
32 Iris Borowy, "Thinking Big—League of Nations Efforts towards a Reformed National Health System in China," in *Uneasy Encounters*, 205–228.
33 LNHO, *Annual Report of the Health Organization for 1929* (July 1930), 15.
34 Bullock, *An American Transplant*, 154.
35 "Co-operation, in Health Matters, between the National Government of the Republic of China and the League of Nations," *Quarterly Bulletin of the Health Organization*, vol. 5 (1936), 1088.
36 M. M. Hamilton to Stanley Hornbeck, "Memorandum," March 10, 1930, file 893.12/2 League Survey, Record Group 29, National Archives, Washington D.C.; Nelson Johnson to Secretary of State, Cordell Hull, Dispatch #237, June 8, 1934, file 893.12/85, Record Group 59, National Archives. Quoted in Bullock, *An American Transplant*, 139, footnote 14.
37 "Co-operation, in Health Matters," *Quarterly Bulletin of the Health Organization*, vol. 5 (1936), 1089.
38 Yang Shangchi, "National Quarantine Service and Dr. Wu Liande," *Chinese Journal of Medical History* 18.1 (1988), 29–32; and Wu Liande and Wu Changyao, *Reports of the National Quarantine Service*, (Shanghai: National Quarantine Service, 1932–1935).
39 Wu Lien-teh, J. W. H. Chun, R. Pollitzer, and C. Y. Wu, *Cholera: A Manual for the Medical Profession in China* (Shanghai: National Quarantine Service, 1934).
40 Ibid., iv.
41 Jin Baoshan, "Hopes on Peiping Health Authority," *Zhonghua yixue zazhi*, vol. 14, no. 5 (1928), 3.
42 "Co-operation, in Health Matters," *Quarterly Bulletin of the Health Organization*, vol. 5 (1936), 1083.
43 "Technical Cooperation with Certain Governments," *Quarterly Bulletin of the Health Organization*, vol. 1, no. 3 (September 1932), 403–414, 404.
44 Roger S. Greene's interview with Dr. Rajchman, December 21, 1930, Folder 155, Box 22, CMB, Inc., RAC.
45 Iris Borowy, *Coming to Terms with World Health: The League of Nations Health Organisation 1921–1946* (Frankfurt: Peter Lang Publishers, 2009).
46 Martin David Dubin, "The League of Nations Health Organization," in *International Health Organizations and Movements, 1918–1939*, ed. Paul Weindling (Cambridge: Cambridge University Press, 1995), 72.
47 Roger S. Greene's interview with Dr. Rajchman, December 21, 1930.
48 The Central Field Health Station was renamed as the National Institute of Health in 1941.
49 "Regulations Governing the Organization of the National Economic Council and its Bureaux, Committees and Offices, 1934," in *Annexes to the Report to the Council of the League of Nations of Its Technical Delegate on His Mission in China from Date of Appointment Until April 1, 1934* (Shanghai, North China Daily News and Herald, 1934).
50 Yip, *Health and National Reconstruction*, 57.

51 "Report of the Central Field Health Station" (Nanjing: Central Field Health Station, 1935); and "Technical Co-operation with Certain Governments," *Quarterly Bulletin of the Health Organization,* vol. 1, no. 3, 412.
52 A. Stampar, "Observations of a Rural Health Worker," *New England Journal of Medicine*, vol. 218, no. 24 (1938).
53 Borowy, *Uneasy Encounters*, 213.
54 Ibid.
55 For the bureaucratic structure of the National Health Administration and its affiliated institutions in 1937, see Yip, *Health and National Reconstruction*, appendix 1.
56 Jin Baoshan, "A Brief History of Health Development of the Republic of China," *Yishi zazhi* [Journal of Medical History] vol. 2 (1948), 18–25. See also Gong Chun, "Health Organization of the Republic of China," *Zhonghua yishi zazhi* [Chinese Journal of Medical History] vol. 19, no. 2 (1989), 80–85, 81.
57 Jin Baoshan, "Rural Health Work Report of NHA," *Zhonghua yixue zazhi* 19.5 (1933), 755–75.
58 Jin Baoshan, "A Brief History of Health Development," 19.
59 Jin Baoshan, "Rural Health Work Report of NHA."
60 In addition to Li Ting-an's survey report, there were other proposals and studies, such as Zhu Dian, *Jianshe sanqian ge nongcun yiyuan* [Building Three Thousand Rural Hospitals] (Society for Rural Medical Reform, 1933); and Xue Jianwu, *Zhongguo nongcun weisheng xingzheng* [Rural Health Administration in China] (Shanghai: Shangwu zhubanshe, 1937).
61 Li Tin-an, "Report of Rural Public Health in China," *Zhonghua yixue zazhi* (1934), 1113–1201. See also T. A. Li, "Summary Report on Rural Public Health Practice in China," *Chinese Medical Journal*, vol. 48 (October 1934), 1086–1090.
62 Jin Baoshan and Xu Shijin, "Current Public Health Facilities in Provinces and Municipalities," *Zhonghua yixue zazhi*, vol. 23, no. 11 (1937), 1235.
63 Jin Baoshan and Xu Shijin, "An Overview of Health Facilities during the War," *Zhonghua yixue zazhi*, vol. 27, no. 3 (1941), 187.
64 Jin and Xu, "Current Public Health Facilities," 1236.
65 Ibid.
66 On Jiangxi and the New Life Movement, see Federica Ferlanti, "The New Life Movement in Jiangxi Province, 1934–1938," *Modern Asian Studies*, vol. 44, no. 5 (2010), 961–1000; James C. Thomson, Jr. *When China Faced West*: *American Reformers in Nationalist China, 1928–1937* (Cambridge: Harvard University Press, 1969), 151–174, 198–220; and Ka-che Yip, *Health and National Reconstruction*, 86–93.
67 "Health Work in Jiangxi," *Chinese Medical Journal*, vol. 48, no. 11 (1934), 1173.
68 Jin Baoshan, "A Brief History of Health Development," 20. These statistics cannot be verified but slightly different data appeared in Jin and Xu, "Current Public Health Facilities," 1235–1248.
69 For the details of their organization and health responsibility, see Ka-che Yip, *Health and National Reconstruction*, appendix 2.
70 Jin and Xu, "Current Public Health Facilities," 1237.
71 "Report by Dr. A. Stampar on His Missions to China," *Quarterly Bulletin of the Health Organization*, vol. 5 (1936), 1090–1126, 1122–23.
72 Ibid., 1091.
73 A. Stampar, "Observations of a Rural Health Worker," *New England Journal of Medicine*, vol. 218, no. 24 (1938), 994.
74 Wu Lien-teh, "Fundamentals of State Medicine," 777.
75 Hsi-ju Chu and Daniel G. Lai, "Distribution of Modern-Trained Physicians in China," *Chinese Medical Journal*, vol. 49 (1935), 542–552.
76 Wu Lien-teh, "Fundamentals of State Medicine," 777–78.
77 "Initial Year of the Medical Education Program," folder 27, box 3, series 601, RG1, RAC.

78 "Report by Dr. A. Stampar on His Missions to China," 1117–1118.
79 Knud Faber, *Report on Medical Schools in China* (Geneva: League of Nations Health Organization, 1931).
80 "Report by Dr. A. Stampar on His Missions to China," 1118.
81 For medical colleges and schools in Nationalist China in 1936, see Ka-che Yip, *Health and National Reconstruction*, appendix 3.
82 Tina P. Johnson, *Childbirth in Republican China.*
83 "Report by Dr. A. Stampar on His Missions to China," 1119.
84 Ibid., 1118.
85 Socrates Litsios, "Selskar Gunn and China: The Rockefeller Foundation's 'Other' Approach to Public Health," *Bulletin of the History of Medicine*, vol. 79 (2005), 295–318.
86 Selskar Gunn, "China Program Progress Report for the Period 1 July 1935–15 February 1937" and appendixes, folder 130, box 12, series 601, RG 1, RAC. The China Program collaborated with the National Health Administration and the Ministry of Education in various aspects of training of health professionals. See Gunn's reports and correspondence at RAC.
87 James Thomson, Jr. *While China Faced West*, 122–150; Bullock, *An American Transplant*, 157–160; and Yip, *Health and National Reconstruction*, 93–95.
88 K. K. Chen and Carl F. Schmidt, *Ephedrine and Related Substances* (London: The Williams & Wilkins Company, 1930).
89 Faber, *Report on Medical Schools in China*, 8, 33.
90 "Comprehensive Report of the Work of the Special Nanjing Municipal Government, 1930," Nanjing Municipal Archives, 1001–1732, p. 175, Second Archives, Nanjing.
91 Yu Yunxiu studied medicine in Japan. His proposal, in a degree, was inspired by the Meiji abolition of *Hanyi* (Chinese medicine) in Japan during its modernization movement. Japan did not abolish the use of Chinese drugs. Instead, it made further studies of the subject. Influenced by their understanding of Japanese Meiji Reforms, some Chinese medical modernizers tended to think of the value of Chinese drugs but not Chinese medicine. In the proposals that the Nanjing Municipal Health Bureau made to the Health Ministry, Hu Ding-An recommended the planting of Chinese herbs in public parks for pragmatic use.
92 Hu Ding-An submitted eight proposals that included the training of health administrators, establishment of criteria for health administrators, registering physicians, prohibiting dissemination of unscientific medical and pharmaceutical information, establishing model health districts in every province and municipality to promote public health, creation of medical material production factories, building a running water system in the capital city Nanjing, and planting Chinese medicinal herbs in public parks. ("Comprehensive Report of the Work of the Special Nanjing Municipal Government, 1930," 175–82, Nanjing Municipal Archives, 1001–1732.)
93 Zhao Hongjun, *Jindai zhongxiyi zhenglun shi* [History of the Debate between Chinese Medicine and Western Medicine] (Hefei: Anhui kexue jishu chubanshe, 1989), 111–121; and Deng Tietao, *Zhongyi jindai shi* [Modern History of Chinese Medicine] (Guangzhou: Guangdong gaodeng jiaoyu chubanshe, 1999); and Cai Jingfeng, Li Qinghua and Zhang Binghuan, eds., *Zhongguo yixue tongshi: xiandai juan* [A Comprehensive History of Medicine in China: Modern volume] (Beijing: Renmin weisheng chubanshe, 1999).
94 Zhao Hongjun, *Jindai zhongxiyi zhenglun shi*, 114–115.
95 Different discussions can be found in Sean Hsiang-lin Lei, *Neither Donkey nor Horse: Medicine and the Struggle over China's Modernity* (Chicago: University of Chicago Press, 2014); and Bridie Andrews, *The Making of Modern Chinese Medicine, 1850–1960* (Vancouver: University of British Columbia Press, 2014). Their works explain, from different perspectives, the changes of Chinese medicine in a modernizing society.

96 Numerous schools of Chinese medicine were established by prominent doctors of Chinese medicine since the 1910s as a way to improve the reputation and practice of Chinese medicine. These schools included Shanghai Chinese Medical School founded by Ding Ganren (丁甘仁) and Xie Liheng (谢利恒) in 1915–1917, Shenzhou Medical School by Bao Shishen (包识生) in 1918, Guangdong Chinese Medicine College by Lu Naitong (卢乃潼) in 1924, Chinese Medicine School in Shanghai by Yun Tieqiao (恽铁樵) in 1925, Chinese Medicine College by Lu Yuanlei (陆渊雷) and Zhang Cigong (章次公) in Shanghai in 1930, Guoyi (national medicine) College by Xiao Longyou (肖龙友) and Kong Bohua (孔伯华) in Beijing, and many other schools in Hubei, Guangxi, Hankou, Xiamen, Hangzhou, Jinan, Suzhou, Wuxi. They printed lots of teaching materials of Chinese medicine and trained Chinese medical specialists, who became key figures of post-1949 Chinese medicine.

97 Chen Guofu and Chen Lifu were brothers and they were powerful men of the Nationalist Party (GMD). They held a balanced view of Chinese medicine as a knowledge system and a proven practice. Chen Guofu's books, such as *Weisheng zhi dao* [The Way of Health], *Yizheng mantan* [Ramdon Thoughts on Health Administration], and *Ertong weisheng ge* [Children's Songs of Hygiene], contributed to the interaction and mutual learning of Western and Chinese medicines in the Nationalist era.

98 Yip, *Health and National Reconstruction*, 60.

99 Zhang Zanchen, *Feizhi Zhongyi an kangzheng zhi jinguo* [The Clash over the Abolition of Chinese Medicine] (Shanghai wenmin shuju, 1929), 21.

100 Propaganda work was an essential element of the Nationalist government to spread new ideas to the public. Public health was one of the areas where much propaganda was done. For the local effort of propaganda work, see Christopher A. Reed, "Propaganda by the Book: Contextualizing and Reading the Zhejiang GMD's 1929 Textbook *Essentials for Propaganda Workers*," *Frontiers of History in China*, vol. 10, no. 1 (March 2015), 96–125.

101 *Guideline for the Propaganda of Health Movement* (Nanjing: Propaganda Department of the GMD Central Executive Committee, 1929), 4, Nanjing Municipal Library.

102 Sun Yat-sen defined the three principles of the people—People's Nation, People's Livelihood, and People's Rights—as the basic goals of the Nationalist revolution.

103 *Guideline for the Propaganda of Health Movement*.

104 Documents on public health practice in counties and village towns, public health, 1001-5-30, Archives of Jiangsu Province, Nanjing.

105 *Shanghai huanjing weisheng zhi* [Shanghai Sanitation and Hygiene], 262, Shanghai Municipal Archives.

106 *Shoudu weisheng* [Hygiene of the Capital], vol. 1, 1929, p. 12, 1001-4-128, Nanjing Municipal Archives.

107 According to the Sino-Dutch agreement, "65 percent of the Indemnity of 1901 Boxer Protocol will be used for conservancy work while the remaining 35 percent shall be devoted to cultural purposes." The half a million came from the 65 percent. "Nanjing Built Running Water and Sewage Systems in 1930–1932." 1001-1-1245, Nanjing Municipal Archives.

108 *Shoudu weisheng*.

109 *Shi nian lai zhi Nanjing* [Nanjing in Ten Years], p. 102, Public Health (1001 (2)–1737: 1, Nanjing Municipal Archives.

110 "Comprehensive Report of the Work of the Special Nanjing Municipal Government, 1930," pp. 214–15. 1001–1732, Nanjing Municipal Archives.

111 *Shi nian lai zhi Nanjing*, pp. 103–104.

112 "Comprehensive Report of the Work of the Special Nanjing Municipal Government, 1930," 214–15.

113 "Smallpox Vaccination Training Centers," documents of the Executive Yuan of Republic of China, 1001- (2)-1562, Second Archives.

114 "Report of Health Movement, October 1928–March 1929," p. 216. 1001–1732, Nanjing Municipal Archives.
115 Beiping Health Bureau, Radio Health Lecture, the 78th week, Feb. 26, pp. 68–72, 1936, J5-3-93, Beijing Municipal Archives,.
116 Beiping Health Bureau, Radio Health Lecture, the 78th week, Feb. 26, 1936, pp. 68–72, J5-3-93, Beijing Municipal Archives.
117 Cover of "Special Edition of the 15th health campaign" (Shanghai: Guangxie shuju, 1936).
118 Document No. 321 of the Special Municipality of Beiping, 1928, J23-2-6, Beijing Municipal Archives.
119 Beiping Health Bureau, "radio lecture on health methods and manuscripts," October 1935–April 1937, J5-1-211, Beijing Municipal Archives.
120 1936 manuscripts for radio hygiene lectures, Beijing Health Bureau, J5-1-178, Beijing Municipal Archives.
121 Health Department of Beiping, 1928, J29-3-875, pp. 14–15, 10–11, Beijing Municipal Archives.
122 Beiping Municipal Health Bureau, "Change of Name from Exhibition Hall to Exhibition Room," 1935, J1-3-67, pp. 5, 46–47, Beijing Municipal Archives.
123 Health Exhibition Institute, 1928, J2-1-4, p. 14–15, Beijing Municipal Archives.
124 *"1929 World Fair at West Lake" Tour Guide*, (Hangzhou, 1929), Nanjing Municipal Library.
125 "On the Society of Health Education in China, Summary Report of 1935–1946," 530–14, Second Archives.
126 "School Hygiene, July 1927," pp. 3–12, Beijing Health Bureau J4-1-266, Beijing Municipal Archives.
127 Beiping Education Bureau document, 1930, p. 1–2, J4-1-380, Beijing Municipal Archives.
128 Beiping Education Bureau, Feb. 1931, J4-1-388, Beijing Municipal Archives.
129 "Statistics gathered in 1931," Beiping Health Bureau, J2-3-232, Beijing Municipal Archives.
130 "General Outline of the Plan for 1933 School Hygiene Practice by the Hygiene Commission of Beiping Social Bureau," Beiping Health Bureau, J2-3-232, Beijing Municipal Archives.
131 "Implementation plan for municipal school hygiene in Beiping," J2-3-232-172, Beijing Municipal Archives.
132 *Nanjing in Ten Years*, chapter 8 "Public Health," p. 102, 1001 (2)–1737: 1, Nanjing municipal archives.
133 Nanjing Health Bureau, 1935–1937, 1001-4-117, Nanjing municipal archives.
134 "Report of Health Movement, October 1928–March 1929," pp. 216–219, 1001–1732, Nanjing Municipal Archives.
135 See Chinese school hygiene posters at https://www.nlm.nih.gov/hmd/chineseposters/hygiene.html.
136 National Beiping University Medical College, Department of Hygiene and Public Health, 1933, p. 82–85, J29-1-881, Beijing Municipal Archives.
137 Beijing Daily publisher, Feb. 22, 1934, Health Bureau, J5-1-37, Beijing Municipal Archives.
138 Barnes and Watt "The Influence of War on China's Modern Health Systems," in *Medical Transitions in Twentieth-Century China,* ed. Bridie Andrews and Mary Brown Bullock (Bloomington: Indiana University Press, 2014), 227–243.
139 For detailed studies of wartime health construction, see John R Watt, *Saving Lives in Wartime China: How Medical Reformers Built Modern Healthcare Systems Amid War and Epidemics, 1928–1945* (Leiden: E. J. Brill, 2014); and Nicole Elizabeth Barnes, "Protecting the National Body: Gender and Public Health in Southwest China during the War of Resistance against Japan, 1937–1945," PhD Diss. (University of California-Irvine, 2012).

140 Jin Baoshan, "A Brief History of Health Development," 21.
141 C. C. Chen, "Report of Szechuan Provincial Health Administration for 1941," box 218, series 3, RG5, RAC.
142 Jin Baoshan, "A Brief History of Health Development," 22.
143 Ibid., 18–25.
144 In 1927, the Jiang Jieshi-led GMD forces attacked and killed CCP members and labor activists in Shanghai, Wuhan and Guangzhou, which effectively ended the United Front of the GMD and CCP, and started the GMD suppression of the Communist movement in China. For a general reading, see Jonathan D. Spence, *In Search for Modern China* (New York: W. W. Norton and Company, 1990), 348–360.
145 Mao Zedong, "Be Concerned with the Wellbeing of the Masses, Pay Attention to Methods of Work," in *Selected Works of Mao Tse-tung*, vol. I (Peking: Foreign Languages Press, 1965), 147–52.
146 John R. Watt, *Saving Lives in Wartime China*, 77–78.
147 Mu Jing, *A Brief Biography of Fu Lianzhang* (Beijing: Kexue puji chubanshe, 1980).
148 Mao Zedong, "Why Is It that the Red Political Power Can Exist in China," *Collected Works*, vol. 1 (Beijing, Foreign Languages Press, 1965), 70.
149 Regarding Fu Lianzhang, He Fusheng, and Dai Jimim, see Feng Caizhang and Li Baoding, *Hongjun Jiangling* [Red Army Generals] (Beijing: Kexue jishu chubanshe, 1991).
150 Chen, *Zhongguo weisheng baojian shi*, 30–32.
151 Ibid., 32.
152 Zhu Chao, *Zhongwai yixue jiaoyu shi* [History of Chinese and Foreign Medical Education] (Shanghai: Shanghai yike daxue, 1988), 135.
153 Tang Yizhen was the first wife of Lu Dingyi, a veteran CCP leader who served as Minister of Propaganda and Culture of PRC.
154 Fan Pu, *Zhongguo yixue shi*, [History of Chinese Medicine] (Guizhou: Guizhou remin chubanshe, 1988).
155 Zhang Ruguang, Guo Laofu and He Manqiu, *Zhongguo gongnong hongjun weisheng gongzuo shilue* [A Brief History of the Health Work of China's Workers and Peasants Red Army] (Beijing: Jiefangjun chubanshe, 1989); and Gao Enxian, *Xin Zhongguo yufang yixue lishi ziliao xuanbian* (1) [Selection of Historical Documents on Preventive Medicine of New China] (Beijing: Renmin junyi chubanshe, 1986).
156 Sun Shuyun, *The Long March* (London: HarperCollins Publishers, 2006).
157 Lillian M. Li, *Fighting Famine in North China: State, Market, and Environmental Decline, 1690s–1990s* (Stanford, CA: Stanford University Press, 2007); and Sun Shuyun, *The Long March.*
158 Li Lixia, "1928–1930 nian nianjin shangxi zaihuang yimin wenti," [Famine and Migrants of Shanxi during 1928–1930], *Fangzai keji xueyuan xuebao*, vol. 8, no. 4 (2006), 27–30.
159 H. M. Jettmar, "Plague in Shansi and Shensi," *Chinese Medical Journal*, vol. 46, no. 4 (April 1932), 429–435.
160 Shanxi Province and Shanxi Social Science Academy of Archives, *Selected Documents of ShanGanNing Border-Region Government*, vol. 3 (Beijing: Dangan chubanshe, 1987).
161 Xi'an Incident: In December 1936 when Jiang Jieshi went to Xi'an to mobilize the soldiers in a campaign against the CCP, the soldiers under the command of Zhang Xueliang and Yang Hucheng kidnapped Jiang in an attempt to force him to unite with the CCP to fight against the Japanese who had invaded China. It was ironic that it was the CCP representative Zhou Enlai who helped negotiate the release of Jiang on Christmas Day after Jiang verbally promised to stop the civil war with the CCP and to fight against the Japanese.
162 See map at http://dangshi.people.com.cn/GB/151935/164962/9786299.html, accessed November 6, 2014.
163 Mark Selden, *China in Revolution: The Yenan Way Revisited* (New York: M.E. Sharpe, Inc., 1995); and Pauline B. Keating, *Two Revolutions: Village Reconstruction and the*

Cooperative Movement in Northern Shaanxi, 1934–1945 (CA: Stanford University Press, 1997).

164 Zhang Qi'an, "Shanganning bianqu de yiliao weisheng gonzuo he yide jianshe," [Shanganning Border Region's Medical and Health Work and Ethics], *Chinese Medical Ethics*, no. 3, (2001)), 57–58.

165 The Dixie Mission was the United States Army Observation Group in Yanan during 22 July 1944–11 March 1947. It was the first effort of the U.S. to establish official relations with the Communist Party of China and its military forces.

166 Gunther Stein, *The Challenge of Red China* (London: Pilot Press, 1945), 216.

167 Agnes Smedley, "Hospitals in China: A Contrast; Progress of the Fourth Army Scientific Methods." *Manchester Guardian*, January 17, 1939.

168 Sydney Gordon and Ted Allan, *The Scalpel, the Sword: The Story of Dr. Norman Bethune* (New York: Monthly Review Press, 1952); Edgar A. Porter, *The People's Doctor: George Hatem and China's Revolution* (Honolulu: University of Hawaii Press, 1997); Sheng Xiangong, *An Indian Freedom fighter in China: A Tribute to Dr. D. S. Kotnis* (Beijing: Foreign Language Press, 1983).

169 Gunther Stein, *The Challenge of Red China*, 217.

170 Ma Haide held a major health advisor position in the CCP throughout the war years. He and his family remained in China after 1949. He held a high health position in PRC and made great contributions to eliminating venereal disease and leprosy in the country.

171 B. R. Deepak, *India–China Relations in the First Half of the 20th Century* (New Delhi: A. P.H. Publishing Corporation, 2001), 126, footnote 32.

172 Chen, *Zhongguo weisheng baojian shi*, 36–37.

173 Ibid., 36–46; and John Watt, *Saving Lives*, 253–298.

174 China Medical University (中国医科大学) was relocated to Shengyang in 1946 and merged with the Manchurian Medical University and the Shengyang Medical College to form a major medical university in northeast China. Wang Bin served as the president for a decade before he was appointed Vice Minister of Health in 1953.

175 On Zhu Lian's discovery, see Kim Taylor, *Chinese Medicine in Early Communist China, 1945–1963* (London: Routledge, 2005); and Ka Wai Fan, "Pavlovian Theory and the Scientification of Acupuncture in 1950s China," *New Perspectives on the Research of Chinese Culture* (Springer, 2013), 137–145.

176 Mao Zedong, "On the United Front in Cultural Work," *Selected Works* III (Peking: Foreign Language Press, 1967), 185.

177 Yang Lifu, *Fenghuo xiaoyan zhong de baiyi zhanshi* [White-Coated Warriors Amidst the Fire of Battles] (Chengdu: Chengdu keji daxue chubanshe, 1991).

178 Mao Zedong, "On the United Front in Cultural Work," 185–186.

179 Mao Zedong, "On Coalition Government," *Selected Works* III (Peking: Foreign Language Press, 1967), 155.

180 On the Communist literacy education programs, see Di Luo, "Reading and Writing Modernity: Rural Literacy Education in the Communist Base Areas in Shanxi in the 1930s–1940s," and Mark McConaghy, "Language, Labor, and Revolutionary Consciousness: Notes towards an Understanding of Mass Literacy Arts in 1940's Yanan," both papers were presented at Association for Asian Studies Conference in Philadelphia, March 2014.

181 Robert Payne, *Journey to Red China* (London: William Heinemann, 1947), 97.

182 Hsu Yung-ying, *A Survey of the Shensi-Kansu-Ninghsia Border Region* (New York: Institute of Pacific Relations, 1945), 49.

183 C. K. Chu, "The Modern Public Health Movement in China," in *Voices from Unoccupied China*, ed. H.F. MacNair (Chicago: University of Chicago Press, 1944).

184 Robert Payne, *China Awake* (London: Dodd, Mead and Company, 1947), 358–61.

185 Chen, *Zhongguo weisheng baojian shi*, 43–44.

186 Gunther Stein, *The Challenge of Red China*, 175.

187 Edgar Snow, *Random Notes on Red China, 1936–1945* (Cambridge: Harvard University Press, 1968), 54.
188 Norman Bethune, "The University in the Caves." *China Today*, 4:13 (September 1938).
189 Jack Chen, *China Today*, 4. September 14, 1938.
190 Jack Belden, *China Shakes the World* (New York: Monthly Reviews Press, 1949), 119.
191 Jin Baoshan, "A Brief History of Health Development."
192 Gunn cited Borčić in his letter to Fosdick, November 5, 1937, folder 180, box 20, series 100, RG1.1, RF, RAC.
193 "Report by Dr. A. Stampar on His Missions to China," 1121.
194 Ibid., 1120–21.
195 Grant recalled the League's advice on land reform in his "Reminiscences," 233.
196 Wu Lien-teh, "Fundamentals of State Medicine," 777.

4 People's health and socialist reconstruction

Introduction

The People's Republic of China (PRC) was founded on October 1, 1949, after the Communists defeated the Nationalists in a civil war during 1946–1949. The Nationalists retreated to Taiwan and the Communists unified the mainland. The period of 1949–1953 was the phase of political consolidation and economic recovery, but the task was complicated and challenged by the Korean War. China was divided into six major administrative regions after the CCP took power, and a tripartite structure of the party, the military and the administration formed the governing system. In the phase of consolidation and unification of China, the CCP-led government carried out major land reforms, nationalization of business enterprises, clean-ups of social vices of prostitution and opium addition, massive sanitation movements and disease prevention campaigns, recovery of economic production, and participation in the Korean War. Local governments mobilized the masses to participate in these programs of reforms to change the society with tremendous national pride and enthusiasm. When the Korean War was over and peace returned in 1953, the government turned its attention to systematic reconstruction of a socialist China. The country was re-structured from the six military regions into twenty-two provinces and five autonomous regions. The central government strengthened its relations with local governments and played the leading role in national economic planning and social reforms. Following the Soviet model, the government created the first five-year plan to guide national economic reconstruction. As the Cold War had shaped the world into a bi-polar system with the United States and the Soviet Union promoting competing ideologies and paradigms of modernization, the Soviet Union exerted broad influence on many fronts of China's socialist reconstruction in the 1950s.

Health occupied an important place of the government agenda as the country tried to recover from the decades-long war devastation and to re-start economic and social reconstruction on every front. The Ministry of Health was established in November 1949, with Li Dequan (Li Teh-chuan,李德全, 1896–1972) serving as the Minister and He Cheng (贺诚, 1901–1992) as the Vice Minister of technical and professional authority.[1] The Ministry of Health included departments and units of medical administration, public health (changed to health and epidemic prevention in 1951), women's and children's health, health planning and examination, health education, technical office, and medical science research committee. Health departments and bureaus were also established at different administrative levels in the six military regions. Additionally, factories, mines and railways established their own health units. After the restructuring of the provinces, municipalities, and autonomous regions in 1953–1954, health departments, bureaus and offices were established at every level—province, prefecture, municipality, city, county and village town, making a national network of health institutions under the Ministry of Health.

National health policies were formulated and health tasks specified at the beginning of the PRC, which laid the ground work for mass campaigns to prevent diseases. In the following decades, China trained vast numbers of medical and health workers at different technical levels, established numerous hospitals of different types and specialties, and created a free healthcare system. This chapter examines people's health and socioeconomic transformations, health campaigns and literacy movement, political commitment to Chinese medicine, mutual learning of Western and Chinese medicines, building of rural healthcare system and barefoot doctors, and medical education and health institutions during the modernization of China through socialist reconstruction.

Laying the foundation: national health policies and tasks (1949–1953)

The PRC strove to integrate health work into the general economic and social reconstruction of the society. People's health was considered vital for a strong new China as well as its economic production and national defense. The government aimed to achieve better health for all, which was a formidable task, given the shortage of health personnel and facilities as well as financial difficulties. This emphasis on providing health service to all people set the CCP apart from the GMD in regard to government commitment to people's health. The immediate health tasks were to concentrate all efforts on preventing major epidemic diseases and consolidating the existing health profession and institutions. The Communist leaders, with their Yanan experience and the health institutions inherited from the Nationalist government, envisioned the reconstruction of a people's healthcare system with limited technical and financial resources. As the competition and rivalry intensified between the two superpowers of the United States and the Soviet Union in the cold-war world, the communist government of China did not have access to the World Health Organization, which worked with the American ally, the Nationalist government in Taiwan. Chinese health workers learned preventive medical practices from the Soviet Union in the 1950s when the Soviet Union was China's ally.

The PRC's health policies, which followed the CCP traditions in Yanan, were formally defined at national health conferences in the early 1950s. Three key principles were specified at the First National Health Conference in August 1950 to guide health work: (1) serving the needs of workers, peasants and soldiers

(面向工农兵), (2) prevention as the first priority (预防为主), and (3) uniting Chinese and Western medicines (团结中西医). The first two principles were formulated in accordance with the goals of the Chinese Communist revolution of serving the people and the general policy of prevention as the priority set forth in 1949 for national health reconstruction. Chairman Mao Zedong wrote to the First National Health Conference: "Unite all the health and pharmaceutical personnel of old and new as well as Western and Chinese medicines, form a solid united front and work hard for the development of the great people's health."[2] Mao's instruction laid the foundation for the third health principle of uniting Western and Chinese medicines, which the health authorities were not so keen about. The very fact that Chairman Mao called for the unity of all medical groups indicated the tensions and divisions existing between different groups, particularly Chinese and Western medicines. Four major areas of health work were defined for the implementation and development of people's health at the First National Health Conference: (1) strengthening and expanding basic health units; (2) re-adjustment of public and private relationships in regard to medical, pharmaceutical and health institutions; (3) unity among medical and pharmaceutical groups for mutual aid and study; and (4) expansion of health education and training of various levels of health workers.[3] These policies and decisions provided the framework of health work for the entire nation in the early stage of the PRC's health reconstruction.

The Korean War (1950–1953) had an unexpected impact on the re-formulation of Chinese national health policy. The year of 1952 was a definitive turning-point for China's national health policy when public health became an urgent national security matter in the midst of the alleged American germ-warfare against China in the Korean War.[4] Chinese state media reported "the heinous crime of germ warfare of American imperialism" and promoted the fight against epidemic diseases as vitally important in combating American germ-warfare and for the defense of the nation and protection of the people from pestilence and disease.[5] The central people's government stated that the goal of the anti-disease campaigns was to defeat the germ warfare and "to use this opportunity to greatly improve our work of public health."[6] The threat of American germ warfare prompted Chinese leaders to seize the crisis and turned it into a great opportunity to rally people for the support of a patriotic health movement that integrated health protection of the people into the defense of the nation. The government urged health workers to combine mass movements with health campaigns (卫生工作与群众运动相结合), which became the fourth principle of national health work. Premier Zhou Enlai (周恩来, 1898–1976) detailed this new approach of mass health movement at the Second National Health Conference in December 1952. Leading newspapers, such as the *People's Daily*, followed up with the promotion of mass health movement as the fourth principle of health work. Thus, the Great Patriotic Health Movement (伟大的爱国卫生运动) was born during the Korean War. The central government's Committee on Disease Prevention was re-named the Patriotic Health Committee. The mass health movement rallied people to unite against enemies. In urban and rural China, men and women, young and old, were mobilized with patriotic enthusiasm to clean up communities and homes and to eliminate flies and mosquitoes in the movement of disease prevention and national defense.

A variety of nation-wide health programs were conducted to prevent epidemic diseases and to improve sanitation and hygiene while the health policies were being formulated. National health work concentrated on fighting major epidemic diseases, protecting women's and children's health, improving ethnic minority people's health service, and protecting industrial workers' health. The government made a special effort to build modern medical and health services for those who did not have access to modern medicine. These health programs had profound implications for economic development as well as gaining support of the new government. People's health would ensure the undertakings of economic recovery and national defense as well as winning the trust of the people. The task of protecting the health of a population of 540 million, however, was a difficult and arduous job for the health workers and the government when the country was terribly limited in financial resources and faced severe shortages of health facilities and personnel.

General sanitary and health campaigns were immediately launched after the PRC was founded. Cities and towns carried out mass movements to clean up the debris and trash left by the wars, and opium addicts and prostitutes were rehabilitated. More than 20 major infectious diseases, such as smallpox, plague, cholera, typhus, typhoid fever, tuberculosis, tetanus, hookworm, schistosomiasis, kala-azar, meningitis, malaria, measles, polio, diphtheria, polio, leprosy, filariasis and venereal diseases, were targeted in the mass health movement where education, propaganda, prevention, and vaccination were coordinated by different departments of the government. Health workers fought the diseases simultaneously with available means of prevention, vaccination, and treatment.[7] This approach of tackling multi-epidemic diseases at once was different from the method of targeting a single-disease campaign often seen in the United States and promoted by the World Health Organization. China's experience indicated that confronting major diseases in a collaborative manner proved effective in reducing and controlling them at low cost while improving people's health and socioeconomic development.

The central government formed a general prevention team with six sub-units that worked in different parts of China. They would converge onto a particular epidemic-affected area when an epidemic broke out. Methods of vaccination and inoculation and sanitation improvement were used to fight smallpox, cholera and plague—diseases that caused rampant epidemic crises and devastating losses of lives. Smallpox vaccination was carried out on an extensive scale. More than 45 percent of the total population was vaccinated in 1949–1951, which was about 29 times the record of GMD vaccination, according to Li Dequan, the Health Minister.[8] As a result, the incidence of smallpox in 1951 was 90 percent less than in 1950. China achieved the eradication of smallpox in 1963 thanks to consistent vaccination and prevention. This achievement was made without the assistance of the WHO because of the Cold War, and was almost twenty years ahead of the world eradication of smallpox in 1980. In preventing cholera, great efforts were made to improve environmental sanitation to protect water sources, clean up garbage, strengthen the quarantine service along the lines of communication and transportation, and to give cholera-preventive inoculations at focal points of contagion. According to a government report, not a single case of true cholera was discovered in China in 1951.[9] In the field of plague prevention, efforts were emphasized on catching rats and eliminating fleas in the mass health movement, together with sanitary campaigns and anti-plague vaccinations. These methods brought about effective control of the disease across the nation, and even complete elimination of bubonic plague in certain areas. In short, bubonic plague was no longer a menace to the lives of Chinese people. Moreover, mobile delousing stations with showers (淋浴灭虱站) were set up in many places to tackle contagious diseases like typhus and relapsing fever. Improvement of environmental sanitation by filling up dirty ponds and ditches and dredging rivers helped reduce other diseases such as malaria, kala-azar, and schistosomiasis.

Despite the top-down mobilization for preventive activities, responses at the lower-level administration did not always appear to be satisfactory as people still held on to the old idea of treatment rather than prevention of diseases. The central government emphasized that educational propaganda work should be further strengthened among the people to make them understand the importance of prevention. In September 1951, after reading He Cheng's report on the preventive work of the past 21 months, Mao Zedong wrote on behalf of the central government that it was a mistake that the party committees did not pay enough attention to health, prevention and general medical work, and that the mistake must be corrected. Mao pointed out that the work of health, prevention and medicine should be conducted as an important political task and be actively carried out. He instructed that cadres should be educated to understand that, in the present situation, national losses of people and livestock caused by diseases and deaths due to lack of health knowledge and health work were no less than the losses caused by natural disasters such as floods, droughts, winds and insects. Hence, health work should be viewed just as important as the work of disaster relief and prevention; and it should never be neglected.[10] Mao's instruction was disseminated to the party committees of every county government, which began to vigorously push the mass health movement.

Women's and children's health was given special attention, as they were regarded fundamental to national advancement. Women and children constituted about two thirds of the Chinese population and women were an important workforce of the nation. However, their health had been given the least attention in old China, despite the Nationalist effort at training modern midwifery. Perinatal care was considered vital in safeguarding maternal and children's health, as puerperal fever and tetanus neonatorum were the top threats to mother and infant lives. The first national women's and children's health conference in 1950 acknowledged that the biggest health threat to women and children was the problems associated with birth delivery. Pre-and-postnatal care was, therefore, made the first priority in improving women's and children's health. The national infant mortality rate was conservatively estimated at 200 per thousand in 1949, but the situation was much worse in rural areas. Yang Chongrui's effort to train modern midwives to reduce the death rates of mothers and infants with aseptic techniques was the first major work toward improving women's and children's health in the 1930s. The number of modern midwives was very small in the Nationalist era and they were available only to the elite in big cities. The PRC government worked with the National Women's Association on a variety of midwifery training programs across the nation, including the re-training of old-style midwives, to vastly increase modern-trained midwives in cities and rural towns. Women cadres promoted: "One pregnancy, one live birth; one live birth, one healthy child."[11] Their methods were to reform the old-style midwives and promote new scientific methods of delivery with aseptic procedures. Long and short programs were created to train large numbers of midwives with new delivery methods (新接生法) and to transform the old-style midwives through education and re-training.

By the end of 1951, more than 17,800 midwifery stations were established, and 127,000 old-style midwives were re-trained and reformed in the entire country.[12] Health workers and women cadres extensively promoted modern scientific methods of delivery and new methods of child care. In the beginning, it was quite challenging to persuade women cadres to engage in promoting modern midwifery because some of them thought it was the affair of old grannies and housewives and not their revolutionary work.[13] The cadres had to be educated about the importance of the work before they would play the activist role. As in the 1920s–1930s, officials who were supposed to lead the health modernization programs had to be educated first. In this regard, the Nationalist health professionals who chose to stay (instead of going to Taiwan) and work with the new PRC government played an important role in the training and education of new medical and health workers because they were fully recruited as experts.

With the directive of the central government, hospitals for women and children were established in significant numbers, and Health Centers for Women and Children (妇幼保健院/所) were gradually established in every city and county across the nation, creating a three-tiered national network of hospitals, institutes and stations for women's and children's health (院、所、站三级妇幼保健网) by the 1960s. All children were given free smallpox and other vaccines across the country, while kindergartens were established in many places. Additionally, special nurses for children were trained via regular and short-term educational programs. All of these contributed to the considerable reduction of infant and maternal mortality. In Beijing, the infant mortality rate was 117. 6 per thousand and the death rate of women in labor was 7 per thousand in 1949; by 1954, the infant mortality rate dropped to 65 per thousand, an almost 50 percent decrease, and the death rate of women in labor dropped to 0.7 per thousand.[14] In rural China, women and children's health also improved when these programs were implemented. The birth rates and death rates of the Liulin village of Pingyuan Province indicated drastic changes in the early 1950s. In 1949, eight out of ten infants born in the village died; in 1950, four out of eleven died; and in 1951 three out of thirteen died.[15] New methods of parenting (新法育儿) were also promoted to emphasize nutrition, hygiene, and infant development and the training of child nurses. As the general health and living standards of the people improved, the birth rate gradually increased across the country. In some areas, the birth rate, which was 30 per thousand before 1949, increased to 45–54 per thousand in 1952. The national infant mortality rate dropped from over 200 per thousand in 1949 to 121 per thousand in 1952. By 1957, the proportion of child births attended by trained health workers was estimated at 60 percent in rural areas and 95 percent in cities, which significantly contributed to the decrease of infant mortality.[16]

The government paid special attention to the health of ethnic minorities as they had historically little modern medical service available and their mortality rate was alarmingly high before 1949. To the regions of Inner Mongolia, Qinghai, Xinjiang, Tibet and Yunnan where ethnic nationalities concentrate, the central government dispatched anti-epidemic and medical service teams to take care of the urgent health needs. Basic health units and anti-venereal disease centers were established. These efforts led to the stabilization of the population growth in minority regions. In places where ethnic minorities constituted more than 50 percent of local populations, health institutions and hospitals were established in the counties, with a total of 1176 medical and health institutions in the early 1950s. During 1950–1951, the government built 94 health institutions and 24 public hospitals, plus 48 mobile medical and anti-epidemic units for the minorities in Xinjiang, Inner Mongolia and Qinghai.[17] In all of these areas, people enjoyed free medical care. Training of ethnic minorities as local health cadres helped overcome the shortage of health personnel. Health work for minorities not only demonstrated the care of the central government for the ethnic groups who used to be ignored, but also tested the governing ability of the new regime and its handling of ethnic relations. The social and political implications of health policy and work towards minorities, therefore, were profound and far-reaching. The CCP government invested significant financial and human resources to develop health, education and the economy in minority regions so that they would advance along with the rest of the country.

Factories, mining districts and railways throughout the country also organized their own basic health units, medical services, and safety and health protection committees. As a result of industrial and mining health protection, injuries and the occupational disease rate of workers and staff members fell from 6.4 percent in 1949 to 1.6 percent in 1951.[18] Apart from this, numerous teams of anti-epidemic and medical service were dispatched to look after the health of the several million workers who were engaged in the great construction works, such as the harnessing of the Huai River, the dredging of the Yi River, the Qing River flood diversion project, and the construction of the Chengdu-Chongqing Railway line. The medical and preventive work ensured no epidemic breakout and the successful execution of those large engineering projects.

In the meantime, cities conducted general campaigns to clean up debris and refuse as well as the transformation of many slums that had been the eyesore of old China. Longxugou (龙须沟) of Beijing and Zhaojiabang (肇嘉浜) of

Shanghai became the symbols of transformation of the old into the new China. In the post-war reconstruction of Beijing, the major challenge to public health was water and sewage problems that affected the health of millions. Longxugou was the worst of the city's shanty towns with filthy water and broken sewage systems. Poverty, filth and disease characterized the area, where laborers, rickshaw pullers and the urban poor constituted the local population. The Beijing municipal government under Mayor Peng Zhen (彭真, 1902-1997) decided to clean up and rebuild Longxugou in 1950, despite a very tight city budget. From May to November 1950, all the filthy ditches and rivers were filled up, pipes were laid for a new sewage system, and broad streets and new houses were built. Many people found jobs to earn a decent living during the transformation of Longxugou. They turned the lower land of reed ponds into a Longtan Lake Park. The poor in Beijing for the first time enjoyed a beautiful living environment with sanitation, clean water, working sewage, and medical and health services.[19] They were deeply grateful and supportive of the new government, as they personally experienced the care of the government for the welfare of the poor. Lao She (老舍, 1899–1966), the famous writer, who had just returned from the United States, was deeply moved by the transformation of his hometown Beijing. He wrote the play "Longxugou [Dragon Beard Ditch]," which vividly depicted the struggles and the enthusiasm of the people in the transformation of the place and themselves.[20] Longxugou embodied the fundamental changes in China under the CCP-led government, where filthy ditches were transformed into broad streets, depressing slums into beautiful communities, and most importantly, people changed from the oppressed nobodies into masters of their own society. The transformation of Longxugou was presented as an allegory of socialist transformation of China.

Zhaojiabang was known as the largest river shanty town in Shanghai, where more than two thousand slum huts occupied the river banks with 8000 people. Under the leadership of Mayor Chen Yi (陈毅, 1901–1972), the Shanghai municipal government allocated a special budget of 75,400 yuan in 1954 to re-build Zhaojiabang. The city government organized the clean-ups of slums and built instead new houses for the residents. They filled up the filthy ditches, laid sewage pipes, and constructed the modern transportation route of Zhaojiabang Avenue with trees on both sides. The whole project took two years to complete. By 1956, an entirely new city district emerged where people lived in modern houses with green trees and clean broad streets.[21] Changes of these former slums showed the sharp contrast of the CCP-led new government and the old regime. The transformation of shanty towns helped establish the CCP image as a people's government that cared about the well-being of the people and won the CCP broad support among the urban population.

In the nationwide health campaigns, healthcare for the people was effectively facilitated by the building of institutional infrastructure of health at the basic level. "The Decision to Fully Build and Develop Basic Health Organizations of the Entire Country (关于健全和发展全国卫生基层组织的决定)" was adopted at the 1950 national health conference. According to the decision, every city district and every rural village must have a medical and health unit. A rural health infrastructure was designed where a county must have a hospital (*weisheng yuan*, 卫生院, later called *yiyuan*, 医院), a sub-district town a health station (*weisheng suo*, 卫生所), and an administrative village a health committee (*weisheng weiyuanhui*, 卫生委员会), and a natural village or hamlet a health worker (*weisheng yuan*, 卫生员). This rural health structure was an obvious continuation of the CCP health work before 1949 but built upon the GMD rural health design as well (see chapter 3). The county hospital was responsible for directing the public health work of the entire county. Basic health organizations were gradually established following the policies and decisions of the central government. By the end of 1951, more than 91.2 percent of all counties had established county hospitals. The total number of public hospitals and hospital beds increased 275.4 percent and 300 percent respectively over the pre-1949 figures. There were 2102 county hospitals and 7961 sub-district health stations by the end of 1952.[22] Sub-district health stations and village health organizations adopted diverse forms of operation with some government-run and others government-private joint run. Many united clinics or medical service cooperatives were operated with government subsidies. In June 1952, the State Council of the Central People's Government promulgated a directive, offering free medical service and free preventive service for all government workers and members of political parties and organizations—a total of several million.[23] The system of free medical and preventive services was gradually extended to other groups in the following years.

Health and Epidemic Prevention Stations (卫生防疫站) were gradually established across the country after the 1952 national health conference. This type of health stations were first established in the northeast based on the Soviet model and China's own experience of fighting plague and other epidemics. The epidemic prevention station was initially a comprehensive technical agency dealing with all epidemic affairs to prevent diseases and safeguard people's health, national security, and economic reconstruction. In 1954 the Ministry of Health issued the administrative guide of "Temporary Methods of Health and Epidemic Prevention Stations," and ten years after in 1964, the Ministry issued the "Rules of the Work of Health and Epidemic Prevention Stations" (the trial draft) and in 1979, another fifteen years after, the Ministry issued the official "Rules of the Work of Health and Epidemic Prevention Stations."[24] The long process of trial and modification of the work and rules for epidemic prevention stations showed the difficult progress of health and epidemic prevention in China.

Tremendous efforts were made to train large numbers of medical, pharmaceutical and health workers at higher, intermediate and basic levels to supply the vast demands of health personnel across the nation. The numbers of medical and pharmaceutical colleges and schools increased significantly along with many short-term training programs and intermediate medical schools and training classes from 1950 through 1952. The enrolment of medical students in 1950 was 176.5 percent of 1949, and the 1952 enrolment was 142.9 percent of 1951. The students enrolled in medical educational institutions in the two years of 1950 and 1951 were 60 percent more than the total number of doctors trained in the past seven decades.[25] The general low literacy rate of the population, however, proved a serious obstacle to health reconstruction, as it was in every other aspect of economic and social reforms. That was why a nationwide literacy movement was launched immediately after the PRC was established.

The outbreak of the Korean War had a significant impact on China, as the country was involved in the war on the side of North Korea. At home, the government tightened political control when the external threat of the war triggered the fear of internal sabotage and resistance.[26] The health campaigns to fight the alleged American germ warfare against China gained a new urgency that combined national health with national defense. The whole country was mobilized to support the fight against diseases and American imperialism simultaneously. Hundreds of thousands of people attended political rallies against germ warfare in cities and towns, which generated emotionally charged demands for international justice against the crimes of American imperialism. Media propaganda and popular posters provided people at work and in communities materials on the meaning of germ warfare and instruction on how diseases were spread by rats, flies, fleas, mosquitoes and bugs.[27] Public health education found a convenient and effective channel of communication at the public rallies to explain the links between disease and vermin. When people of all walks of life were mobilized to fight diseases in a political movement to defend their country, they stopped being passive recipients of medical treatment but became instead active forces of public health work. The changing roles of people in the society proved the political rhetoric that they were now the masters of the new China.

The Patriotic Health Movement, literacy, and scientific socialist reconstruction

The Great Patriotic Health Movement energized nationwide anti-epidemic campaigns with the call to defend the motherland and to fight American imperialism. In urban and rural China, people were mobilized to clean up communities and homes, and to kill fleas, flies, and mosquitoes in a mass health movement. To the masses, the movement was a personal experience of health modernization and socialist reconstruction. People were eager to show patriotic enthusiasm and learn scientific ideas of disease and health. In cities, health campaigns were organized by work units (工作单位) and street committees (街道居委会) as routine sanitary work. In rural China, health campaigns were combined with land reclamation, irrigation construction, and environmental improvement of sanitary conditions for humans and livestock. The movement promoted the political discourse of socialist revolution and injected national pride and political significance into the activities of disease prevention and health work. It popularized scientific knowledge of disease through public health education to change people's traditional attitude and health behavior to socialist ideas and values. Health education and propaganda were carried out in the mass literacy movement as well. The anti-tuberculosis and anti-malaria campaigns, which are discussed later in the chapter, showcased the Patriotic Health Movement in relation to the transformation of individual citizens and the society during the reconstruction of a socialist China.

The government regarded people's health an obligation of the state to the well-being of citizens as well as the foundation of economic productivity and national development. The Patriotic Health Movement was launched throughout the country in 1952 with Mao Zedong's encouragement: "Mobilize the people to emphasize hygiene and reduce diseases, improve people's health to smash the enemy's germ warfare."[28] Local activists and organizers used popular slogans to promote the movement, where adults and children learned the rudiments of public health, sanitation and personal hygiene. There were the "eight cleans"—clean children, clean bodies, clean interior of homes, clean courtyards, clean streets and lanes, clean kitchens, clean toilets, and clean pens; and there were also the "five kills" and "one catch"—kill flies, kill mosquitoes, kill lice, kill fleas, and kill bedbugs, and catch rats. The movement advanced the national slogan: "Killing one housefly is equivalent to destroying one American imperialist."[29] Hundreds of thousands of tons of garbage were removed, hundreds of thousands of sewage lines and drains were cleared and restored, and vast numbers of dirty water pools and ponds were filled up. The movement aimed to promote people's power and science in addressing environmental sanitation and personal hygiene and public health.

People's health was promoted as vitally important to economic production and national development. China's first Five-Year Plan (1953–1957) outlined the construction of a socialist economy and elaborated new health programs and services, which demonstrated the long-term commitment to people's health in national programs. It stated that as industrial production developed, factories would provide labor insurance and health protection, government employees would have free medical care, and health facilities would be strengthened to protect people's health in cities and countryside. The government policies were widely disseminated via popular education and propaganda programs and visual education material on diseases such as the series of anti-tuberculosis health posters.[30] Improvement of people's health meant increased national productivity, stronger national defense, and faster economic development. The social and economic drains caused by widespread epidemic diseases were on the minds of CCP policy makers when they deliberated on the state planning of economy and national development.

Good health was publicized as a significant part of the socialist transformation of people and society. People were mobilized with the exultation that under the leadership of the Communist Party they had become masters of new China and that they should take an active role in reconstructing a socialist society and replacing traditional views with socialist values. They were encouraged to "transform social traditions and re-create the world (移风易俗，改造世界)" with their own hands. Various government ministries, such as Education, Culture, Propaganda, Labor, and Agriculture, cooperated with the Health Ministry and the Patriotic Health Committee on multiple-fronts to coordinate health campaigns at every level of administration. Professional and social organizations, such as the Red Cross, the National Federation of Women, and the Labor Union, also participated in the movement to mobilize people of all walks of life and school children to fight against epidemic and endemic diseases. The campaigns purported to turn the masses from passive recipients of healthcare into active agents to detect and prevent diseases. Ka-che Yip used the term "mass mobilization model" to characterize Chinese health campaigns in the 1950s–80s.[31]

The Patriotic Health Movement emphasized sanitation and hygiene, clean water sources, food safety, and elimination of pests. Sanitation and hygiene campaigns were regularly held in every spring, summer, autumn and winter, and during major holidays such as the Chinese Spring Festival, Labor Day, and National Day. Mass campaigns against four pests (除四害运动)—rats, mosquitoes, flies, and sparrows—started in the mid-1950s with the concerns that people's health and agricultural production were harmed by these pests. Major newspapers, such as *The People's Daily*, explained that elimination of rats, mosquitoes and flies would effectively stop the spread of acute epidemic diseases and therefore reduce the threat to people's health. Rats and sparrows ate grains and caused the reduction of harvest, even though farmers worked very hard at increasing yield. It was important to eliminate the pests that harmed agricultural production.[32] The list of pests later expanded to include bedbugs, fleas, roaches, and snails in the fight against parasitic diseases.[33] Sparrows were spared after people realized that they were natural enemies of insects and they actually helped farmers. The anti-pest movement was often combined with sanitation campaigns and the collection of animal manure as fertilizers in rural areas.

Educating the masses to be effective participants in the movement was a major task for health workers and political activists. People needed to understand both the preventive and curative aspects of diseases if they were to fight effectively. The reality was China had a population of 563 million in 1950 with an illiteracy rate of more than 80 percent. The overwhelming majority of the population (about 88 percent) lived in rural villages, where the illiteracy rate was even higher, traditional views much stronger, and illnesses more widespread. The health campaigners and organizers, such as local officials, political activists and health workers, were encouraged to disseminate scientific knowledge among the masses to help them understand diseases scientifically and to change their views of illnesses from superstitious fatalism to a positive scientific can-do attitude. The change of people's health behavior and attitude was considered part and parcel of the fundamental transformation of the society as a whole. Without changing the old views and values and replacing them with new scientific beliefs, the populace would not be able to act as effective fighters against diseases, nor would they be able to contribute to the general reconstruction of a socialist China. It was a daunting task for the Chinese public health workers, local officials, and the campaign activists to teach a largely illiterate population about modern scientific knowledge of epidemic diseases and the methods of prevention.

Literacy was a key element of transforming Chinese people and society. Since 1950, China had been conducting a national illiteracy elimination movement (扫盲运动, literacy movement) to help peasants, workers, and soldiers to learn to read and write. Party officials and political activists mobilized people at work units, urban communities, and in rural villages to attend illiteracy elimination classes (扫盲班, literacy classes), which were usually held in the evenings after work. Millions attended such classes, learning government laws and policies, scientific knowledge of industrial and agricultural production, and health knowledge of epidemic diseases. There was such a severe shortage of literate adults that even elementary school pupils were recruited to take up the job of teaching. The movement emphasized serving the needs of the masses of workers, peasants and soldiers and increasing their scientific knowledge (面向工农兵大众，提高工农兵科学知识). Mass meetings were regularly held for political struggles as well as for reading newspapers and learning new knowledge. Mass meetings aimed to encourage people to get rid of old ideas and values of selfishness and individualism and to learn socialist values and goals of collective good. The literacy movement continued into the 1970s, benefitting hundreds of millions of Chinese. From 1949 to 1956, approximately 294 million people attended literacy classes with the majority of them being peasants, and 20.76 million acquired literacy.[34] By 1964, the illiteracy rate in China dropped to 37 percent, compared with over 80 percent in 1949.[35] Literacy classes taught people not merely the skills of reading and writing and calculation, but more significantly, they raised the political consciousness of the masses with socialist values and visions. The literacy movement helped disseminate scientific knowledge of diseases while at the same time introduced socialist ideas to the vast population as a transformative force.

Chinese modernizers had been promoting science as a fundamental tenet to guide China's national development since the early twentieth century. The PRC government continued to emphasize science as the yardstick of social progress and advancement. In the effort to transform people's mentality, the government employed the media and educational means to persuade people to discard old superstition and folk beliefs. People were encouraged to learn science and develop a scientific world outlook. The dissemination of scientific knowledge of disease effectively helped popularize germ theory and strengthen the concept of "scientific medicine" in China.[36] Although germ theory was initially introduced to Chinese urban residents in the 1910s through public health education campaigns and school hygiene education, it was understood mainly by the educated elite.[37] The literacy movement brought modern scientific concepts and ideas of germ theory to the vast Chinese population, via the use of visual materials such as posters, charts, and pictures to help them understand what germs looked like and how they spread diseases.

Visual materials were an effective medium to transmit modern scientific knowledge to the general public, particularly the abstract concepts of science to the less literate. The colorful and vivid images were attractive to people and easy for them to understand in actual practice.[38] The thinking was, if people understood germs causing diseases, they would use scientific methods to fight them. The use of visual materials intended to achieve immediate impact, as literacy took time for individuals to acquire. Publishing houses printed out various book series on science with extensive use of images. Pictorial books, magazines, health posters, and wall bulletins became popular educational materials for the public. Visual communication has the distinct advantage of containing a large quantity of information within limited space. Visual messages are straightforward, eye-catching, and easy to follow. Little wonder Chinese health educators made good use of visual images in the health campaigns.

First-hand experience proved that teaching scientific ideas and subjects in professional jargons and chemical formulae only put the masses to sleep. The common folks liked to hear vivid stories and learn things that they could directly apply to their needs. In rural China, peasants were more interested in learning how to deal with head scratches and bleeding than CPR (Cardio-Pulmonary Resuscitation) first aid because head scratches and bleedings were very common and the need for CPR was small. In teaching nutrition to the un-schooled peasants, a health worker warned that one should avoid using jargon such as "carbohydrate" and "source of energy" because they meant nothing to them. Instead, one should say whole grain was better than the refined flour for you to live a long life.[39] In order to make scientific knowledge accessible to the ordinary people, science had to become something understandable by the masses. Campaign mobilizers urged people to write scientific subjects in popular and colloquial language.

Uniting Chinese and Western medicines: a difficult road in the 1950s

Chinese medicine had been challenged by the health modernizers since the early twentieth-century. The failed attempts to abolish Chinese medicine in 1914 by the Yuan Shikai government and in 1929 by the Nationalist health authority led to increased animosity between Chinese and Western medicines. Chinese medicine received limited recognition but continuous discrimination in the Nationalist health system (see chapter 3). In contrast, the CCP made full use of Chinese medicine during the war years of revolution. The CCP leaders, such as Mao Zedong, Zhou Enlai, Liu Shaoqi and many others, who had personally experienced the benefits of Chinese medicine during the years of military battles, recognized the value of Chinese medicine and its essential role in re-building people's health in the new China. In 1949 there were a total of 542,401 medical workers, out of which more than 500,000 were of Chinese medicine, 38,875 of Western medicine, and 300 of dental medicine.[40] Only about 40,000 physicians of Chinese medicine practiced in cities while the rest practiced in rural towns and villages. Those of Western medical and dental services almost exclusively practiced in cities, with the majority concentrating on coastal cities. People in rural China relied on Chinese medicine and traditional folk healings. It was estimated that more than 80 percent of patients in rural areas had no access to medical assistance in 1950 mainly because practitioners of Chinese medicine were not put to full use.[41] The policy of uniting Chinese and Western medicines, which was formulated with the instruction of Chairman Mao Zedong, intended to fully use the old-style Chinese medical doctors to serve the people. The policy also gave practitioners of Chinese medicine a great hope of gaining back their respect in society after being oppressed and discriminated by previous health authorities. The old divide of Western and Chinese medical doctors and their mistrust forged over the past decades, however, did not fade simply because the CCP leaders adopted a more encouraging and supportive policy towards Chinese medicine. Health leaders of PRC, such as Wang Bin (王斌) and He Cheng (贺诚), had different views of Chinese medicine from the CCP political leaders. In their opinion, Chinese medicine was a product of the old society, unscientific and inferior to Western medicine, which would be weeded out in the new society. Their views obviously continued the ideas that were articulated by the medical elite of Western medicine since the early twentieth century, despite the fact that they were PRC health leaders and the CCP government policy emphasized the unity of Chinese and Western medicines. In the name of raising quality, the Health Ministry standardized the training programs and issued regulations on Chinese medicine in early 1950s. These measures, however, were used to restrict the practice of Chinese medicine and marginalize Chinese medical practitioners.

Many doctors of Chinese medicine were surprised that Yu Yunxiu (余云岫), the champion of Chinese medicine abolition, was invited to the First National Health Conference in 1950. In the new political climate of uniting Chinese and Western medicines, Yu continued his advocacy against Chinese medicine, but he changed "abolition" to "reform" in regard to handling Chinese medicine. He proposed to reform Chinese medicine by eliminating the majority of the old-style medical doctors and retaining a few to be reformed and transformed into medical assistants. He suggested that the government accept his idea of eliminating Chinese medicine via registration and prohibition of training of Chinese medicine.[42] Although there was no evidence available that the Health Ministry ever adopted Yu's proposal of "reforming" Chinese medicine into elimination, the regulations on licensing and qualifying practitioners of Chinese medicine in 1951–1953 would basically have achieved the same goal.

Wang Bin (王斌, 1909–1992), Health Minister of the Northeast People's Government and President of the China Medical University (Vice Health Minister in 1953), argued from a sociopolitical perspective against Chinese medicine. He published in the journal *Northeast Health* (东北卫生, vol. 1, no. 9) in 1950 an article, "On the Certain Medical Health Organizations and Styles of Thoughts Produced on the Basis of Certain Political and Economic Structures." Wang made a speech on the same topic at the Fourth Health Meeting of the Northeast that year. His main argument was that traditional Chinese medicine was created during the feudal time and therefore it was a "feudal medicine" that had to be eliminated now that the feudal society was already done away with. He also argued that Western medicine was produced in the bourgeois society and therefore it was a "capitalist medicine" that had to be revolutionized to serve the people. Wang's interpretation of medicine was apparently guided by the Marxist theory that economic basis shaped the development of superstructure. He criticized Chinese medicine as unscientific and that Chinese medicine had no real effect in treating illnesses but the comfort for the peasants that they were having medical treatment. He even claimed that the reason to let Chinese medicine exist for the time being in new China was because not enough scientific health workers were trained yet to replace the practitioners of Chinese medicine.[43] Wang proposed that all Chinese medical practitioners be given short-term training to learn scientific medical knowledge and that those who qualified would be given the status of medical assistants. Chinese medicine, in the meantime, was not allowed to train future practitioners. The result of Wang's scheme of handling Chinese medicine would be little different from what Yu Yunxiu wished. The ultimate goal was to eliminate Chinese medicine in China. In order to train large quantity and qualified health workers, Wang proposed a new scheme of training methods, quite revolutionary in terms of approaches and innovation. He explained that modern medical education should be revolutionized by shortening the training time and focusing on specialties to produce competent medical workers to solve real health problems. With the training focused on specialties (专科重点制), Wang promoted a new teaching method of using visual images (形象教学法) and real objects instead of the abstract teaching with lots theories. His method emphasized the "combination of listening, seeing, and doing" (听、看、做合一) so that students would learn things much faster.[44]

He Cheng (贺诚, 1901–1992), Vice Health Minister, held the opinion that Chinese medicine would eventually be replaced by Western medicine because of its inferiority. He predicted that Chinese medicine would be weeded out via a process of natural selection from the city to the countryside.[45] The common understanding of the leaders of the Health Ministry, however, was that Chinese medicine had accumulated lots of valuable clinical experiences over thousands of years but its theories lacked scientific foundation. It needed transformation to become scientific lest it stayed unreformed and unable to carry out the work of preventing and treating diseases. The Ministry called for efforts to combine the experience of Chinese medicine with modern science and to make Chinese medicine scientific to improve its quality. In short, Chinese medicine must be scientized (中医科学化). By scientization, it meant Chinese medicine must learn modern medical sciences and use modern science to analyze the nature of secret pharmaceutical recipes (秘方). In short, the Health Ministry had critical eyes focused on the Chinese medicine as a flawed medicine, and purported that only modern science would be the reforming force to improve Chinese medicine. Some scholars argued that the goal, in the minds of the Health Ministry leaders, was to transform Chinese medicine with Western medical theories and techniques to make it effective in serving people's health.[46]

Schools were set up to re-train Chinese medical doctors with scientific knowledge and theories. They were required to learn the basic medical sciences, such as physiology, anatomy, germ theory, pathology, and management of infectious diseases. They were also expected to work with medical scientists in the study of Chinese herbal medicine to analyze the secret recipes and ascertain their functions. Moreover, the clinical effect of Chinese acupuncture was to be studied with science to make it scientific.[47] With such an agenda to scientize Chinese medicine, the Ministry of Health issued "Temporary Regulations on Chinese Medical Practitioners" (中医师暂行条例) on May 1, 1951.[48] The regulations specified that the Health Ministry would not accept those as qualified who had obtained their training in Chinese medicine via the traditional method of apprenticeship and correspondence. Only those who had graduated from three-to-four year public or private schools of Chinese medicine would be licensed physicians of Chinese medicine (中医师). Licenses issued before the said regulations by the central Health Ministry and regional governments as well as by the Nationalist government would continue to be valid. The Health Ministry also issued details on the implementation of the regulations and rules for the qualification examinations in 1951–1952. In the written examination of Chinese medicine, candidates had to answer questions far beyond the knowledge of Chinese medicine. For instance, the required part of the examination included knowledge of physiology, anatomy, germ theory, and infectious diseases; and the elective part had internal medicine (including gynecology and obstetrics and pediatrics), surgery, and ophthalmology.[49]

In this new effort to strengthen the quality of Chinese medical practice and to make Chinese medicine scientific, local governments began to register and examine Chinese medicine practitioners. In the northeast, 2347 Chinese medicine practitioners took the exams in 1949 but only 173 passed.[50] In 1950–1951, Jiangxi province registered 8728 Chinese medicine practitioners, only 424 (less than 5 percent) were given official recognition of license.[51] In 1953, practitioners of Chinese medicine in 92 cities and 165 counties were registered and examined. As a result, about 14,000 were considered qualified and the majority were banned from practice on the grounds of being unqualified.[52] These actions of health administration seriously undermined the medical and health services across China when the country was already suffering severe shortages of medical personnel. Moreover, restriction of Chinese medicine was also implemented in healthcare institutions. For instance, physicians of Chinese medicine could not practice in hospitals nor write prescriptions. People who wanted to use Chinese medicine for treatment had to get approval of their work unit's medical committee before they could go to the united Chinese medicine clinics or acupuncture clinics for treatment.[53] Those restrictions seriously limited the health service of Chinese medicine in the society. Professionally, no physicians of Chinese medicine were accepted as members of the Chinese Medical Association (中华医学会), the national organization of medical professionals. Medical colleges and universities offered no courses on Chinese medicine and Chinese pharmacy.[54]

There was wide spread resentment about the restriction and marginalization of Chinese medicine, which caused serious concerns among the CCP leaders. In early 1953 the political director of the Health Department of the Central Military Commission, Bai Xueguang (白学光，1914–), wrote a report on the various problems existing in the military health department, which Mao Zedong read with deep concerns. Mao immediately instructed Zhou Enlai, Xi Zhongxun, Hu Qiaomu, Peng Dehuai, He Cheng and others that the report be printed and sent to all members of the Central Committee and to party committees of the Central Government. Mao was furious:

> Those departments that do not carefully administer their professional work but indulge in gain and power as lords of the bureaucratic officialdom probably are not the Health Department of the Military Commission alone but other departments as well. In the struggle against bureaucracy, I encourage you to tear apart the face [meaning not to stand on ceremony] and fundamentally transform these agencies into competent work places.[55]

He asked Xi and Hu to thoroughly investigate the work of the Health Ministry and to find methods to solve the problems. It was during the investigation of the bureaucratic problems of the Health Ministry that the discrimination and restriction of Chinese medicine were revealed. It was determined that such dealings of Chinese medicine by the Health Ministry obstructed the true intention of the health principle of uniting the Chinese and Western medicines emphasized by the central government.

Under the pressure of the CCP leaders, the Health Ministry began to reflect on its work and examined its mistakes in handling Chinese medicine. It also provided specific information on how to fight bureaucracy and improve its work. The Government Administration Council (政务院, it became the State Council in 1954) conducted a three-month investigation of the Health Ministry and sent its report to the Central Government and Chairman Mao. When the Central Political Bureau discussed national health work in November 1953, Mao Zedong made the speech:

> China has made great contributions to the world, Chinese medicine being one of them, in my opinion. We have very few doctors of Western medicine. The great many people, particularly the farmers, relied on Chinese medicine for treating illnesses. We must therefore do well in uniting the workers of Chinese medicine . . . It is wrong to look down upon Chinese medicine, it is also wrong to say Chinese medicine is all good and very good. Chinese and Western medicines must unite. Western medicine must break down factionalism.[56]

In July 1954, Liu Shaoqi met with the department and bureau chiefs of the Health Ministry and discussed the problems associated with the mishandling of Chinese medicine. He criticized those who despised Chinese medicine as being enslaved by bourgeois thought. He pointed out that the discrimination and exclusion of Chinese medicine revealed a despicable bourgeois mindset.[57] Premier Zhou Enlai also pointed out in his report on government work that the health department at every level should unite, educate, and use the several hundred thousand Chinese medicine workers and that they should work together to compile and carry on the useful knowledge and experience of Chinese medicine.[58] Mao Zedong positively commented on the values of Chinese medicine that "Chinese medicine synthesized the thousands of years of experiences of our people in struggling against diseases and Chinese medicine was a great treasure house."[59]

A Temporary Work Team on the Problems of Chinese Medicine (中医问题临时工作组) was formed in July 1954, composed of members of the Central Propaganda Ministry, the Cultural and Educational Commission, and the Health Ministry. Health administrators across the nation began to study the instructions of the CCP Central Committee on Chinese medicine. Meetings were held for doctors of both Chinese and Western medicines to discuss topics such as the studying and researching on Chinese medicine, the expansion of health service of Chinese medicine, and the publishing of books on Chinese medicine. The work team submitted to the central government a "Report on Correcting the Mistakes and Improving the Work of Chinese Medicine" on October 26, 1954, after three months of investigation of the problems associated with the so-called scientization of Chinese medicine. The report recommended that a research institute of Chinese medicine be established, and Chinese medical doctors be allowed to work in major hospitals to expand and improve their health service. It also recommended that advanced training of Chinese medicine be improved and the management of Chinese pharmacy be strengthened. The central government approved these recommendations for implementation on November 5, 1955, which stopped the discrimination and exclusion of Chinese medicine.[60] A fundamental shift of attitude towards Chinese medicine began to take place afterwards. Doctors of Chinese medicine were admitted, for the first time, as members of the Chinese Medical Association, which had been exclusively serving doctors of Western medicine. Major hospitals in Beijing, Shanghai and Tianjin began to set up outpatient and in-patient departments of Chinese medicine; and the free healthcare service also reimbursed the costs of Chinese medicine and drugs. Even hospitals of Chinese medicine (中医医院) were gradually established across the country. By 1958, more than 300 hospitals of Chinese medicine were established.[61] In December 1955, the China Academy of Chinese Medicine (中国中医研究院, renamed as China Academy of Chinese Medical Sciences, 中国中医科学院) was established. Premiere Zhou Enlai wrote the inscription to celebrate the new academy: "To carry forward our medical heritage, and to serve the construction of socialism."[62] Provincial and municipal research academies of Chinese medicine were also established in the following years. By 1960, China had 83 such research institutions of Chinese medicine.[63] All the previous restrictive regulations on Chinese medicine were repealed to guarantee the development of Chinese medicine.[64]

The People's Daily, in the meantime, published editorials on implementing the correct policies regarding Chinese medicine. The newspaper, very much the voice of the central government, examined how the scientization of Chinese medicine (中医科学化) went astray to become Westernization of Chinese medicine (西医化). It pointed out that Chinese medicine should be developed by using modern scientific methods to sort out Chinese medical theories and to summarize its clinical experiences so as to keep its essence and to discard its dross (取其精华，去其糟粕). It advocated that Chinese medicine must be integrated into modern medical science to become an important part of medical science.[65] The Health Ministry called on health administrators at every level to study Chairman Mao's instructions on Chinese medicine and government policies regarding Chinese medicine. Immediately afterwards, in places such as eastern China, Shanghai, Tianjin, Sichuan, Xikang, and Shangxi, conferences and discussion meetings were held for the representatives of Chinese medical practitioners to discuss how to organize and bring into play the power of Chinese medicine in health service, and how to carry out the research and advanced training of Chinese medicine. Even the Chinese Medical Association called for the strengthening of the work on Chinese medicine and pointed out that Chinese medicine was an important part of Chinese cultural heritage. It acknowledged that the great majority of Chinese people relied on Chinese medicine for treating illnesses and that the work of Chinese medicine was fundamentally important to people's health.[66] The efforts directed by the instructions of the central government brought about changes of attitude among health administrators and medical leaders toward Chinese medicine in the mid-1950s.

In the endeavor to correct the mistakes in scientization of Chinese medicine, doctors of Western medicine were called upon to learn Chinese medicine, instead of the previous one-way street of requiring doctors of Chinese medicine to learn Western medicine. In 1956, the Health Ministry decided that Western medicine must study Chinese medicine and that a university of Chinese medicine be established in each of the cities of Beijing, Shanghai, Guangzhou, and Chengdu. On December 19, 1955, the day the China Academy of Chinese Medicine opened, a selected group of 76 best doctors of Western medicine began the study of Chinese medicine in Beijing under the directive of "systematic study, comprehensive understanding, and synthetic improvement (系统学习，全面掌握，整理提高)."[67] They were given leave of work so that they could concentrate on their study. They learned to master the essential knowledge of Chinese medicine, such as the theories, methods, formulas, and pharmacy (理、法、方、药) and became the pioneering leaders in the field of integrated Chinese and Western medicine (中西医结合, integrative medicine), the third force of medicine in China. The Health Ministry issued a report in 1958 that summarized the experience of arranging doctors of Western medicine on leave to study Chinese medicine. The central government approved the report with the expectation that Western medical doctors, after learning Chinese medicine, would become brilliant theorists of Chinese medicine so as to contribute to its scientization. It predicted that such an achievement would have unusual significance for the modern development of Chinese medicine.[68] With the support and encouragement of the government, more and more doctors of Western medicine began to study Chinese medicine nationwide. Medical journals published increasing numbers of articles on the events and experiences of Western medicine doctors learning Chinese medicine. According to the 1960 data, about 2300

Western medicine doctors were on leave to study full-time Chinese medicine at 37 classes nationwide, and about 36,000 Western medical professionals were studying Chinese medicine while working in their posts.[69] Students at higher and intermediate levels of medical colleges were also studying Chinese medicine. Many of them became the leading doctors in the field of Chinese medicine or the integration of Chinese and Western medicine.[70] The emphasis on doctors of Western medicine to study Chinese medicine continued in the following decades. The result was the emergence of a third type of medicine in China, the integrated Chinese and Western medicine, apart from Chinese medicine and Western medicine. After Tu Youyou (屠呦呦, 1930–) received the Nobel Prize in medicine in 2015, she has been cited as the best example to represent this integrated Chinese and Western medicine. Tu started as a student of Western medicine at the Medical College of Beijing University. Upon graduation, she was assigned to work at the China Academy of Chinese Medicine. With her training in Western medicine, Tu began studying Chinese medicine and pharmacology at the academy. The reason she was able to achieve what she did was exactly because of her medical bilingualism in both Western and Chinese medicines.[71]

Vice Health Ministers Wang Bin and He Cheng were criticized for leading astray the scientization of Chinese medicine into the wrong direction of exclusion and marginalization. They were dismissed from their positions in the Health Ministry in 1956. Wang was even accused of being a counter-revolutionary and jailed for a few months in the intense days of Anti-Rightist political movement. He was released when no evidence was found to support the accusation. Wang Bin and He Cheng were two pioneering CCP medical leaders, who started their career in the CCP movement during the Jinggang Mountain days and survived the Long March. Wang and He were both educated in Western medicine. Wang Bin was a graduate of Chengdu Medical School in 1932 and joined the CCP revolution at the Jiangxi soviet base in 1933. He Cheng was a graduate of the National Medical College of Beijing in 1922 and joined the CCP in 1925. He came from a family of practitioners of Chinese medicine. Prominent as they were as medical authority of the CCP, they were not immune from a nation-wide criticism of their mistakes. Their views of Chinese medicine and their failure to faithfully carry out the unity of Chinese and Western medicines as the central government expected were criticized as expressions of bourgeois thought that undermined socialist reconstruction. For quite some time, *Jiankangbao* (健康报, the Health Newspaper), a newspaper of the Health Ministry, carried on the criticisms of Wang and He by publishing articles written by different health administrators and officials to make sure that the health field was to be cleansed of their harmful influence and that their mistakes were corrected. The criticisms emphasized that the medicial and health work was responsible for people's health, their productivity and their happiness, which was important in the endeavor of socialist reconstruction. The encroachment of bourgeois thought in the field of medical and health was regarded as enemy's attempt to undermine socialist reconstruction, and therefore it must be defeated.[72]

The establishment of Chinese medicine colleges and schools and the creation of Chinese medicine hospitals fundamentally transformed the training of Chinese medicine personnel from traditional apprenticeship to modern classroom study and residency, and the status of Chinese medicine doctors. Both the education of Chinese medicine and the physicians of Chinese medicine were officially lifted to the same level as that of Western medicine, though social and professional bias against Chinese medicine as inferior to Western medicine did not disappear in the society. The traditional method of apprenticeship, however, was allowed to continue in the training of Chinese medicine, but the standardization established by medical colleges and schools to train Chinese medicine soon replaced traditional methods of training. The general quality of Chinese medicine was no doubt improved as a result. However, some senior physicians of Chinese medicine felt that the college education of Chinese medicine had rooms for improvement. With the graduation of the first class of students at the Chinese Medicine College of Beijing (北京中医学院) in 1962 after six years of study, five prominent physicians of Chinese medicine who were teaching at the college sent a letter to the Health Ministry with recommendations for improvement. The five physicians were Yu Daoji (于道济), Chen Shenwu (陈慎吾), Qin Bowei (秦伯未), Li Chongren (李重人), and Ren Yingqiu (任应秋). This was the well-known incident of the "Letter from Five Elders" (五老上书). Their major argument was that students were weak in the foundation studies of the classic texts of Chinese medicine, though they had grasped the knowledge of treating illnesses. They urged the increase of study of classic texts in the modern curriculum of Chinese medicine so as to strengthen the scholarly quality of Chinese medicine education. They recommended that students spend four and a half years studying Chinese medicine and one and a half years studying general medical knowledge and Western medicine.[73] The Health Ministry paid attention to their recommendations and directed the discussion of their recommendations across the nation. However, the beginning of the Cultural Revolution in 1966 ended all possible adoption of their ideas, and the "Five Elders" suffered brutal attacks and persecution from their former students in the political movement of the Cultural Revolution.

Despite the difficult road of the modern development of Chinese medicine, new generations of Chinese medicine doctors were produced at modern colleges and schools of Chinese medicine. There were 339,291 Chinese medicine personnel in 1963 and 368,462 in 1990 after a decrease in the 1970s and 1980s caused by the Cultural Revolution.[74] The numbers also indicated that Chinese medicine, in comparison with Western medicine, expanded at slower speed to replace the older generations. In 1979 the All China Association of Chinese Medicine (中华全国中医学会) was established, which signified the professional unity of Chinese medicine personnel as a modern medical group. In 1980 the Health Ministry reiterated the policy of "continuing the development and long-term coexistence of Chinese medicine, Western medicine, and the integrated Chinese and Western medicine."[75] The plurality of medical development benefited the Chinese people by offering diverse ways of diagnosing and treating diseases and providing different types of drugs. Medical plurality characterizes current healthcare practices and medical education in China.[76]

Healthcare in urban and rural China

The PRC created a system of hospitals and clinics to provide state-run medical services to the people. Medical professionals of private practice were gradually organized through programs of united clinics (联合诊所) and united hospitals (联合医院) after 1949. The government set forth basic standards for hospitals and clinics by issuing the "Provisional Regulations on the Management of Hospitals and Clinics" in March 1951.[77] Workers and state employees and members of organizations began to enjoy free medical treatment when the Labor Insurance Regulations was promulgated in February 1951 and the Government Administration Council issued the directive on the provision of medical treatment and disease prevention at public expense for state employees, political parties, organizations, and their subordinate business units in June 1952.[78] As socialist reconstruction deepened with the first Five-Year Plan, hospitals and clinics were gradually changed into state-run institutions, although some form of private practice of medical service remained for a while, particularly in rural China. The government invested heavily in building comprehensive hospitals, which constituted over 90 percent of all hospitals in China, to make them key health institutions of medical service. The hospitals and clinics, which included a variety of comprehensive and specialized types, not only provided curative treatment but also actively led preventive medicine in local and industrial health campaigns. In urban communities, there were basic-level community health stations and clinics that provided rudimentary medical service and disease prevention. Factories and companies had their own hospitals and health clinics. A hierarchical structure of hospital system was gradually formed with the best doctors working at the top tier hospitals, which were usually designated as the provincial or municipal hospitals. Then came the second tier of hospitals at the prefectural or city level, and the third tier were the county hospitals (县卫生院、县医院). Although county hospitals were at the lower-end of the urban comprehensive hospital system, they occupied a unique place in the chain of urban and rural healthcare system because they provided technical guidance and support to the work of rural health institutions. They were the top health centers of the county that reached down into the countryside to connect with health institutions and offices in rural towns and villages.

A three-tiered healthcare network was gradually established in rural China, with the county hospital at the top, the rural town and district hospital in the middle, and the medical room in village at the end. The rural healthcare network developed along with the phases of social and economic transformation of the countryside. The period of 1949–1955 saw land reform and mutual aid of peasants when land was distributed to and owned by peasants. The medical service was a private practice during this time, where Chinese medicine men and various types of healers worked individually at home or as a group in united clinics.

They were encouraged to join the local medical workers' association and form united clinics voluntarily. The united clinic was a medical service provider formed by a few medicine men working together to create an organized medical service in the rural community. Those who wished to continue practicing medicine by themselves were allowed to practice individually and they were respected by local government.

The united clinics and hospitals started after the Health Ministry issued the "Decision on the Adjustment of the Public and Private Relations in Medical and Pharmaceutical Enterprises" in 1951. The Ministry called on individual medical practitioners to collaborate and form united medical enterprises. It emphasized that local health administration should encourage, guide and assist private-run united medical enterprises and mobilize individual medical practitioners to form united hospitals or united clinics to expand health service to people. Many individual practitioners of Chinese and Western medicines began to form united hospitals and clinics in cities, even though individual practices of medicine were allowed to co-exist. The policy demonstrated the flexibility of the government in regard to diverse types of public and private medical practices in the early 1950s. The government paid special attention to the development of basic-level health and medical services in rural towns and villages and in minority regions where medical services were historically scarce. The Health Ministry gave specific instructions on the formation and operation of united health facilities with the directive "On the Measures of Forming United Medical Organizations." The united medical service was the government's initial step in transforming individual medical practice into an organized healthcare service, in parallel to the economic transition from private enterprises to national entities.

Many individual practitioners of Chinese medicine in rural China began to form town or district health stations and united clinics that were privately run with government sponsorship. These operations reminded people of the practice of health cooperatives in the Yanan era. In rural China, the majority were Chinese medicine practitioners, in addition to some folk healers such as herbalists and bonesetters. The diverse medical and healing practices continued even as increasing numbers of Chinese medicine practitioners formed united clinics. Fang Xiaoping's studies showed that when the Hang County formed an association of medical practitioners and workers, the majority of Chinese medicine men joined the association. However, about one fifth of them did not because either they had no interest or they were disqualified professionally and politically.[79] The association was a venue of sorting out the qualified and the unqualified medical personnel in local area. A few doctors of Chinese medicine formed a united clinic to provide medical service to the community. This organized effort changed their ways of medical practice. In the past, they stayed at home to offer medical treatment; now they provided a medical service at a professional place called a clinic. The doctors ran their clinic as a private enterprise. They charged fees and paid their own salaries, but they were cooperative partners of the government in healthcare during the agricultural mutual aid phase. Doctors made medical service tours to nearby villages to reach out to places that had no medical service. They also promoted and conducted sanitation and epidemic prevention programs in the Patriotic Health Movement.

The Health Ministry's "Decision on Strengthening and Developing the Basic-Level Public Health Organizations" in April 1951 directed the strengthening of existing health institutions at the *xian* (county) level and the creation of health facilities in regions that did not have them. Major industrial and mining areas were also to establish full staff of medical and public health personnel.[80] In order to achieve the goal, the government systematically trained health workers with special attention to increasing paramedics and maternal nurses to meet the urgent needs. As a measure to standardize the operation and organization of county hospitals, the Health Ministry issued the "General Rules for the Organization of County Hospitals" in 1952. These measures helped strengthen the service of health institutions at the basic level. The county hospital was the medical and health protection center that engaged in curative treatment as well preventive medical activities. It was the leading force in the mobilization and propaganda of local health campaigns and sanitation movement.

Healthcare in rural areas began to expand and move closer to collective medical service when agricultural collectivization went from mutual aid to higher cooperative phase after 1955. Rural town and district health stations expanded and changed into district hospitals with some beds, and the village united clinics developed into health stations. A new type of medical cooperative enterprise of collective ownership began to emerge in different parts of rural China during the high stage of agricultural cooperatives of communes. When the people's communes were established across China as the new rural system in the late 1950s, particularly during the 1958 Great Leap Forward, rural towns (*xiang*, 乡) became communes (*gongshe*, 公社), villages (*cun*, 村) became production brigades (*shengchan dadui*, 生产大队), and hamlets became production teams (*shengchan xiaodui*, 生产小队). The town health station became the commune hospital funded and administered by the commune, whereas the rural district hospitals became state-owned health institutions. Mishan town of Gaoping county in Shanxi province (山西省高平县米山乡) was a pioneer in integrating medical service into the agricultural cooperative system to provide an insured medical service to farmers. In the early 1950s, ten doctors and three Chinese medicine shops joined together to form a private-owned united clinic in Mishan town, and in 1955 this private united clinic changed into a collective-owned medical cooperative called the Mishan Town United Health Protection Station (米山乡联合保健站). The health station was under the local town government with funds coming from the sources of the agricultural production cooperative (农业生产合作社), farmers, and medical doctors. The agricultural production cooperative took 15–20 percent of its common fund and added medical income from drug fees as contribution, and each farmer paid 0.2 yuan of health fees (2角钱的保健费) to enjoy the benefits of free preventive health service and free medical diagnosis and treatment. The health station offered treatment of diseases, conducted medical service tours and each doctor was responsible for the health and disease prevention of a particular area in the town. To take advantage of Chinese medicine and to reduce expenses of the cooperative, the station carried out the program of three locals and four selves (三土四自), namely, local medicine, local drugs, and local recipes/formulas (土医、土药、土方), and self-plant, self-collect, self-make, and self-use herbal medicine (自种药、自采药、自制药、自用药). Doctors of the health station were paid with a combination of work points and cash. Thus, as agricultural collectivization moved from mutual aid phase of private ownership to high cooperative phase of collective ownership, the medical clinics also underwent a parallel change from private to collective ownership. Counties in different provinces, such as Neijiang of Sichuan (四川内江), Zhengyang of Henan (河南正阳), Zhaoyuan of Shandong (山东招远) and Macheng of Hubei (湖北麻城) had similar transformation of rural medical clinics from private to collective ownership sponsored by the agricultural cooperatives. The collective health service of Mishan town caught the attention of local and national leaders. It was hailed as a great success of rural healthcare development because the health station had created a reliable organizational foundation of socialism in rural healthcare and disease prevention. The Health Ministry promoted the Mishan town health station as a model for the whole nation in 1955, and immediately a trend to create cooperative healthcare service swept across rural China. A year after, more than 10,000 health stations had been established with the sponsorship of their agricultural cooperatives. More than 100,000 health workers worked at these health stations, covering about 10 percent of rural China with medical mutual aid and relief.[81]

Another successful story of rural health innovation was Jishan county of Shanxi province (山西省稷山县). Its impressive work earned the county the fame, “a red flag in rural health,” meaning a model in rural health.[82] In the early 1950s, the county took an active part in the nationwide patriotic health movement and every household pledged hygiene with the slogans of “clean person, clean house, clean courtyard, and clean street” and “elimination of flies, fleas, lice, rats, and mosquitoes.”[83] The county had 25 united clinics and 14 health stations. In 1955, the 25 united clinics were re-organized into 13 town health protection stations (乡保健站), each supported by their respective agricultural cooperatives. The county had 1229 health rooms each in a village, and 226 baby delivery stations and nurseries. Every village had a health worker. A health protection organization was thus formed in every agricultural cooperative.[84] Taiyang village (太阳村), for instance, had maternal and children’s healthcare since 1952. When the agricultural cooperative was established in 1955, it took 30 yuan out of the collective common fund to create a health protection room (保健室) and to train midwives and health workers. Farmers each contributed 0.3 yuan (三毛钱) of health fees to receive four types of free healthcare service at the health room—free registration, diagnosis, injection and house call. This basic free medical service excluded drugs. In 1958 during the Great Leap Forward, the Taiyang village health room was expanded into a health station when the agricultural cooperative became a people’s commune.

The commune created a common health fund for the provision of free medical service for farmers (大家集资、治病免费). Thus, a commune-sponsored free cooperative medical service (合作医疗) was formed.[85] The experiment of collective rural healthcare in Jishan county was highly praised by local government as an exemplary health model.

The Health Ministry described Jishan county's work in its report on the progress of rural health to the central government, whereby the central government decided to support the practice of people's commune's collective cooperative medical service. Accordingly, the Health Ministry encouraged the communes to build cooperative medical service but cautioned that they should take into account the following factors: the level of local agricultural production, the degree of people's willingness, the appropriate reduction of people's economic burden, the proper compensation for health workers, and the gradual development of healthcare. The well-off communes could continue to experiment with commune-sponsored free medical service (社办公费医疗), but the communes that had been using self-pay method of medical care did not have to rush into a commune-sponsored free medical service. Communes should develop their collective healthcare gradually according to their production level and people's willingness. The pay for health workers should not be, in general, below their pre-commune level.[86] Those suggestions on rural health development were sent to every level of local government as a reference of guidance. As Jishan county was hailed as the model by newspapers and promoted by the government, communes rushed to create cooperative medical service across the country. Communes provided funds to organize free cooperative medical service and few liked to be left behind. The enthusiasm in creating collective medical service reflected the revolutionary passion in building a better socialist society during the people's commune movement. Macheng county of Hubei province (湖北省麻城县), for instance, saw all of its 96 communes set up collective medical service in 1958.[87] With the help of county hospital and mobile medical teams from cities, rural cooperative medical services trained their own health workers to treat minor illnesses so that farmers did not have to travel far for medical needs.

Rural health workers served as local activists in health campaigns that tackled devastating epidemic and endemic diseases such as schistosomiasis, filariasis, malaria, hookworm, cholera, typhoid, dysentery, etc. Collaborating with mobile medical teams, they provided free vaccinations and led people in sanitation and anti-pest campaigns. Public health and disease control was integrated in the national plan of agricultural development. The 1956 National Guideline of Agricultural Development (全国农业发展纲要) specified the goals of eliminating more than a dozen major epidemic and endemic diseases in the next twelve years (1956–1967). Management of water and waste was the center of attention in rural health movement. People were mobilized to dig wells for clean water, and collect human and animal waste to turn them into fertilizer. In the efforts to improve hygiene and sanitation, people were encouraged to change their wood stoves to chimney stoves, to enlarge their windows to keep the kitchens bright, clean and ventilated, and to build sanitary latrines, pigsties and animal sheds. In short, people tried to achieve "two managements and five improvements (两管五改)"—management of water and waste, and improvements of latrines, animal sheds, wells, environment and stoves. With the political mobilization of people to participate in the transformation of the society, land reclamation and irrigation projects were combined with disease prevention. The most extensive and well-known campaign was the eradication of schistosomiasis and land reclamation, where people dredged rivers, filled up ponds and ditches, and killed snails that spread the disease.[88] The preventive campaigns and the cooperative medical service, coupled with the increase of agricultural production, in the communes significantly improved people's health and living standards. The life expectancy of the Chinese population increased dramatically in the first two decades of the PRC, approximately from 38 in 1949 to 45 in 1955, 50 in 1960, and 60 in 1965.[89]

Rural health development relied on the availability of health personnel, and the government paid special attention to the training of rural medical and health workers to strengthen healthcare at the basic level. According to the Health Ministry's "Specific Implementation Measures for the Work of Rural Basic Organizations (draft)" issued in 1951, basic health personnel included health workers, midwives (and assistants) and assistant nurses (卫生员、妇幼保健员、护士助理员). Health workers were recruited from "sons and daughters of peasants and workers, elementary school teachers including rural elementary school teachers and private school students without gender discrimination." "Midwives and assistant nurses should be recruited from village old-style midwives, female elementary school graduates, female factory workers, rural women and elementary school teachers."[90] It was clear that educational level and ability was the foundation of the requirement of the recruits, though political consideration was taken into account. As a rule, the recruits would undergo a short training program without taking leave of work. Village health workers were to be trained by the town/district health station or by the county hospital if the town/district health station was not established yet. Midwives and assistant nurses were to be trained by the county hospital. The Health Ministry provided the training curriculum and defined half a year as the training time for midwives and assistant nurses and eight weeks for health workers. The health workers learned preventive medicine, first aid, maternal and children's health. Sometimes, the training took much shorter courses just to get the health workers familiar with the most basic knowledge to meet local needs. In Zhejiang province, local training centers in 1955 provided a five-day training for 1100 village health workers about the handling of schistosomiasis (a devastating endemic in the region), first aid for external injuries, common knowledge of disease prevention, and maternal and children's healthcare.[91] In 1962, the Health Ministry instructed that county hospitals should have good plans with specific emphasis on providing technical guidance and training to rural health organizations.

As the healthcare system evolved in the socialist reconstruction of China in the 1950s and 1960s, county health institutions included county hospital, county health and epidemic prevention station, and county maternal and children's healthcare station. Some counties established Chinese medicine hospitals, county health education schools, drug examination offices, and special disease prevention stations. Rural towns/communes had health centers and hospitals, and village/production brigade had health stations, thus forming a three-tiered healthcare network with the county hospital at the top, the town/commune hospital in the middle, and the village/brigade health station at the bottom.

When the agricultural sector suffered major setbacks in the three years following the 1958 Great Leap Forward, many communes could not sustain the cooperative medical expenses. As a result, rural medical services began to decline. By 1964, only about 30 percent of communes and brigades continued to operate cooperative medical service in the entire country.[92] It was a major setback of rural health work. In the meantime, the majority of college trained medical and health personnel stayed to work in city hospitals including county hospitals. Few of them worked in commune hospitals, not to mention village health stations. According to the data of 1964, the distribution of medical personnel was in strong favor of cities, with 69 percent of high-level (college educated) medical personnel in cities and 31 percent in counties and their rural communities (10 percent in rural communes). Regarding the intermediate-level (school educated) medical personnel, 57 percent were in cities and 43 percent in counties and their rural communes (27 percent in rural communes).[93] The majority of medical workers in rural China continued to be the traditional practitioners of Chinese medicine, although the newly trained health workers and paramedics began to fill the ranks of rural health. In terms of medical expenditure, 30 percent of national health budget was spent on free healthcare (公费医疗) for state employees, whereas 27 percent was spent on the countryside that included counties and their rural communities (16 percent for the rural population in the communes). The data indicated that those who enjoyed state free healthcare (about 8.3 million) cost more than that spent on the 500 million (五亿) farmers in 1964.[94] Apparently, two types of healthcare co-existed in China: one was the state-sponsored free healthcare, and the other was the commune collective-sponsored free healthcare. The 1964 data revealed a huge gap between urban and rural China in terms of access to medical service and health protection. It was in this context that Chairman Mao Zedong made the call in June 1965: "Put the emphasis of health work in the countryside."[95] Mao was upset about the work of the Health Ministry after he read about the health situation. With Mao's criticism of the Health Ministry, leaders of the central government, such as Zhou Enlai, Liu Shaoqi, and Lu Dingyi, worked with leaders of the Health Ministry and gave specific instructions on how to improve rural health work.

Rural health and barefoot doctors during the Cultural Revolution

In January 1965, Qian Xinzhong (钱信忠, 1911–2009) was appointed as Health Minister at the third People's Congress. During the meeting of the Congress, Mao Zedong met Qian and complained that medical colleges took too long to produce doctors. He quizzed Qian: "Does your health ministry want to open up to serve the workers, peasants and soldiers? I see it doesn't."[96] Changes in medical education came soon afterwards. The Health Ministry added a three-year curriculum to the existing medical education and increased the enrollment in 15 medical colleges to produce more doctors for the countryside. It also decided that city doctors be organized as mobile medical teams to go to rural areas on regular basis and high-level doctors like chief physicians take turns to participate in the mobile medical teams to provide medical treatment and training in the countryside. By April 1965, more than 1520 mobile medical teams with 18,600 doctors were already in the countryside. With hundreds of millions of farmers needing medical service, that number was too small to make a significant difference. In August 1965, the Health Ministry proposed to reduce medical education from 6 to 5 years at college and pharmacy education from 5 to 4 years.

In the meantime, large numbers of young rural farmers were trained as part-time health workers (半农半医). They would return to their rural communities after training to serve their fellow villagers.[97] Their work was compensated with work points, and therefore, would cost nothing extra for the commune and production brigade. The part-time health workers, who gained the endearment of "barefoot doctors" in 1968 during the Cultural Revolution, would participate in farming work while providing rudimentary health services to peasants in the field. The Health Ministry proposed to achieve the goal that within the next 3–5 years each production brigade would have a midwife and each production team a health worker. It provided local health administration with the guideline of strengthening the training of part-time rural health workers and midwives. In general, rural health workers were required to learn the following: (1) knowledge about 20–30 types of the most common local diseases, treatment of minor illnesses and injuries, use of simple first aid, prescription of commonly used drugs, and basic methods of acupuncture; (2) knowledge of how to eliminate the four pests, how to provide hygienic treatment of water and waste, and how to carry out patriotic health movement and health education; and (3) knowledge of how to report epidemics and use simple methods to prevent contagious diseases such as using vaccination injection. Requirements for midwives included the ability to use new delivery methods, conduct prenatal examinations, provide care for the puerperal mother and baby, and conduct family planning education.[98] These specific requirements of rural health workers and midwives provided a standard of health work and the basic quality of healthcare in rural China. Rural health workers and midwives would receive repeated training to update their knowledge and new requirements of health work. Different from the health assistants of Dingxian in the 1930s that C. C. Chen innovatively trained, the rural health workers and barefoot doctors were trained to function independently in treating and preventing diseases and even providing prescription of drugs, a much more important responsibility than merely assisting doctors.

In some rural areas, there was a differentiation of health workers of production team (生产队卫生员) and health protection workers of production brigade

(生产大队保健员) after a three-tiered network of prevention and health protection was established in the mid-1960s. Health protection workers were selected from health workers of a production team, who would receive advanced training in understanding and treating the most common local diseases from a few to a dozen types. They were also trained in the skills and knowledge of medical emergency and first aid. They were responsible for the health work of the entire production brigade, handling serious medical cases of common and infectious diseases and making referral to hospitals if necessary. They reported the health conditions of the production brigade to the commune and county hospitals and received training there on a regular basis. Free vaccinations were carried out in rural China from the 1950s in collaboration with sanitation and hygiene movement that emphasized clean water and better management of waste to prevent diseases. When the city mobile medical teams came to rural communes, literate young farmers were selected to receive training from the doctors of the mobile teams. For instance, the second Hangzhou mobile medical team conducted short-training sessions in communes and production brigades in 1965, which included anatomy, pathology, common diseases and medicine, preventive medicine, handling injuries, emergency and first aid, acupuncture, basic nursing, family planning, etc. The entire training session lasted for two months, with 20 days for classroom studies and the rest for practice. During the five-month mobile medical service in rural Hangzhou, the team trained 165 health workers for four communes and one rural town. Another mobile medical team offered part-time trainees 11 courses, such as human physiology, microbes, common medicine, medical skills, rural health management of parasitic and infectious diseases, surgery, acupuncture, the five sense organs (ears, eyes, lips, nose and tongue), skin disease, maternal and infant health and family planning, and first aid for external injuries. The trainees learned the prevention and treatment of 68 types of common diseases, 15 types of diagnosis and treatment skills, more than 60 acupunctural points, and the application of over 70 types of Western drugs and 57 types of herbal medicine.[99] The rural health workers were expected to function as general practitioners of medicine with constant attention to disease prevention. Both Western and Chinese medicines were taught at the training sessions of rural health workers and the use of Western medicine apparently made ways into rural China during this time. Peasants loved the quick effect of Western medicine and often sought the treatment of Western medicine, particularly the injection of penicillin and other antibiotics.[100]

A new movement of rural health gained momentum after Chairman Mao's instruction on rural health work was widely promoted by newspapers and the government. From leaders of the central government to the cadre of rural communes, attention was turned to building up a rural cooperative medical system. Premier Zhou Enlai and Party Secretary Liu Shaoqi talked with Health Minister Qian Xinzhong and other health leaders, urging them to send more urban doctors, including ophthalmologists and dentists, to the countryside, by half of or at least one third of urban health work force. Premier Zhou asked: "Wouldn't it be better that the Health Ministry send half of its own personnel to the countryside as well, doing what it had done during the war time by going to whatever places it was most needed?" Zhou explained: "When Chairman (Mao) said to serve the great numbers of people, he meant to serve the peasants."[101] Major newspapers, such as *The People's Daily*, *Health Newspaper*, and the party magazine *Red Flag*, published series of articles in 1968–69 about rural cooperative medical services as the type of healthcare welcomed by the peasants. Media popularization and promotion provided the political rhetoric to a mass movement to develop a rural cooperative medical system (农村合作医疗制度). Meanwhile, the Cultural Revolution was reaching its peak in encouraging the masses to destroy the old and to create the new. Rural cooperative medical services were promoted as a new socialist creation and expanded across China. Barefoot doctors, the rural part-time paramedic health workers, were hailed as the new thing (新生事物) of the Cultural Revolution.

When Chairman Mao saw the newspaper report in 1968 that Leyuan Commune of Changyang county in Hubei province (湖北省长阳县乐园公社) had organized a free cooperative medical service for the peasants, he praised it as a good thing. Immediately, Leyuan Commune became the model for rural health of the entire country. Leyuan Commune organized its cooperative medical service in December 1966 with each person contributing one yuan a year, and the production team, out of a common welfare fund, contributing 0.1 yuan for each participant member. In this way, farmers would enjoy complete free medical treatment and free drugs after paying only a five fen (0.05 yuan) registration fee each time they sought medical service. The commune hospital had a medical staff of 12 people; only two of them received a regular salary while the rest received their pay by earning work points, as did the production brigade cadres and barefoot doctors, with additional monthly cash compensation of 3–5 yuan. Ninety-nine percent of the farmers joined the cooperative medical program, and they were happy that it solved their problems of medical service and drugs.[102] From 1969 onwards, the whole China went through a new enthusiastic movement to develop a rural cooperative medical system. By 1980, 90 percent of production brigades had established cooperative medical services to provide free healthcare for 85 percent of the rural population.[103]

In the prevention of diseases, free vaccinations were given in collaboration with the sanitary movement of "two managements and five improvements" (两管五改), which had been promoted in the 1950s. People conducted sanitary management of water and waste and the improvement of latrines, animal sheds, wells, environment, and kitchen stoves. All of these activities were part of the effort to get rid of the pests—flies, fleas, bedbugs, and mosquitoes. Health measures were integrated into agricultural development and the transformation of rural lifestyle in the socialist modernization program. Health posters were popular educational tools to instruct people where and how to build cow sheds and pigsties with modern sanitary standards, and the effective ways of managing animal and human waste and converting it into fertilizer. Often, the health messages in posters were written in the traditional style of rhymed couplets to make it easy to remember.[104] As in the 1950s, health education encouraged people to change their small wood stoves into bigger chimney stoves so that the smoke would go out of the house though the chimney, and to change the old small windows into large ones to let in more fresh air and light. To make sure that water was clean and convenient to use, villagers were instructed to dig wells close to homes and far away from toilets, and to change old latrines into modern toilets. These methods aimed to achieve better sanitation and health, and to increase agricultural production at the same time. The importance of rural cooperative medical services, together with epidemic prevention and sanitary movement, in protecting people's health and preventing diseases was seen in the drastic decrease of epidemic diseases and the increase of life expectancy in those years. The life expectancy of the Chinese increased from 60 to 68 years old during 1965–1980.[105]

The Cultural Revolution (1966–1976) was a time when the rural cooperative medical system was established with a significant increase of rural health workers and barefoot doctors. The barefoot doctors played a vital role in rural healthcare, though their services varied from place to place depending on the type of training they received and the ability of individuals. During the Cultural Revolution, the political quality of the recruits for barefoot doctors was emphasized: they were expected to be born with a good family background like a poor peasant family, loving rural China and willing to serve the people whole-heartedly. Training was carried out in local county and commune hospitals, with re-training or rotation of training to improve their knowledge and skills continuously. Women were promoted as the image of health workers in socialist China, even though more female doctors were seen in cities than in the countryside. In fact, only one third of barefoot doctors were female because there was a lack of educated females in villages to qualify for the literacy expectations (quite a number of barefoot doctors were the sent-down youth). The majority of rural parents still held the traditional ideas of educating the sons rather than the daughters, despite the CCP's revolutionary efforts to transform people's thoughts.

Training of barefoot doctors varied from region to region and even from county to county. The general principle of training was to teach them prevention and treatment of the most common epidemic and endemic diseases with both Chinese and Western medicines. The content of study was tailored to local conditions, with emphasis on combining Chinese and Western medicines and relying on local resources. Attention was given to the integration of medical treatment and prevention, and planting and producing herbal medicine. Barefoot doctors were expected to know how to create a sanitary village by managing water, waste, and kitchens, and eliminating pests. They were also expected to have knowledge of modern contraception and methods of midwifery. Methods of training included short courses of a few months or a year, repeated training, advanced training and internship at different levels of hospitals, working together with experienced doctors, and taking classes at local health schools. Barefoot doctors were trained to provide basic medical diagnosis and treatment on their own as independent paramedics and health educators in rural China.

The Cultural Revolution also saw a transfer of medical resources from cities to the countryside when doctors as well as many other urban professionals were sent down to rural communes for re-education. Those people, due to their professional expertise, were immediately asked to work as doctors or teachers in the production brigade instead of working in the field. The doctors were soon recruited to work in the county and commune hospitals, whose quality of medical service was strengthened as a result. Many more part-time barefoot doctors were trained in those years and put to work in their own production teams due to the availability of the sent-down doctors to train them. By the end of 1975, the number of barefoot doctors reached more than 1.5 million, with another 3.9 million health workers (卫生员) and midwives (接生员) working in production teams, totaling the number of rural health personnel at more than 5 million. More than 65 percent of the national health budget was spent on rural China, with rural health institutions and hospital beds increased from 40 percent of national totals in 1965 to 60 percent in 1975.[106] The development of a rural cooperative medical system and the increase of barefoot doctors were mutually dependent on each other in the operation of a rural collective healthcare. They were both integral parts of the collective agricultural system of the people's communes.

Disease control and social transformation: cases of anti-tuberculosis and anti-malaria campaigns

The anti-tuberculosis and anti-malaria campaigns were two examples of how health campaigns aimed to change people more broadly than just health improvement. Tuberculosis (TB) affected urban residents more than those in the countryside, whereas malaria affected people in rural villages more than those in cities in the 1950s–1980s. Using these two types of diseases as case studies, I hope to demonstrate that the measures taken to address public health problems were incorporated in the general economic development and social transformation of the people and the nation. Disease prevention started with the change of individual behavior and the transformation of the community not only in terms of health but also in terms of the social and moral expectations of citizens in socialist China.

The anti-tuberculosis and anti-malaria campaigns were integral elements of the Patriotic Health Movement that targeted simultaneously more than a dozen major epidemic and pandemic diseases as aforementioned. In order to bring the epidemic diseases under control, the government sent mobile medical teams to urban communities and rural villages to treat the sick, while mobilizing the public to participate in preventive health campaigns. As a measure to coordinate health work with the anti-germ warfare campaign during the Korean War, the central government proposed the establishment of Health and Epidemic Prevention Stations as a priority in 1952. The stations were created in every city district and rural county and functioned as the professional and technical centers of health education and preventive services including vaccinations in a national network. By 1957, China had established 1626 health and epidemic prevention stations; and in 1985 the number of the stations increased to 3410 with a total staff of 144,998.[107] Hundreds of thousands of Chinese health professionals were being trained in the new medical educational system that had been influenced by the Soviet model in the 1950s. China trained more than 100,000 doctors in 17 years (1949–1966), with a total of 150,000 doctors of Western medicine by 1966, about one for 5000 people.[108]

Poverty, unsanitary conditions, malnutrition, and unhealthy habits all contributed to the spread of epidemic diseases. The socioeconomic problems of diseases were addressed through the integration of health programs into the national economic development plans. The approach of treating health as integral to general socioeconomic development shaped China's health policies that battled all major epidemic and endemic diseases at once in a coordinated manner across regions and provinces. Moreover, specific committees were established to deal with individual diseases with targeted research and preventive methods, although they were not separated from the overall health movement. The methods proved effective in fighting the widespread epidemics and endemics. Cholera was eradiated by 1951; plague was under basic control by 1955; venereal diseases were basically eradicated by 1959; and smallpox was eradicated in 1963. Other major epidemics such as typhus, typhoid, polio, measles, relapse fever, and hookworm were also eradicated or under basic control.[109] The health campaigns brought an enormous decrease of tuberculosis and malaria across China, with eradication in many places, but they have returned with the expansion of industrialization and urbanization since the 1990s. The anti-TB and anti-malaria campaigns of the 1950s–1980s illustrated how the Chinese actually carried out their health movement when striving to build a socialist country.

The anti-tuberculosis campaign emphasized the promotion of changing people's behavior from unhygienic to civilized and cultured manner. Tuberculosis has a long history in China. Its Chinese name, *xulao bing* (虚劳病, exhaustive disease), and the description of its symptoms first appeared in the Yellow Emperor's Classic of Internal Medicine (*huangdi neijing*, 黄帝内经), compiled between 403 and 221 BC. Tuberculosis became a leading killer in the early twentieth century as China suffered from constant wars, widespread poverty, poor sanitation, and the health hazards of industrial factories in port cities. More than 27 million Chinese suffered from TB and over one million died of it in the 1930s.[110] Organized efforts to fight the disease took a major step forward on 21 October 1933 when the Tuberculosis Prevention Association of China (中国预防痨病协会, renamed as Chinese Anti-Tuberculosis Association, 中国防痨协会, in January 1948) was established in Shanghai. The sanatorium was the only way of treating tuberculosis, and it was limited and localized, available only to those who could afford it before 1949. The Nationalist government did not include tuberculosis in the list of notifiable diseases, nor did the government take active measures to treat and prevent the disease. Much of the anti-TB work was carried out by the Tuberculosis Prevention Association.[111] Even the anti-TB education and propaganda appealed to urban middle class in the 1930s–1940s, with poster images promoting Western-style homes of spacious rooms and decorative paintings.[112] The major groups who suffered from TB, such as industrial workers and the urban and rural poor, were left out on their own.

Things began to change when the PRC government started the public health campaigns to fight all major diseases that harmed people's health and weakened the nation. Tuberculosis incidence was estimated at 4 percent of the population in 1950, which meant over 25 million of a population of 563 million suffered from tuberculosis in China.[113] Urban residents were particularly affected as poverty, overcrowding and industrial pollution contributed to the spread of the disease. Major cities like Shanghai, Tianjin, and Beijing were notorious for TB epidemics. In Shanghai alone, about 11,000 people died of TB in 1951, with a mortality rate of 208 per hundred thousand.[114] After years of coordinated measures of comprehensive anti-TB campaigns of treatment and prevention and improvement of living standards, China's TB incidence dropped from 4 percent in 1950 to 1.5 percent in 1965, and the mortality rate decreased from 280 to 40 per hundred thousand in the same period.[115] In Shanghai, both incidence and mortality rates dropped significantly by 1965 when the number of TB deaths was about 2000 and the mortality rate was 31.1 per hundred thousand. In 1986, the number of deaths from TB in Shanghai decreased to 176 and the mortality rate was 6.06 per hundred thousand.[116] The major reason for such significant success against TB lay in the energetic campaigns of combined treatment and prevention, coupled with extensive public health education in a continuous anti-TB movement powered by political motivation and patriotic discourse.

The PRC government first tackled TB in the campaign to improve workers' health at factories and mines, where incidence of the disease was high. Methods included treatment of TB patients in hospitals and sanatoria and education of the masses about prevention by taking BCG (Bacille Calmette-Guérin) vaccine and X-rays and by maintaining sanitation and personal hygiene and healthy habits. In addition to TB hospitals and clinics, factories and mining companies established their own sanatoria and resting rooms for TB patients. Labor unions of the railway system, for instance, set up their own sanatoria with 150–200 beds each, which were administered by a small staff and a few TB health specialists.[117] The sanatorium approach was most active in the early 1950s when the campaign concentrated on bringing TB patients to treatment and preventing them from spreading the disease. Sanatoria reduced the pressure on TB hospitals, which did not have the capacity to handle all the TB patients. Sanatoria admitted the less acute cases and helped them recover in a relaxed and pleasant environment with lots of fresh air, sunshine, nutritious food, and good sleep. The goal was to recover the physical strength and well-being as well as to restore the productivity of the sick so that they would return to society as healthy and productive workers.[118]

TB hospitals and clinics were the centers of treatment. In 1949, there were only 13 TB hospitals with 600 beds and 5 TB treatment and prevention stations in the entire China. By 1985, the number of TB hospitals increased to 117 with a total of 27,821 beds and a staff of 26,640, whereas TB clinics and stations grew to over 400 nationwide.[119] TB clinics, which worked with TB hospitals and municipal governments, often served as a training ground for health workers of local factories and schools. In Shanghai, district TB clinics maintained relations with doctors in workplaces and the municipal disease control facilities. They were also training grounds for workplace doctors to carry out primary, secondary, and tertiary prevention.[120] Nationwide, these TB clinics played a vital part in the implementation of local anti-TB activities and gathering statistical data for the health administrators and agencies.

The Chinese Anti-Tuberculosis Association started its publication, *Anti-Tuberculosis Newsletter* (防痨通讯, later changed to *Chinese Journal of Anti-tuberculosis*,中国防痨杂志) in 1950 as a national communication platform to publicize government anti-TB policies and programs. The *Newsletter* introduced medical advances in the field, reported international anti-TB meetings and events, and shared anti-TB experiences and methods of individual factories and cities. The content of the *Newsletter* from 1950 through to 1970 indicated interesting shifts of strategies in the anti-TB movement. In the beginning, much attention was given to sanatorium and medical treatment of TB, but the focus shifted to preventive measures of BCG vaccination and X-rays after 1953. From the late 1950s into the 1960s, the *Newsletter* published articles on Western medicine learning from Chinese medicine and the discussion of Chinese medicine in the treatment and prevention of TB. The increased attention to and elevated status of Chinese medicine apparently reflected the new attitude and policy of the Health Ministry after the central government criticized its mishandling of Chinese medicine in the early 1950s. The Soviet influence was significant in the mid-1950s as articles of Soviet authors (translated into Chinese) were conspicuously published in the *Newsletter*.[121]

Preventive education and service characterized the activities of the anti-TB movement throughout the 1950s–1980s. Major efforts included free BCG vaccinations and free X-rays, and instructions for people not to spit. People were encouraged to maintain good health and a strong immune system with enough sleep, good nutrition and regular exercises. Mobile medical teams brought BCG vaccines to factories, schools, urban communities and rural villages. People lined up to receive free BCG injections provided by the government in workplaces and schools, and even on the streets where the mobile vaccination station was set up. China has produced its own BCG and other vaccines since the 1950s. Workers were encouraged to take X-rays at hospitals and at mobile X-ray vehicles, which was part of the detection and prevention effort. These preventive activities were, in fact, not so different from what post-war Britain did where the National Health Service provided similar preventive check-ups for children and adults.

Visual materials, particularly colorful anti-TB posters, used simple and straightforward images to promote methods of TB prevention and treatment. Many posters contained multi-images, detailing the cause of the disease, its treatment and prevention, while some emphasized a simple message of taking BCG and not spitting on the ground.[122] In 1953–1954, the Shanghai Anti-Tuberculosis

Association created a series of 28 posters that elaborated on anti-TB methods. The series started with two cover posters that carried the guiding instruction of national health work. The first one summarized the health policies and programs specified in the First Five-Year Plan (1953–1957) and the second reiterated the four health principles of the national policy. Following the two cover posters, the series began the pictorial explanation of the cause of TB—tubercle bacillus—and the channels of transmission such as the respiratory and digestive systems. For the treatment of TB, the posters visualized fresh air, sunshine, good nutrition, and good rest as the basic methods, though medicine and surgery were presented as useful possibilities as well. On detection and prevention, the posters urged people to pay attention to personal hygiene and environmental sanitation, take the BCG vaccine and X-rays, not to spit on the ground, disinfect TB patients' belongings, separate patients' utensils, have exercise and maintain a regular lifestyle to boost the immune system. The images encouraged people to disseminate anti-TB knowledge to help eradicate the disease. They also emphasized the relation between an individual's good health and productivity. An interesting significance of the series was that the two cover posters were added last to the set in 1954, which clearly indicated that health workers tried to keep up with the most current political rhetoric and policy in the changing society. Images of health posters and anti-TB materials were constantly recycled throughout the decades from the 1930s to the 1950s.[123]

Children benefitted from the BCG vaccinations as medical teams came to schools and kindergartens to give regular vaccine shots against TB and other infectious diseases. In Beijing, for instance, 86.7 percent of infants aged 4 years old received the BCG vaccination in 1954; and in 1973, it was 96.9 percent.[124] School pupils were often led and mobilized by their teachers to disseminate anti-TB instructions in urban communities, urging people to take BCG and X-rays and to develop a good health habit of not spitting on the ground. Children actively promoted personal hygiene and environmental sanitation at home and in public parks. They also competed in contests to see who caught and killed the most flies and mosquitoes. In the public health campaigns against TB, spitting became a focus of prevention not only for health reasons but also for social and cultural reasons. Spitting was considered unhygienic and dangerous in spreading diseases such as TB. It was also described as an uncivilized behavior socially and culturally unacceptable. If TB carried the social stigma of incurability and death in the old days, spitting now signified a person's barbaric and uneducated traits. Disease prevention intended to transform people and change their behavior. Hence, a model citizen would be both healthy and civilized in social behavior, and be a cultured citizen as well. It was commonplace to see signs of "Do not spit on the ground! Splitting is uncivilized!" in Chinese parks and public places, at work units and schools. China's omnipresent fixation on spitting as the cause of spreading diseases was not unique if we put it in an international context. The anti-TB movement in the United States at the turn of the twentieth century carried a comparable zeal in targeting spitting as an immoral and barbaric behavior. Fighting tuberculosis helped generate a germ gospel in American households and society where anti-TB activities gained a serious moral stake as well as a health awakening.[125] For the Chinese, a civilized behavior such as not spitting on the ground indicated a person's healthy and cultural behavior as well as the person's socialist moral virtues.

The anti-malaria campaign was promoted to improve people's health and physique as well as to make them better productive citizens. Anti-malaria programs were integrated and coordinated in the national Patriotic Health Movement against all major diseases. However, specific preventive measures were taken and implemented against malaria. Chinese scholars divided the post-1949 anti-malaria campaigns into three phases.[126] The first ran from 1949 through 1955, when investigations of malaria incidence and prevalence were carried out across China and services of treatment and prevention were provided in the most severely infected regions. The second phase covered the period from 1956 to 1977 when treatment and prevention were conducted in nationwide anti-malaria campaigns. Consequently, malaria declined from 102.8 per ten thousand in 1955 to 21.6 per ten thousand in 1958, a drop of 80 percent. In the 1960s and the 1970s, however, malaria made a comeback, resulting in one widespread outbreak in early 1960s and another one in early 1970s. By 1982, malaria incidence was finally brought down to the level of 1959. The third phase was the 1978–1990s when anti-malaria work was carried out persistently, using different methods that fit local environment and circumstances, with the help of new drugs such as antimalarial tablets (止疟片). The result was the achievement of basic control of malaria by the early 1990s. In 1998 when China's population was 1.3 billion, only 31,000 malaria cases were reported, with a morbidity of 0.25 per ten thousand, a drop of 99 percent compared with 1954.[127]

Malaria, like tuberculosis, has a long history in China. Its symptoms were recorded in the Yellow Emperor's *Internal Medicine*. Medical scientists started investigation of malaria in China in the 1930s, with limited surveys of the heavily infected south and central regions.[128] In the 1940s a few local health centers were established to study and treat malaria with the sponsorship of the Rockefeller Foundation. In 1950, more than 30 million Chinese people were reported suffering from malaria and 1 percent of them died.[129] Since there was no vaccine against malaria and there was a severe shortage of medicine, anti-malaria campaigns concentrated on preventive measures. The Health and Epidemic Prevention Stations played a key role in getting anti-malaria work started in rural villages in the 1950s, despite limited resources. Xuyi county (盱眙县) of Northern Jiangsu served as an example. The county was located on the banks of Hongze Lake, a very poor region. It suffered badly from malaria and other epidemic diseases such as typhoid, cholera, measles, schistosomiasis and filariasis. The county's epidemic prevention station had a staff of six people in the mid-1950s, who were responsible for the anti-epidemic work of the entire county's 300,000 people. The six staff members were divided into medical teams to go to villages to give vaccinations, and to conduct investigations of schistosomiasis, filariasis and malaria—diseases that had no vaccines available at the time. The station had only one microscope, and each staff member a protective suit and a sprayer for insecticide. But they were gung-ho about their work and not afraid of hardship. They walked tens of miles to villages with beddings on their back. They lived with peasants for days with 0.3 yuan (三毛钱) per diem, and captured mosquitoes at night under the beds of villagers for medical research. After analyzing the different types of mosquitoes, they would select the appropriate insecticide to achieve the best effect.[130] The situation improved over the next decade when China's economy improved and the number of health professionals increased. The station had more staff members as more health workers were trained, and new drugs were made available through development and production. More importantly, a cooperative healthcare system was being established in rural areas to provide medical services.[131]

Anti-malaria campaigns were integrated in the state-planning of economic and social development by the central government. In fact, disease control was never separated from the overarching goals of transforming China and building a better society. The national program of agricultural development of 1956 made clear that China aimed to achieve the basic eradication of diseases that harmed people the most, including malaria. In the same year, a national conference was held to discuss specific guidelines and measures to eradicate malaria within seven years.[132] The ambitious program to eradicate malaria in a short time of seven years did not materialize, though it achieved significant progress in reducing malaria. The difficulty in bringing malaria under control indicated the profound challenge in fighting the disease when no vaccine was available.

A major effort of the anti-malaria campaigns was to educate the public about malaria and teach them the methods to prevent it. Visual materials, such as health posters and pictorials, became an important popular educational tool and especially useful for the less literate masses.[133] They depicted the cause, the symptoms, the preventive methods and curative treatment of the disease. An anti-malaria poster generally had two essential components: (1) illustrations of scientific information of the disease, and (2) methods of prevention. Scientific knowledge of the disease included information about the mosquito's life cycle and how it spread malaria from the sick to the healthy. Methods of prevention focused on two types. One was to clean up the sources and environment that produced mosquitoes such as standing water, by covering water jars, filling up shallow ponds and ditches, pulling out weeds and raising fish to feed on mosquito larvae. These activities involved the improvement of environment, which were incorporated in land reclamation and irrigation construction for agricultural production. The other method was to kill or drive off mosquitoes by using bed-nets, window and door screens, spraying DDT and the traditional method of burning mosquito repellent incense. The anti-malaria messages were easy to understand and the images realistic to imitate and practice in real life. Health education and dissemination of information on the disease influenced people's views and change of health behavior. They voluntarily carried out the preventive work of spraying to kill mosquitoes and using bed-nets to keep mosquitoes away when they realized the benefits of the actions.

Some anti-malaria posters directly targeted the rural population with more traditional tactics of appeal. In one health poster, the traditional form of literary style of *sanzi jing* (三字经, an easy-to-remember rhymed three-character style) was used to sum up the harm of malaria on people and farm production. The health text reads:

> malaria harms people, it comes from plasmodium, spread by mosquitoes; after their bites, you get the disease, you feel chill, and then fever, headache and sweat; July and August, easy to get, once infected, four limbs weak, face yellow, and spleen swollen, busy farming time, labor is lost.[134]

Images of anti-malaria posters usually portrayed peasants actively engaged in collective efforts to eradicate malaria and improve their lives. Peasants were sometimes depicted in colorful traditional attire doing various jobs of prevention. Visual images highlighted people dredging rivers and filling up ditches in the rural community, working together to eliminate the breeding grounds of mosquitoes. Barefoot doctors, the paramedics in rural China, took blood samples and gave patients timely treatment. People were instructed to report malaria to health workers for immediate action of treatment and prevention. The anti-malaria activities brought changes in people's health behavior, improved the environment, increased production, and modernized the rural community with electricity and new farmland. Health improvement, therefore, was part of the modern transformation of people and society.[135]

China developed anti-malarial drugs, such as chloroquine (氯奎), pyrimethamine (乙胺嘧啶), and primaquine Kui (伯氨奎), in late 1950s and manufactured them in large quantities from the early 1960s. As anti-malarial drugs were increasingly available free to ordinary people, they became an indispensable element of anti-malaria campaigns. The strategies of fighting malaria shifted when medicine was available to treat patients. Anti-malaria education and propaganda began to disseminate information of different types of malaria drugs, in addition to promoting preventive measures. Malaria patients were urged to get timely treatment for their own good and for the people around them. Those who had suffered malaria in the previous two years were now registered and given medicine to prevent relapses. In 1972, Chinese medical scientists successfully extracted artemisinin [*qinghaosu*, 青蒿素], which was more effective in treating malaria.[136] The new medicine, which has helped save millions of lives in the world, eventually helped China achieve the basic control of malaria in the early 1990s. Chinese scientist, Tu Youyou (屠呦呦, 1930–), a key member of the science team that discovered artemisinin, was awarded the Nobel Prize in 2015 for her significant role in the discovery.[137]

Conclusion

People's health was an integral part of socialist modernization of China. The health movement offered a broad view of China's transformation in the

1950s–1980s when anti-disease campaigns were incorporated into the overall sociopolitical and economic reconstruction of Chinese society. The CCP-led government emphasized the health work of serving the people under the guidance of socialist ideology and patriotic nationalism. Built upon the institutional structure of state medicine that the Nationalist modernizers had established, the PRC government created a national healthcare system, extending modern health facilities and services to the vast rural villages and minority regions. Organized health and medical services in the form of state-run hospitals and clinics became the feature of health provider in socialist China. A universal free healthcare system was gradually built in the 1950s–1970s where people of state-owned enterprises (全民所有) enjoyed free healthcare with state support and people of collective-owned enterprises (集体所有, all rural communities and some urban business enterprises) enjoyed free healthcare with collective sponsorship. The establishment of the Health and Epidemic Prevention Stations and the Maternal and Children's Health Protection Stations in every city, urban district, county, and village town created a national network of a preventive mechanism and the basic care for women and children, two of the most urgent tasks of health work. With the emphasis on prevention, people were mobilized to participate in the health campaigns as active agents to protect their own health, defend their country, and increase economic production. Large numbers of health workers of different levels of professional expertise were trained to meet the enormous demands, particularly the need of rural health work. In 1978 the peak time of rural healthcare, about 5 million rural health workers including barefoot doctors and midwives provided basic health service to the rural population of about 800 million.

The mass movement of patriotic health campaigns demonstrated how an external event, such as the Korean War, exerted an unexpected influence on China's national health policy and work, especially when the event threatened public health and national security at once. The alleged germ warfare by America during the Korean War became a catalyst in the formation of the Patriotic Health Movement to turn health campaigns into a mass movement. The health movement was a political movement that rallied people to fight disease and defend the nation with patriotic pride and national urgency. It was estimated that 90 percent of urban residents and 60 percent of rural population participated in the Patriotic Health Movement of mass campaigns in the mid-1950s. The sanitary and cleanliness campaigns not only aimed to prevent diseases but also the transformation of former shanty towns into beautiful neighborhoods of modern houses and roads. The patriotic health movement was a continuous national reconstruction movement to improve people's health and to advance the overall socioeconomic development throughout the 1950s–1980s.

Movements to eliminate illiteracy and to popularize science swept across the nation from 1950 onwards, which provided opportunities to spread health education beyond health campaigns. People learned scientific knowledge of health and disease when they attended literacy classes. Visual materials, such as posters, pictorials, and wall bulletins, were popular means of education for the masses with low costs. Visual images served to illuminate specific health problems and inform the viewers of useful methods of fighting diseases. The goal was to achieve the maximum effect in a short time by visually explaining scientific knowledge to solve health problems in real life. In the mass movement to learn scientific knowledge, science was popularized in vivid images and colloquial language. Political ideas of socialism were also imparted to the masses in the learning process where new social values and attitudes were forged. The rich content of visual health educational materials often captured the distinctive social and political lives of China in those decades.

Chinese medicine, after undergoing a brief difficult road of integration, finally secured its place on a par with Western medicine in the people's health system, thanks to the promotion and support of the central government. The CCP leaders, such as Mao Zedong, Zhou Enlai, and Liu Shaoqi, appreciated the value of Chinese medicine and considered it an important national heritage. They not only supported Chinese medicine but also determined to update it scientifically by emphasizing the unity of Chinese and Western medicine. The attempt to marginalize Chinese medicine by the leaders of Health Ministry in the early 1950s, nonetheless, demonstrated the deep-rooted bias against Chinese medicine among the medical elite of Western medicine, no matter what political party and ideology they might hold. How Chinese medicine was treated had not been a medical matter but a political matter throughout the twentieth century. The CCP, out of its own experience in the hardest days of revolution, learned the value of Chinese medicine but confirmed it needed to be updated with science. The PRC's effort to scientize Chinese medicine, amazingly, led to the development of a third force of medicine in China, i.e. the integrated Chinese and Western medicine (also called "integrative medicine"), which has become a significant part of the Chinese medical system today.

Rural healthcare developed in parallel with the agricultural collectivization that transformed rural China economically and socially. During 1949–1955, the land reform swept across rural villages and mutual aid teams were formed among peasants to help each other in farming when land was privately owned. Individual medical practitioners were encouraged to form united clinics to provide medical service and promote anti-disease health activities in villages. When collectivization developed into the higher cooperative stage in 1955–1958 with people's communes being established and land becoming collectively owned, cooperative medical services began to be formed and sponsored by individual communes out of collective resources to provide free healthcare for participating members. The rural cooperative medical system developed as an integral part of the commune system and was economically dependent on the communes. Part-time health workers of the rural cooperative medical services relied on the economic distribution system of the communes for their pay. This dependent relation was tested and made vulnerable when the agricultural sector suffered setbacks in the three years immediately following the Great Leap Forward of 1958. Rural cooperative medical services declined due to the inability of communes to support the services. When agricultural production of the communes recovered to a normal pattern of growth in 1962, rural cooperative medical services began to revive as well.

A three-tiered rural healthcare network was established with the county hospital at the top, the commune hospital in the middle, and the production brigade health station at the bottom in the village. Structurally, there appeared a similarity between this three-tiered rural healthcare system and the three-tiered health structure that Chen Zhiqian created in Dingxian in 1930s and the Nationalist government tried to create before the Japanese invasion. A close examination, however, indicates fundamental differences in that the post-1949 three-tiered rural healthcare system was constructed as an integral component of the new rural economic system of communes and that rural health workers were trained to function as independent paramedics, not as assistants to doctors as in the 1930s, to treat illnesses, to prevent epidemics, and to provide midwifery service. The county hospital functioned as the major medical and health service center for the entire county, and it also provided technical guidance and training to rural health workers at commune and brigade levels. The commune hospital served the middle link between the county hospital and the production brigade health station, where basic illnesses were treated without having to send patients to county hospital. Rural educated youth were recruited and trained as part-time health workers and midwives to work alongside their fellow villagers in the farming fields and provide medical service. Peasants called them "barefoot doctors" because they went down to work in the rice paddies bare-footed just like the peasants. With Chairman Mao's instruction of emphasizing the health work in the countryside, hundreds of thousands of health workers and barefoot doctors were trained and some city medical professionals were sent down to the countryside during the Cultural Revolution to serve the millions of rural people. The rural cooperative medical system and barefoot doctors made healthcare, for the first time, free and accessible to people in rural villages. People's lives improved due to the improvement of living standards, medical access and healthcare, and the socioeconomic transformation in general. Chinese life expectancy increased from 38 in 1949 to 68 in 1980, a huge increase in a very short time.

Notes

1 Li Dequan was active in national women's and children's affairs during the war and firmly supported the anti–Japanese war efforts. He Cheng was the Health Minister of the People's Liberation Army's General Logistics Department while serving as Vice Minister of Health. He was one of the founding leaders of the CCP health work in the Jiangxi soviet era.

2 Chen Haifeng, *Zhongguo weisheng baojian shi* [History of Health Care in China] (Shanghai: Shanghai kexue jishu chubanshe, 1992), 81.

3 Li Teh–chuan, "The People's Health Services" in *Culture, Education and Health in New China* (Peking: Foreign Language Press, 1952), 38–39.

4 Works on China and the Korean War include Shu Guang Zhang, *Mao's Military Romanticism: China and the Korean War, 1950–1953* (University Press of Kansas, 1995); Chen Jian, *China's Road to the Korean War* (New York: Columbia University Press, 1996); Allen Whiting, *China Crosses the Yalu: The Decision to Enter the Korean War*

(Stanford University Press, 1960); and William Stueck, *Rethinking the Korean War: A New Diplomatic and Strategic History* (Princeton, New Jersey: Princeton University Press, 2004).

5 Different perspectives on the germ warfare include Yang Nianqun, "Disease Prevention, Social Mobilization and Spatial Politics: The Anti–Germ Warfare Incident of 1952 and the 'Patriotic Health Campaign,'" *The Chinese Historical Review*, vol. 11, no. 2 (2004), 155–182; Ruth Rogaski, "Nature, Annihilation, and Modernity: China's Korean War Germ–Warfare Experience Reconsidered," *Journal of Asian Studies*, vol. 61, no. 2 (2002), 381–415; Kathryn Weathersby, "Deceiving the Deceivers: Moscow, Beijing, Pyongyang, and the Allegations of Bacteriological Weapons Use in Korea," *Cold War International History Project Bulletin*, vol. 11 (Winter 1998), 176–184; and Stephen Ednicott and Edward Hageman, *The United States and Biological Warfare: Secrets from the Early Cold War and Korea* (Bloomington: Indiana University Press, 1998).

6 *Zhou Enlai Nianpu* [Chronicle of Zhou Enlai's Life], vol. 1 (Beijing: Zhongyang wenxian, 1997), 233.

7 Chen, *Zhongguo weisheng baojian shi*, 107–127.

8 Li Teh–chuan, "The People's Health Services," 31.

9 Ibid., 32.

10 Gao Enxian, "Jianguo chu Mao Zedong zhuanpi de weisheng gongzuo wenxian [Instructions and Comments on Health Work by Mao Zedong in Early PRC]," *Zhonghua yishi zazhi* [Chinese Journal of Medical History], no. 1 (2000), 44–46.

11 Zhonghua quanguo minzhu funu lianhe hui, ertong fuli bu (中华全国民主妇女联合会儿童福利部 [Children's Welfare Department of the All–China Women's Democratic Association] "Xuanchuan puji xinfa jiesheng he yuer zhishi [Disseminating and Popularizing New Delivery Methods and Parenting Knowledge]" *Xin Zhongguo funu* [Women of New China] November 1949, 5.

12 Li Teh–chuan, "The People's Health Services," 32.

13 Stories of the challenges and experiences were published in the magazine *Women of New China*. The deplorable situation of rural women and birth deliveries in the 1950s was so widespread that it took time to tackle the problems, as documented by Gail Hershatter who wrote a chapter titled "Birthing Stories: Rural Midwives in 1950s China," in *Dilemmas of Victory: The Early Years of the People's Republic of China*, eds. Jeremy Brown and Paul G. Pickowicz (Cambridge MA: Harvard University Press, 2007), 337–358.

14 Chen, *Zhongguo weisheng baojian shi*, 122.

15 Li Teh–chuan, "The people's Health Services," 33.

16 Lim Kahti, "Obstetrics and Gynaecology in the Past Ten Years," *Chinese Medical Journal* 79.5 (November 1959), 375–83.

17 Huang Guangxue, ed., *Dangdai Zhongguo de mingzhu gongzuo* [Ethnic Work of Contemporary China] (Beijing: Dangdai zhongguo chubanshe, 1993), vol. 1, 75.

18 Li Teh–chuan, "The People's Health Services," 34.

19 Qu Wanlin, "Guancha xin Zhongguo de yige shijiao—shixi Longxugou zhili yu xin Zhongguo xingxiang [A Perspective of Observing the New China: An Analysis of the Transformation of Longxugou and the Image of New China]," *Dangdai Zhongguo shi yanjiu* [Contemporary China History Studies] vol. 14, no. 2 (March 2007), 46–51.

20 Lao She, *Long Xu Gou* (Beijing: Foreign Language Press, 1956.)

21 Lou Chenghao, "San zhang zhaopian jianzheng Zhaojiabang de jubian [Complete Changes of Zhaojiabang Seen through Three Pictures]," September 18, 2009, Shanghai Municipal Archives. http://www.archives.sh.cn/shjy/scbq/201203/t20120313_5692.html

22 Chen, *Zhongguo weisheng baojian shi*, 90.

23 Li Teh–chuan, "People's Health Services," 34–35.

24 Chen, *Zhongguo weisheng baojian shi*, 108–109.

25 Li Teh–chuan, "People's Health Services," 36.

26 Corresponding to the Korean War in 1950–1953, China carried out a Patriotic Health Movement and three major political campaigns against political enemies, economic abuses, and corruption. They were the Campaign of Suppression of Counterrevolutionaries, the Five–Anti Movement (against bribery, tax evasion, theft of state property, cheating on government contracts, and stealing of state economic information), and Three–Anti Movement (against corruption, waste, and obstructionist bureaucracy). These three political campaigns ended when the Korean War was over, but the Patriotic Health Movement continued into the 1980s to fight diseases and improve people's health.

27 Liping Bu, "Korean War Anti–Germ Warfare Posters," in *Hidden Treasure: The National Library of Medicine*, ed. Michael Sappol (New York: Blast Books, 2012), 198–199.

28 Mao Zedong's inscription to the Second National Health Conference, December 1952.

29 Li Dequan, "San nian lai Zhongguo renmin de weisheng shiye [Chinese People's Health in the Past Three Years]," *Xinhua yuebao* [Xinhua Monthly], October 1951, 47.

30 The health policies and programs were presented on the cover posters of a series of anti–TB posters produced by Shanghai Anti–Tuberculosis Association, 1954. See online exhibit at National Library of Medicine: http://www.nlm.nih.gov/exhibition/chineseantitb/fourseries4.html.

31 Ka–che Yip, *Disease, Colonialism, and the State: Malaria in Modern East Asia* (Hong Kong: Hong Kong University Press, 2009), 8.

32 "Chu si hai [To Eliminate the Four Pests]," *Renmin ribao* [The People's Daily], January 12, 1956.

33 On the anti-four pest movement, see Zhao Sheng and Su Zhiliang, "Xin Zhongguo de chu si hai yundong [The Anti–Four Pest Movements in New China]," *Dangdai Zhongguo shi yanjiu*, vol. 18, no. 5 (September 2011), 28–35.

34 Liu Yingjie, *Zhongguo jiaoyu dashiji* [Major Events of Education in China] (Hangzhou: Zhejiang jiaoyu chubanshe, 1993), 1831; and Liao Qifa, *Dangdai Zhongguo saomang he nongcun chengren jiaoyu de huimo yu qianzhan* [Literacy and Adult Education in Contemporary Rural China] (Chongqing: Xinan shifan daxue chubanshe, 2002), 10–11.

35 Yu Bo and Xie Guodong, *Zhongguo saomang jiaoyu* [Literacy Education in China] (Harbin: Dongbei linye daxue chubanshe, 1998), 6.

36 "Scientific medicine" was a term constantly used by the medical professionals of Western medicine in China to attack Chinese medicine as superstitious and to promote Western medicine in China.

37 Liping Bu, "Public Health and Modernization: The First Campaigns in China, 1915–1916," *Social History of Medicine*, vol. 22, no. 2 (2009), 305–319.

38 For images of germs and parasites displayed in Chinese health posters, targeting specific diseases, see the website http://www.nlm.nih.gov/hmd/chineseposters/prevention.html. The National Library of Medicine of the National Institutes of Health at Bethesda, Maryland, USA has a large collection of Chinese public health materials including posters, pamphlets and books.

39 Ma Longrui, "Xiangcun weisheng yuan de xunlian ji weishengshi de jianli [Training of Village Health Workers and the Establishment of Village Clinics]," *Huadong weisheng* [East China Health], vol. 1, no. 2 (February 1951), 22.

40 Zhu Chao and Zhang Weifeng, *Xin Zhongguo yixue jiaoyu shi* [Medical Education in New China] (Beijing yikeda Zhongguo xiehe yikeda lianhe chubanshe, 1990), "Preface," 2.

41 He Cheng, "Zhongxiyi jiehe yu zhongyi de peixun [Unity of Chinese and Western Medicines and the Training of Practitioners of Chinese Medicine]," *Renmin ribao*, June 13, 1950.

42 Yu Weiliang, "Opinions on 'The Profile and Chronicle of Mr. Yu Yunxiu's Life'," *Zhonghua yishi zazhi* [Chinese Journal of Medical History] no. 3 (1955), 161–163.

43 Zhu Chao and Zhang Weifeng, *Xin Zhongguo yixue jiaoyu shi*, 98–99.

44 Ibid., 100–101.
45 Ibid., 105.
46 Tian Gang, "Xin Zhongguo chengli chuqi 'tuanjie zhongxiyi' fangzhen de queli [The Establishment of the Principle of "Uniting Chinese and Western Medicines" in Early New China]," *Dangdai Zhongguo shi yanjiu*, vol. 18, no. 1 (January 2011), 78.
47 "Zhongyang renmin zhengfu weisheng bu zai diyici quanguo weisheng huiyi shang de baogao (jiexuan) [Report of the Health Ministry of the Central People's Government at the First National Health Conference (excerpts)]," *Xin zhongyiyao* [New Chinese Medicine], vol. 1, no. 7 (1950), 6.
48 On the movement to scientize Chinese medicine in the Nationalist era and on the phenomenon of using science as a verb in China (and in Japan and Korea), see Sean Hsiang–lin Lei, *Neither Donkey nor Horse: Medicine in the Struggle over China's Modernity* (Chicago: University of Chicago Press, 2014), chapter 7.
49 Li Honghe, "Xin Zhongguo chengli chuqi 'zhongyi kexuehua' de lishi kaocha [A Historical Exploration of the 'Scientization of Chinese Medicine' in Early New China]," *Dangdai Zhongguo shi yanjiu*, vol. 18, no. 4 (July 2011), 74.
50 Deng Guangren, "Cong dongbei weishengbu de moxie dangan zhong kan Wang Bin sixiang de wuihai [The Harm of Wang Bin's Thought as Seen Through Some of the Archives of Northeast Health Department," *Zhongyi zazhi* [*Journal of Traditional Chinese Medicine*] vol. 1, no. 8 (1955), 1–4.
51 *Zhongyi gongzuo ziliao huibian* [Collections of Materials on Chinese Medicine Work], vol. 3 (Zhonghua renmin gongheguo weishengbu, October 1956), 30.
52 Zhonghua renmin gongheguo weishengbu zhongyisi [Chinese Medicine Bureau of the Health Ministry of the People's Republic of China], *Zhongyi gongzuo wenjian huibian (1949–1983)* [Collections of Documents of Chinese Medicine Work, (1949–1983)] (Health Ministry of People's Republic of China, July 1985), 216.
53 *Beijing shi zhongyao wenxian xuanbian* (1952) [Selected Important Documents of the Beijing Municipality, 1952] (Zhongguo dang'an chubanshe, 2002), 629.
54 Zhonghua renmin gongheguo weishengbu zhongyisi, *Zhongyi gongzuo wenjian huibian (1949–1983)*, 46.
55 *Jianguo yilai Mao Zedong wengao* [Manuscripts of Mao Zedong since the Founding of People's Republic of China], vol. 4 (Zhongyang wenxian chubanshe, 2000), 176–179. It was during the high time of the Three Anti Movement that the report was written; hence, Mao made the reference to the struggle against bureaucracy. The Three Anti Movement started in 1951 and ended in 1954 and aimed at eliminating corruption, waste, and obstructive bureaucracy among party members, government administrators and factory managers.
56 *Dangdai Zhongguo weisheng dashi ji (1949–1990)* [Major Events of Health Work in Contemporary China, 1949–1990] (Renmin weisheng chubanshe, 1993), 39.
57 Wang Zhipu and Cai Jingfeng, *Zhongguo zhongyiyao wushi nian* [Fifty Years of Chinese Medicine and Pharmacy] (Fujian kexuejishu chbanshe, 1999), 9; and Zhu Chao and Zhang Weifeng, *Xin Zhongguo yixue jiaoyu shi*, 41.
58 *Jianguo yilai zhongyao wenxian xuanbian* [Selected Important Documents since the Founding of the PRC], vol. 5 (Zhongyang wenxian chubanshe, 1993), 605.
59 *Mao Zedong shuxin xuanji* [Selection of Mao Zedong's Correspondence and Letters] (Zhongyang wenxian chubanshe, 2003), 503.
60 Zhonghua renmin gongheguo weishengbu zhongyisi, *Zhongyi gongzuo wenjian huibian (1949–1983)*, 42–53.
61 Zhu Chao and Zhang Weifeng, *Xin Zhongguo yixue jiaoyu*, 43.
62 Cover page, *Xin Zhongyiyao*, January 1956.
63 Zhu and Zhang, *Xin Zhongguo yixue jiaoyu,* 43.
64 Li Honghe, "Xin Zhongguo chengli chuqi 'zhongyi kexuehua' de lishi kaocha," 76.
65 "Guanche duidai zhongyi de zhengque zhengce [Implement the Correct Policies Regarding Chinese Medicine]," *The People's Daily*, October 20, 1954.

66 "Zhonghua yixue zhonghui fachu jiaqiang zhongyi gongzuo de zhishi [Office of the Chinese Medical Association Issued Instructions on Strengthening the Work of Chinese Medicine]," *The People's Daily*, October 22, 1954.
67 Zhu and Zhang, *Xin Zhongguo yixue jiaoyu shi*, 44–45.
68 The successful discoveries of new Chinese drugs, new interpretations of acupuncture and many other integrated techniques and productions of Chinese and Western medicine in the following decades vindicated their expectations. See the website of China Academy of Chinese Medical Sciences, http://www.catcm.ac.cn/.
69 Zhu and Zhang, *Xin Zhongguo yixue jiaoyu shi*, 45.
70 Zhonghua renmin gongheguo weishengbu zhongyisi, *Zhongyi gongzuo wenjian huibian (1949–1983),* 173.
71 Marta Hanson coined the term "medical bilingualism" in her discussion of Tu Youyou's success. She elaborated that medical bilingualism meant the ability to not only read in two different medical languages but also to understand their different histories, conceptual differences, and the potential value for therapeutic interventions in the present. See her article at http://asianmedicinezone.com/east–asia/is–the–2015–nobel–prize–a–turning–point–for–traditional–chinese–medicine/.
72 Gong Yuzhi and Li Peishuan, "Pipan Wang Bin zai yixue he weisheng gongzuo zhong de zichan jieji sixiang [Criticism of Wang Bin's Bourgeois Thought in Medicine and Health Work]," *Zhongguo yaoxue zazhi* [Chinese Journal of Pharmacy], 1955 (10).
73 Liu Lixiang and Zhang Qicheng, "Cong 'wulao shangshu' lun jianchi zhongyi jiaoyu de zhuti xing [The 'Letter of Five Elders' and the Core Course of Chinese Medicine Education]," *Zhongyi jiaoyu* [Education of Chinese Medicine], no. 6 (2006),13–16. See also Ren Yingqiu, *Ren Yinqiu lun yi ji* [Collections of Ren Yingqiu's Writings on Medicine] (Beijing: Renmin weisheng chubanshe, 1984).
74 Chen Minzhang, ed., *Zhongguo weisheng nianjian* [Health Yearbook of the People's Republic of China] (Beijing: renmin weisheng chubanshe, 1997), 294–95.
75 Chen, *Zhongguo weisheng baojian shi*,102.
76 For a detailed account of Chinese medicine since 1949, see Volker Scheid, *Chinese Medicine in Contemporary China: Plurality and Synthesis* (Durham and London: Duke University Press, 2002); and Kim Taylor, *Chinese Medicine in Early Communist China, 1945–1963* (Routledge, 2005).
77 The Health Ministry issued many policies and directives and some of them were introduced by Dr. Tao–Tai Hsia, in his chapter "Laws on Public Health" in *Medicine and Public Health in the People's Republic of China*, ed. Joseph R. Quinn (U.S. Department of Health, Education, and Welfare, Public Health Service, National Institutes of Health, 1973), 113–140.
78 Tao–Tai Hsia, "Laws on Public Health," in *Medicine and Public Health in the People's Republic of China*, 131. There was a timetable of target dates for the free medical service to be implemented, given the uneven development and limited medical facilities in certain parts of the country; and other measures to cover medical expenses were also offered.
79 Xiaoping Fang, *Barefoot Doctors and Western Medicine in China* (Rochester, New York: University of Rochester Press, 2012), 23.
80 Tao–Tai Hsia, "Laws on Public Health," in *Medicine and Public Health in the People's Republic of China*, 128.
81 Cao Pu, "1949–1989: Zhongguo nongcun hezuo yiliao zhidu de yanbian yu pingxi [A Critique of the Transformation of Chinese Rural Medical Cooperative System, 1949–1989]." http://www.usc.cuhk.edu.hk/PaperCollection/Details.aspx?id=6511, accessed November 22, 2015.
82 "Henan tuixing hezuo yiliao zhidu [Henan Province Expands Cooperative Medical System]," *The People's Day*, September 24, 1958.
83 Yue Qianhou and He Puyan, "Shanxi sheng Jishan xian nongcun gonggong weisheng shiye shuping (1949–1984)—Yi Taiyangcun (gongshe) wei zhongdian kaocha duixiang

[A Review of the Rural Public Health of Jishan County, Shanxi Province, 1949–1984: A Case Study of Taiyangcun (Commune)]," *Dangdai Zhongguo shi yanjiu* 14.5 (September 2007), 63.

84 Yue Qianhou and He Puyan, "Shanxi sheng Jishan xian," 64.

85 Ibid.

86 Ibid.

87 Xia Xingzhen, "Nongcun hezuo yiliao zhidu de lishi kaocha [A Historical Exploration of the Rural Cooperative Medical System]," *Dangdai Zhongguo shi yanjiu*, vol. 10, no. 5 (September 2003), 111.

88 Schistosomiasis was one of the most devastating diseases that affected more than half of China. Some villages suffered such heavy losses of population to the disease that few people were left to register for land when the land reform movement took place in 1949–1950. Li Honghe, "Ershi shiji wushi niandai guojia dui xuexicongbing de fangzhi [The Anti–Schistosomiasis Movement in the 1950s]," *Dangdai Zhongguo shi yanjiu*, vol. 19, no. 4 (July 2012), 63–69; Miriam Gross and Kaiwai Fan, "Schistosomiasis," in *Medical Transitions in Twentieth–Century Chia*; and Miriam Gross, *Farewell to the God of Plague: Chairman Mao's Campaign to Deworm China* (Berkeley, CA: University of California Press, 2016).

89 World Population Prospects, the 2008 Revision. United Nations, Department of Economic and Social Affairs (DESA), Population Division, New York. See: www.unpopulation.org. China Profile, Analyses, Tables, Figures and Maps. http://www.china–profile.com/data/fig_WPP2008_L0_1.htm. Accessed December 13, 2015.

90 Weishengbu jicheng weisheng he fuyou baojian si [Bureau of Basic Health and Maternal and Children's Health of the Health Ministry], *Nongcun weisheng wenjian huibian (1951–2000)* [Collections of Documents on Rural Health Work, 1951–2000] (Ministry of Health, PRC, 2001), 247–248.

91 Li Decheng, "Xin Zhongguo qian sanshi nian nongcun jicheng weisheng renyuan peiyang moshi tanjiu [An Exploration of the Training of Basic–level Rural Health Personnel in the First Thirty Years of PRC]," *Dangdai Zhongguo shi yanjiu*, vol. 17, no. 2 (March 2010), 67–68.

92 Wang Sheng and Liu Yingqin, "Jitihua shiqi nongcun hezuo yiliao zhidu Pingxi—Yi Hebei sheng Shenze xian wei ge an [An Analysis of the Rural Cooperative Medical System during the Collectivization: A Case Study of Shenze County of Hebei Province," *Dangdai Zhongguo shi yanjiu*, vol. 16, no. 2 (March 2009), 26.

93 "Guanyu ba weisheng gongzuo zhongdian zhuanxiang nongcun de baogao [Report on Turning the Emphasis of Health Work towards the Countryside," in *Nongcun weisheng wenjian huibian (1951–2000)*, 27.

94 Ibid.

95 It became known as the June 26 instruction, because it was published on that date in *the People's Daily*. Some argued that Mao's attention to rural health was also influenced by his concerns over national security as the Soviet Union and the United States both put pressure on China at the time. See Yao Li, "'Ba yiliao weisheng gongzuo de zhongdian fangdao nongcun qu'—Mao Zedong 'liu er liu' zhishi de lishi kaocha ['Put the Emphasis of Health Work in the Countryside'—A Historical Investigation of Mao Zedong's June 26 Instruction]," *Dangdai Zhongguo shi Yanjiu*, vol. 14, no. 3 (May 2007), 99–104.

96 Zhu and Zhang, *Xin Zhongguo yixue jiaoyu shi*, 113.

97 Ibid., 113–14.

98 Zhang Kaining, *Cong chijiao yisheng dao xiangcun yisheng* [From the Barefoot Doctor to the Village Doctor] (Yunnan renmin chubanshe, 2002), 17; and Li Decheng, "Xin Zhongguo qian sanshi nian," 68.

99 Li Decheng, "Xin Zhongguo qian sanshi nian," 69.

100 Xiaoping Fang, *Barefoot Doctors and Western Medicine in China*.

101 Zhu and Zhang, *Xin Zhongguo yixue jiaoyu shi*, 115.

102 "Shengshou pingxia zhongnong huanying de hezuo yiliao zhidu [A Cooperative Medical System Deeply Welcomed by Peasants]," *The People's Daily*, December 5, 1968.
103 *Nongcun weisheng wenjian huibian (1951–2000)*, 533–534.
104 See posters at https://www.nlm.nih.gov/hmd/chineseposters/prevention.html. See also Liping Bu, "Anti–Malaria Campaigns and Socialist Reconstruction of China, 1950–1980," *East Asian History*, issue no. 39 (2014), 127–128.
105 World Population Prospects, the 2008 Revision, www.unpopulation.org. China Profile, http://www.china–profile.com/data/fig_WPP2008_L0_1.htm. Accessed December 13, 2015.
106 *Collections of Documents on Rural Health Work, 1951–2000*, 420.
107 Chen, *Zhongguo weisheng baojian shi*, 109.
108 Victor Sidel, "Medical Personnel and Their Training," in *Medicine and Public Health in the People's Republic of China*, edited by Joseph R. Quinn (Washington, D.C.: U.S. Department of Health, Education, and Welfare, Public Health Service, National Institutes of Health, 1973), 153–172, 156.
109 *Dangdai Zhongguo de weisheng shiye* [*Health of Contemporary China*], vol. 1 (Beijing: Zhongguo shehui kexue chubanshe, 1986), 10–13.
110 Chen, *Zhongguo weisheng baojian shi*, 111. Little national statistics on TB was available at that time, and the figures should be taken as estimated numbers.
111 Rachel Core, "Tuberculosis Control in Shanghai: Bringing Health to the Masses, 1928–Present," in *Medical Transitions in Twentieth–Century China*, 126–145,
112 Liping Bu, "Chinese Anti-Tuberculosis Flyers," in *Hidden Treasures*, 166.
113 Chen, *Zhongguo weisheng baojian shi*, 111.
114 Mark Elvin and Liu Ts'ui–jung, eds., *Sediments of Time: Environment and Society in Chinese History* (Cambridge University Press, 2006), 526.
115 Chen, *Zhongguo weisheng baojian shi*, 112.
116 Mark Elvin and Liu Ts'ui–jung, *Sediments of Time*, 526.
117 Tu Changliang, "Feijiehe liaoyangyuan de guimo duomo da heshi [On the Proper Size of Sanatorium," *Fanglao tongxun* [*Anti–Tuberculosis Newsletter*], no. 4 (1956), 24–27.
118 Liping Bu and Elizabeth Fee, "Get Well and Go Back to Work!" *American Journal of Public Health*, vol. 101, no. S1 (2011), S165.
119 Chen, *Zhongguo weisheng baojian shi*, 112.
120 Rachel Core, "Tuberculosis Control in Shanghai," 126–145.
121 *Anti–Tuberculosis Newsletter*, Chinese Anti-Tuberculosis Association, Beijing, 1950–1970.
122 See the website "痨病—Consumptive Disease": Chinese Anti-Tuberculosis Posters, 1950–1980," at the National Library of Medicine, http://www.nlm.nih.gov/exhibition/chineseantitb/index.html.
123 Ibid., and https://www.nlm.nih.gov/hmd/chineseposters/
124 Chen, *Zhongguo weisheng baojian shi*, 112.
125 Nancy Tomes, "Moralizing the Microbe: The Germ Theory and the Moral Construction of Behavior in the Late Nineteenth Century Tuberculosis Movement," in *Morality and Health*, eds. Allan Brandt and Paul Rozin (Routledge, 1997), 271–298. See also her book, *The Gospel of Germs* (Cambridge, MA: Harvard University Press, 1998).
126 Qian Huilin and Tang Linhua, "Prevention and Control of Malaria in China in the last 50 Years," *Chinese Journal of Epidemiology*, vol. 21, no. 3 (2000), 225–227.
127 Tang Linhua, "Progress in Malaria Control in China," *Chinese Medical Journal*, vol. 113, no. 1 (2000), 89–92; and Qian Huilin and Tang Linhua, "Prevention and Control of Malaria in China in the last 50 Years," *Chinese Journal of Epidemiology*, vol. 21, no. 3 (2000), 225.
128 Daniel Lai, Yu-Jen Li, and Wei Chang, "Hygiene and Public Health: A Malaria Survey in Kao–Chiao, Shanghai," *Chinese Medical Journal*, vol. 49, no. 5 (1935), 462–469; Stephen M. K. Hu, "Notes on the Relative Adult Density of Anopheles Hyrcanus Var. Sinensis Wiedemann During 1933 with Reference to Malaria

Incidence in Kaochiao, Shanghai Area," *Chinese Medical Journal*, vol. 49, no. 5 (1935), 469–474; and Lan–Chou Feng, "Malaria and Its Transmission in Kwangsi China," *Chinese Medical Journal*, vol. 50, no. 12 (1936), 1799–1814.

129 Zhongguo nueji de fangzhi yu yanjiu bianweihui [Editorial Committee on Malaria Prevention and Research in China], *Zhongguo nueji de fangzhi yu yanjiu* [Malaria Prevention and Research in China] (Beijing: Remin weisheng chubanshe, 1991), 1. Statistics on malaria in China were sporadic and limited until after 1950. For statistics on malaria from 1950 to 2008, see *Zhongguo weisheng tongji nianqian* [Annual Medical Statistics of China] (Beijing: Zhongguo xiehe yike daxue chubanshe, 2009).

130 Author's interviews in 2009 with physicians, Drs. Bao Wenjie, Li Quanchang, Tao Zige, and Zhang Xuebing at Nanjing Gulou Hospital who participated in the health campaigns in the 1950s–1970s.

131 On a case study of rural healthcare in Zhejiang province of China, see Xiaoping Fang, *Barefoot Doctors and Western Medicine in China.*

132 China's anti–malaria campaign was not related to the WHO's worldwide malaria eradication program that was launched in 1955 because of the Cold War. The WHO's program emphasized house spraying with residual insecticides, drug treatment and surveillance, and successive steps of preparation, attack, consolidation, and maintenance. Drug resistance, insecticide resistance, massive population movements, lack of sustained funding, and inadequate community participation were cited as the difficulties in maintaining the long–term effort of eradication. The WHO abandoned the eradication campaign in 1968 and began a program of malaria control instead (Center for Disease Control and Prevention, Department of Health and Human Services, http://www.cdc.gov/Malaria, accessed August 15, 2009).

133 See the online exhibition on Chinese anti–malaria campaigns and posters at the National Library of Medicine, National Institutes of Health, http://www.nlm.nih.gov/exhibition/chineseantimalaria/introduction.html.

134 Health Poster "Prevent and Treat Malaria," produced by the Health and Epidemic Prevention Station of Jiangxi Province, n. d., ca. 1960. The Chinese Public Health Collection, National Library of Medicine, National Institutes of Health, Bethesda, Maryland, USA. https://www.nlm.nih.gov/exhibition/chineseantimalaria/images/2329.jpg.

135 Liping Bu and Elizabeth Fee, "Communicating With Pictures: The Vision of Chinese Anti-Malaria Posters," *American Journal of Public Health*, vol. 100, no. 3 (March 2010), 424–425; and "Unite to Fight Malaria," *American Journal of Public Health*, vol. 100, no. 4 (April 2010), 608.

136 Elisabeth Hsu, "Reflections on the 'Discovery' of the Antimalarial Qinghao," *British Journal of Clinical Pharmacology*, vol. 61, no. 6 (2006), 666–670.

137 Tu Youyou (屠呦呦)and her team worked on the project named "523" to find a better and more effective drug to treat malaria in the late 1960s. The background story was that the Vietnam War was waging on and many North Vietnamese died of malaria due to lack of effective medicine. The North Vietnamese leaders asked China for help, and the Chinese government asked the scientists to work on it with utmost urgency. The success led to the treatment of malaria in China and all over the world, saving millions of lives.

5 Economic reforms and new healthcare

Introduction

In December 1978 the Third Plenum of the Eleventh Congress of the CCP Central Committee adopted the pivotal decision to structurally reform the Chinese economy. Chinese leaders were determined to push the country forward with the four modernizations of industry, agriculture, national defense, and science and technology. This new paradigm of modernity had a long process of development but was publicly promoted as a comprehensive program of national development in the last years of Mao Zedong and Zhou Enlai. After Deng Xiaoping became the paramount leader of China in the late 1970s, the CCP Central Committee took the decisive step to implement a structural change of the existing system to speed up economic growth to achieve national prosperity. Internationally, China significantly increased economic and cultural interactions with Western nations after the Sino-U.S. relations took a dramatic turn for the better with American president Richard Nixon's visit to China in 1972. The opening-up of doors of the West to China offered Chinese leaders opportunities to observe personally the actual economic and technical advancements in developed nations. Moreover, active educational and cultural exchanges with Western nations contributed to the dissemination of scientific and technological knowhow in China. With first-hand observations abroad, Chinese leaders and scholars felt a deep sense of the huge gap between China and developed nations in terms of economy and technological advances. China was still a poor country, lagging far behind the West, with a large population of over one billion, despite the significant accomplishments of national reconstruction after 1949. How to speed up economic growth and raise people's living standards became the urgent task for Chinese leaders. The desire to modernize China into a strong country on a par with the West had been the dream of the Chinese since the late nineteenth century, but the Cultural Revolution had cost China 10 precious years of economic development to catch up with the West. For the leaders of China, there was no time to be lost in deciding on the new path of modernity and national prosperity. The fast population growth appeared to outpace economic growth, however, and it became a serious concern for state economic planners. To coordinate the plan of national economic growth and technical advancement, new policies of family planning were formulated to encourage late marriage and fewer children to slow down the population growth. The government issued the one-child policy in 1978 and vigorously enforced it as an important component of the overall state planning of economy and national development.[1]

Marketization became the new driving force of economic reforms. People were encouraged to seek market forces such as privatization and commercialization to boost business operation and profit-making. In the short span of 30 years, marketization completely transformed the landscapes of urban and rural China, where people's attitudes and values have profoundly altered along with economic behavior. The reforms not only reshaped economic enterprises but also changed the operation of professional institutions of education, arts and culture, and health. The transformation of economic foundation has led to significant changes in the realms of superstructure, to put it in a Marxian term. While national wealth increased dramatically, the Chinese healthcare system fell into crisis when marketization was applied to the health sector. The formerly world-renowned model of low-cost healthcare has been turned into a high-cost medical care system not affordable for many Chinese. Most significant of the national health crisis was the collapse of the rural cooperative medical system when de-collectivization of the people's commune system was completed by the household responsibility system. This chapter discusses the broader social implications of economic reforms in Chinese society and the collapse of the socialist healthcare system. It examines the various efforts of the government to reform and re-create a new health system that would fit the market economy with Chinese characteristics, which is still undergoing its own evolution and transformation.

Marketization of economy and the collapse of socialist healthcare

China's economic reforms began with tentative experiments of private enterprises in the Special Economic Zones of a few selected cities such as Shenzhen (next to Hong Kong) and Shanghai. Private investments and management were actively invited and sought after, particularly from abroad, to come and join the new economic development. The 1980s witnessed the drastic rise of a new industrial structure that consisted of private companies of Chinese and foreign ownership, joint ventures, and state enterprises, all operating in a dynamic economic expansion of infrastructure construction and new industry creation. Privatization and commercialization, the two key elements of marketization, gained momentum in the 1990s with many state enterprises going private or bankrupt, and millions of workers became unemployed, losing their wages along with healthcare and other social benefits at the same time. Acceleration of urbanization and industrialization severely encroached upon farmland and caused the worse environmental pollutions in Chinese history that gave rise to new health hazards and diseases. In the meantime, millions of rural youth migrated to cities to join the industrial labor in the economic boom. These patterns appeared familiar in the industrialization of many countries such as Europe and America in the nineteenth century and Japan in the 1970s.

In rural China, a household responsibility system replaced the people's commune system as a mode of production by mid-1980s. The de-collectivization of rural production started in 1978 when a small number of people of a poor production team in Anhui province contracted land and output quotas to individual households to simulate productivity. By going off the collective production mode to put responsibility squarely on the individual households, the production team saw an increase of farm yields much faster than the collective production teams. The remarkable changes initiated by the farmers caught the attention of local and central government leaders. Deng Xiaoping welcomed the farmers' initiative with the household responsibility contract and praised it as a great invention of farmers. High remarks of government officials soon led to a nationwide promotion of a household responsibility system in rural areas.[2] The household responsibility contracts allowed farmers to use but not own farmland. Each household had complete control over production and management through long-term contracts. Farmers were free to keep everything for themselves for use or for sale after they paid off the quotas to the state and the collective reserves to local government. Incentives of material gains were powerful motivations for people to work harder and be creative. Newspapers reported in the early 1980s that some rural households had accumulated ten thousand yuan (a rich status in rural China at that time) by diversifying their agricultural production and animal husbandry. To further stimulate agricultural production, the state raised the price for quota grains above market price and reduced the price of farming machinery, chemical fertilizers, and insecticides. By 1985, the household responsibility system had replaced 90 percent of the people's communes and completely reversed the collective system into a private rural economy. According to government data, China's agricultural production increased at an average annual rate of 6.7 percent and the annual growth rate of grain production was 2.7 percent, with total grain output exceeding 500 billion kilograms in 1996, making China the largest grain producer in the world. Output of cotton, cereals, oil, sugar, meat and milk products had increased several times over in the same time period.[3] The household responsibility system not only released the rural productive power but also freed large amount of rural labor from land cultivation to go into businesses and factory work. Tens of millions of rural farmers migrated to cities to work as cheap laborers at construction sites and industrial companies.

Great wealth was created and people's living standards increased significantly over the past three decades. China was transformed into the second largest economy in the world, lifting hundreds of millions of people out of poverty. However, inequality widened and deepened in both urban and rural China. Significantly affecting people's lives negatively was the loss of free healthcare and free education that they used to enjoy before the economic reforms. In terms of healthcare, farmers and urban workers who lost their jobs were hit the hardest free as the healthcare service was not available any more. In rural areas, health workers, including barefoot doctors, had to adapt to the changes of the system by working as individual village doctors and charging fees for services. Private practice became the trend and the way of making a living for rural health workers when the household responsibility system prevailed. The former model rural cooperative medical service, such as that of the Taiyang commune of Jishan county discussed in chapter 4, transitioned from a collective entity to private practice with fees charged for service and drugs. By 1984, the Taiyang commune was renamed back to Taiyang village, and the health office of the production brigade was renamed village health office.[4] A diverse pattern of health services emerged during the transition period, with some being fee-based and others relying on a combination of different payments.

Rural cooperative medical service dropped from 90 percent of rural China in 1978 to 5 percent in 1984, a drastic decline in parallel with the de-collectivization of the commune system. The 5 percent that continued the cooperative medical system were mostly well-to-do rural communities in southern Jiangsu province and Shanghai area. Well-to-do communes and brigades, such as the Huaxi Brigade (华西大队) of Jiangsu, formed their own village company instead of going down the household responsibility road, to keep everyone and everything including land and the health office of the brigade intact under the name of the company to creatively develop in the market economy. The government was flexible about local people's decisions and Huaxi blazed a unique road of its own with collective prosperity only for Huaxi locals.[5] But cases like Huaxi were rare, constituting a very small segment in the entire rural China.

When marketization was applied to diversifying forms of industrial and agricultural production by private, collective, state, and multinational business enterprises (企业单位), professional institutions (事业单位) such as those of education, arts and culture and healthcare, were encouraged to adopt market forces in their operation as well. What this meant was commercialization of their services with individual institutions taking on increased responsibility of revenue generation and management while the government reduced its subsidies. The purpose was to use market forces as leverage to stimulate productivity and profitability. In the health sector, the Ministry of Health tried, at first, to uphold the four major principles of national health policy that had been guiding health work throughout the 1950s–1970s. There was, however, a shift of emphasis when the Ministry of Health made it clear in 1979 that city health work should be strengthened in order to be more effective in guiding rural health development. The Health Ministry also declared that diversity of medical practices should be allowed for the basic health service. Health institutions in cities and countryside could have a variety of enterprise-run, collective-run, and individual-run private health practices. Employees of business enterprises could get healthcare through labor insurance; and farmers, though the majority enjoyed healthcare through the rural cooperative medical system, could have access to a paid service as well.[6] The Ministry of Health clearly encouraged private and profitable medical practice by the mid-1980s, but it stated at the same time that healthcare was a form of socialist welfare for the people that should not be for profit, though not to cause deficit either.

How to solve the problems of compensating the barefoot doctors when the sponsoring communes were replaced by the private household responsibility system? In 1981, the Health Ministry required all barefoot doctors to take qualifying exams after the State Council approved its "Report on Solutions to Proper Compensation for Barefoot Doctors." The exams were a measure of quality control over rural healthcare but also a way to weed out large numbers who were considered unqualified. Those who passed the exams at the intermediate level of medical education would receive licenses as village doctors, while those who failed the exams could continue to work as health assistants under village doctors. Consequently, the number of barefoot doctors—now called village doctors—was reduced more than half, from 1.5 million in 1978 to 640,000 in 1984.[7] In January 1985, the Health Ministry issued the directive to abolish the term "barefoot doctor" altogether as it was a product of the Cultural Revolution and not appropriate for the new era of reforms.[8] While the barefoot doctors were being transformed and reduced, the sent-down youth and professionals also began to return to cities, which further weakened rural health and educational force as some of them worked as barefoot doctors and teachers in rural areas. In short, the negative effect on rural health came from a combination of different factors—the de-collectivization of the commune system, the drastic reduction of the rural health workforce, and privatization and commercialization of the health service that drove the costs of healthcare significantly higher than the growth of income. The market forces employed in health reforms ultimately accelerated the disappearance of rural cooperative medical system and the collapse of rural healthcare.

The central government did not seem to have foreseen the coming of the collapse of rural health even as the foundation of the cooperative medical system was being rapidly dismantled by the household responsibility system. It continued to advocate the rural cooperative medical system without providing the necessary financial support to keep it functioning. In fact, government funding for rural healthcare decreased during the same time period. In 1979 the state subsidized the rural cooperative medical system with 0.1 billion yuan, but that amount decreased to 35 million in 1992, which was only 0.36 percent of the entire national health budget and an average of 0.04 yuan per farmer.[9] In other words, the state subsidy for each farmer in healthcare was not even enough to buy a chicken egg in the year 1992. Because of the decrease of state health subsidies and the dismantling of people's communes, over 8000 village town/commune hospitals disappeared, 240,000 hospital beds were lost, and 129,000 rural health staff members were reduced during the years 1980–1990.[10] The 1980s witnessed the increasing hardship of people seeking healthcare in both urban and rural China, but the rural population of 800 million made the problem extremely poignant. Field studies indicated that people's health status (measured by infant mortality, immunization coverage, and rate of infectious diseases) decreased in areas where the rural cooperative medical service declined even though the per capita income increased.[11]

Instead of working on contingent plans to remedy the increasingly serious problems of rural health, the Health Ministry moved forward with the overall economic reform scheme of the central government to push marketization in the entire health sector. The Health Ministry issued policies to encourage state-owned hospitals and health centers to increase the responsibility of their own budgets by charging user fees. The central government, in the meantime, reduced its role in financing health institutions by providing subsidies to cover only the basic salaries of employees and capital investment. Provincial and local governments were asked to shoulder a larger share of health finance, which was not always faithfully followed. The new health policies also encouraged private construction and ownership of medical institutions and supported the private practice of doctors to charge fees for services; all the while there was little supervision and enforcement of standards of practice. With government financing being reduced to about one third of hospital expenditures, public hospitals needed to generate more revenue to pay for their own operations and employees' benefits, including a new bonus system that aimed to stimulate greater productivity. To achieve more economic efficiency with technical advancement, hospitals began to purchase more high-tech equipment to enhance their reputation and competitiveness. Hospitals came up with all sorts of creative methods of marketization to make profits, namely, encouraging patients to use high-tech machinery for physical examination, which would result in more costs for the patients, instead of providing careful personal observation and diagnosis as they used to do. Another major way of generating more revenue was to prescribe more and expensive drugs and install expensive medical devices for patients. There was a personal incentive to prescribe expensive drugs and to use expensive machinery and medical devices because the more revenue a person generated for the hospital the higher his/her bonus would be. Talking about applying a personal responsibility system into the profit-making scheme of hospitals, China became the fertile land of healthcare providers to wantonly charge fees and abuse professional power at the expense of patients simply because of the laissez-faire practice of marketization. William Hsiao made an insightful analysis of the uncoordinated chaos of financing, pricing, and organizational policies in the health sector in the first decade of China's health reforms and pointed out the lessons to be learned.[12]

Not surprisingly, violation of professional ethics became a serious problem in the health sector. The attitude of medical doctors and nurses changed from thinking for the patients to thinking for their own bonus gains when marketization was applied to the health service. Health professionals, in fact, were not alone or unique in any sense in their change of behavior and attitude because the social values of the entire Chinese society have shifted to focusing on profit-making and getting rich. The Health Ministry became concerned about the problems arising in hospitals and issued the directive that hospitals should stick to the correct principles of medical treatment by paying attention to the proper use of drugs and avoiding waste that was motivated by profit-making. Such statement, however, had little effect on checking the abuse of drug prescription and service charges, as long as hospitals had to use market forces to generate more profits to take care of their own budgets.

Moreover, marketization and delegation of power to local governments actually led to new structural problems in China. The reduced role of central government resulted in a decentralized and fragmented health system, as Yuanli Liu pointed out.[13] It weakened the communication between the central and local governments and the control of central government over local affairs. Variation in capacities and performance of the healthcare diverged further as provinces, cities, and private entities made different investments in health. In the marketization of economy and health sector, public health education and campaigns faded. Some of the epidemic and endemic diseases that had been brought under basic control began to return in parts of China as a result of lax prevention and control. Malaria and tuberculosis, for instance, became serious health threats to millions of Chinese people again in the late 1990s.[14] Regarding malaria, China achieved basic control in 1990. But the resurgence caused concerns of China as well as the World Health Organization. In collaboration with the WHO, the Chinese government carried out consistent anti-malaria programs and saw a decrease of 85 percent in reported malaria cases between 2000 and 2011. But tuberculosis was more difficult to control as air and environmental pollutions rose along with industrialization, and worse still, drug-resistant cases increased. China now has the world's second largest number of tuberculosis cases, after India. The challenges of public health and disease prevention in a fragmented health system were manifested in the initial handling of SARS (severe acute respiratory syndrome) in 2003 when the government had difficulty in making quick and coordinated efforts to fight the spread of SARS.

The number of people with any type of health insurance decreased significantly nationwide in the 1990s when medical costs rose sharply. According to National Health Service Surveys conducted by the Ministry of Health, the urban population with health insurance was 53 percent in 1993 but dropped to 42 percent in 1998, whereas the rural population with health insurance was 12 percent in 1993 but dropped to 9 percent in 998.[15] The gap between the urban and rural health insurance rate further indicated the dire conditions of health for rural population. Life quality between urban and rural China widened, which was particularly hard for rural women. The maternal death rate was a case in point. In 1990, the maternal mortality rate was 49.9 per hundred thousand in cities but 114.9 per hundred thousand in rural areas. Half of the rural maternal deaths were caused by bad transportation conditions and a lack of immediate access to medical service.[16] As people had to pay high medical costs, more and more farmers fell into poverty due to medical bills. The national health survey data indicated that nearly 45 percent of rural poverty was caused by medical expenditures. Some people simply gave up medical treatment because of their inability to pay. About 80 percent of hospital discharges happened because of the patients' inability to pay. High medical costs not only kept many patients out of healthcare but decreased the utilization of healthcare facilities. This was particularly significant in rural areas. The bed occupancy rate of town health centers dropped from 46 to 33 percent during the period of 1985 to 2000, and for county hospitals, the rate dropped from 83 to 61 percent in the same period. In the meantime, total hospital beds in China increased from 2.4 to3.2 million during the period of 1985 to 2001, and the total health professionals increased from 3.4 to 5.5 million in the same period.[17] Many of the newly created healthcare facilities were private-owned (some were public ones sold to private owners) and located in urban cities or county centers. From the economic perspective, the under-utilization of healthcare facilities was a waste for the nation and individual health institutions. Such waste should not happen if the purpose of economic reforms was to achieve more efficiency and productivity. Additionally, the more people fell ill and diseased, the more loss of labor and productive power there would be for the nation. From the health perspective, marketization of health-care seriously undermined the basic purpose of healthcare and health profession: to save the dying and care for the sick. Was national health still relevant to national strength at the end of twentieth-century China?

Government efforts to reform and re-build the health system

The high medical costs made healthcare a serious social problem as well as a health crisis. The government was aware of the serious situation of health sector and attempted to develop programs to deal with new challenges. At the request of the Health Ministry, the State Council issued in 1991 the policy that local government at every level should steadily promote a rural cooperative medical system to achieve healthcare for everyone. There was a new push to re-build a rural cooperative medical system but farmers had to contribute the lion's share of costs. In order to reduce the economic burden of farmers, the Ministry of Agriculture stopped all programs that required farmers to pay, including the cooperative medical program.[18] The contradictory policies of the Agricultural and the Health ministries indicated a lack of thoughtful and coordinated planning of the central government at the time to deal with new challenges of rural health after the commune system was gone. The CCP Central Committee confirmed the value of the rural cooperative medical system and the State Council outlined the objectives of re-building a New Rural Cooperative Medical System (NRCMS, 新型农村合作医疗制度) in 1994.[19] The purpose of the NRCMS was to improve the primary healthcare and to reduce problems of poverty that were associated with medical expenditures. The NRCMS was defined as nonprofit with voluntary membership, to be formed according to local economic conditions and the income status of local population. The State Council designated the Ministry of Health, the Ministry of Agriculture, and the State Council Research Office to work with the WHO on an initial pilot program in 14 counties of 7 provinces to test the feasibility of the NRCMS. The 14 counties represented developed areas of Jiangsu, Zhejiang and Beijing, less developed areas of Hunan and Hubei, and least developed areas of Jiangxi and Ningxia.[20] The NRCMS, different from the previous collective rural cooperative medical system, followed the model of a health insurance scheme with the individual, the local government, and the central government each making a certain percentage of contribution to the premium. The insured would receive reimbursements of a certain percentage of costs for various *major* medical services. There was no mention of providing primary healthcare that the NRCMS was supposed to achieve. A complicated calculation system was also introduced along with the health insurance program that included copayments, deductibles and other restrictions. This insurance scheme was apparently modeled on the American health insurance programs and it did not work well in China with all the complicated components. As a result, the reimbursement rates were quite modest and not able to effectively solve the problems of people's medical costs.[21]

The government continued to encourage the formation of NRCMS while further exploring ways to improve the design of NRCMS by addressing the issues of increasing population coverage and level of insurance, and the expansion of insurance benefits and improvement of reimbursements. The key problem for ordinary people was the fact that increases of medical expenditures significantly outpaced their income growth. In 1990–1999 when average farmers' annual income grew from 686 to 2210 yuan per capita, the average medical expenditures per capita for outpatients jumped from 10 to 79 yuan and for inpatients from 473 to 2891 yuan.[22] People could not afford to see doctors in China ironically when the country's economy was creating enormous amounts of wealth. Facing widespread complaints and resentment, the government had to address the serious problems of healthcare lest social discontent and unrest undermine political stability. In January 2003, the State Council, after long months of deliberations with ministries of Health, Finance, and Agriculture on the proposals of reconstructing rural healthcare work, issued the "Guideline of Establishing New Rural Cooperative Medical System" to direct the rural healthcare reform. In the NRCMS, the government was to play the key role in organizing, leading, and sponsoring the program. The NRCMS emphasized voluntary participation with the household as a unit and used reimbursements for major medical services to reduce the high medical costs of farmers.[23] The program basically adopted the aforementioned pilot NRCMS that had been tested in 14 counties. The NRCMS mainly insured farmers against the high costs of serious and catastrophic illnesses to reduce their economic burden, far from solving the problem of providing a primary healthcare service to everyone.

As a health insurance scheme, the NRCMS was to be financed by multicontributors such as individuals, collectives, and the government at every level in accordance with local economic conditions. Although government of different levels—central, provincial, city, county, and town—was supposed to make contributions to the NRCMS, the more developed eastern part of China received less or no subsidies from the central government and was able to offer higher reimbursement rates, whereas the less developed western part of China received significant subsidies from the central government and was able to offer low reimbursement rates. Generally speaking, rich regions could not only afford to forgo the central government subsidies but also set a higher premium to offer higher reimbursement rates. As the operation of the NRCMS is closely tied to local financial resources and economic conditions, variations of the NRCMS program have developed across China due to different levels of economic development and financial ability in different regions.

In reality, the NRCMS was organized and implemented by the county (县) or city (市) as a local unit, and the local government, therefore, had the utmost responsibility of NRCMS operation. The local government of county or city, in fact, designed and managed the NRCMS by following the general policy of the central and provincial governments, but each local government had the authority to set up the specifics, such as the premium and the reimbursement rates, in line with local financial conditions. As a result, reimbursement rates varied significantly from one place to another. For instance, in order to administer the

NRCMS, the county government set up a NRCMS administration that consisted of an NRCMS committee, an office of the NRCMS, and a supervision committee to manage the NRCMS in every village (乡) and town (镇) of the county. During the implementation of NRCMS, a county usually first tested a pilot program in a designated rural town with several villages involved before the program was expanded in the entire county. The following two cases from Jiangsu (江苏) province offered a close-up look at the operation of NRCMS at the micro level with the contrast of significantly different economic conditions. Jiangsu is a prosperous province on the east coast of China, where the average annual income of farmers was 6480 yuan per capita in 2007. The level of economic development within the province was not even, however, with the north lagging behind the south. Guannan (灌南) is a relatively poor county in northern Jiangsu, where the average annual income for farmers was about 5000 yuan per capita in 2007.[24] Changshu (常熟) is a highly developed city in southern Jiangsu, where the average annual income of farmers was 12,000 yuan per capita in 2007.[25] Examinations of the two places offer a useful understanding of the different operations of NRCMS in the context of local economic development and financial conditions.

Guannan county government established the NRCMS across the rural villages in 2004 after having tested a pilot program in Huayuan town in 2003. The county office of NRCMS conducted educational workshops in villages and towns to disseminate information about the program and the benefits. It also investigated the actual operation of NRCMS at village clinics and town hospitals. In the early stage of expansion, the program was baffled by local government's focus on making profits, a characteristic behavior of market economy reflected in government bureaucracy as well as in healthcare institutions. The rural town government cared only about the profits they were to make out of the NRCMS and neglected the supervision of NRCMS service. The town government set up a new office to administer the NRCMS but the staff did not document well the registration of NRCMS participants. The lax attitude of work led to the confusion of different people using the NRCMS benefits. Village doctors, intent on making profits for themselves, tended to distribute expensive antibiotics and a larger quantity of drugs than necessary to patients. The abuse of drug prescription and distribution put more economic burden on the farmers who had to pay, but the practice simultaneously fleeced the NRCMS funds when reimbursements were made to the participant farmers for the medical costs. In response to the problems, the county government used administrative tactics and regulations to improve the supervision of NRCMS operation at village and town levels. The county government demanded that the town NRCMS administration office look into the service of village clinics every week and report their findings to the county office. The town government was also asked to put regular staff members in the NRCMS administration office and submit to the county office documented registrations of participants for verification. In an effort to improve work ethics and responsibility, staff salaries were tied to factors such as moral virtues, ability, diligence, and accomplishments in work. Another punitive mechanism was also put in place to discipline those who did not follow the proper procedure or who abused the new rural cooperative medical system.[26] With little data available, it was not possible to evaluate how effective these measures were and who was checking on the county government in this regard. Supervision and evaluation of the NRCMS was and still is a serious matter to make the program work effectively.

The county's Supervision Committee conducted surveys among farmers about the NRCMS program. Answers to the questionnaires indicated that farmers showed basic understanding of the NRCMS policies and they were basically satisfied with the operation of the NRCMS at the levels of village, town and county. They supported the idea of reimbursing the medical costs of both serious and minor ailments in the NRCMS insurance program, but that had to be decided by the central government as it concerned the general policy of the NRCMS. Farmers did not support the county proposal that the village clinic give up the reimbursement of medical costs in order to increase the reimbursement rates at town and county hospitals. The county government, therefore, did not change the reimbursement scheme, due to farmers' objections. This meant that the county government listened to farmers' opinions. But it did not always work that way. When the county government proposed the creation of a family account for an outpatient service, farmers did not support the proposal. The proposed family account required each family to deposit a certain amount into the account with the possibility of rolling over the money into the next year if the account was not depleted, but farmers had to pay out-of- pocket for the service if the account was used up before the end of the year.[27] Despite farmers' objections, the county government went ahead to create the family account for the outpatient service in 2005 anyway, with each participant in the household paying 10 yuan a year.[28] The responses of the county government indicated that farmers' opinions mattered only to a certain extent, and the county government did not always follow people's opinions in the execution of the NRCMS program.

For the year 2008, the standard premium of NRCMS was 100 yuan per person in Guannan county. The contribution came from the following sources: 60 yuan by provincial government, 2 yuan by city government, 18 yuan by county government, and 20 yuan by the individual. For the very poor individuals, their share of contribution was paid by the county bureau of civil affairs. The NRCMS program in Guannan allowed people to contribute more than the standard premium for higher reimbursement rates. The policy stipulated that the more one contributed the higher reimbursement rates one received for medical costs. Over 90 percent of the county's rural population of 500,000 had joined the NRCMS by 2008. Under the standard premium, people who incurred large amounts of medical costs for serious and catastrophic illnesses such as cancer, acute hepatitis and organ transplantation would receive reimbursement of 40 percent of their medical bills. The minimum pre-payment by patients for inpatient treatment was set as follows: none for staying at town hospitals (a way of encouraging people to seek treatment locally), 300 yuan for staying at county hospitals, and 800 yuan for staying at hospitals outside the county (usually at hospitals of higher level in big cities). For the reimbursement of inpatient costs, the standards were set at these levels: 40–45% for costs below 3000 yuan, 50% for costs between 3001 and 10,000 yuan, 55% for

10,001 to 30,000 yuan, 60% for above 30,000 yuan, with the maximum reimbursement of 45,000 yuan.[29] A few random cases in April 2008 illustrated how much patients were actually reimbursed in Guannan. Ms. Yang had a caesarean birth at her town hospital, and she was reimbursed 630 yuan for her inpatient (medical and hospital stay) costs of 1290.47 yuan, a 48.8 percent reimbursement. Ms. Chen had a regular birth at her town hospital and she was reimbursed 170 yuan for her inpatient costs of 348.76, a 48.7 percent reimbursement. Mr. Jiang was treated for cerebral hemorrhage at his town hospital and he was reimbursed 2702.40 yuan for his medical and hospital costs of 5704.79 yuan, a 47.4 percent reimbursement. Ms. Han had a tumor removed from her abdomen in her town hospital and she was reimbursed 1762.49 yuan for her medical and hospital costs of 3824.98 yuan, a 46 percent reimbursement.[30] These cases indicate that reimbursement rates for inpatient (medical and hospital stay) costs at town hospitals were just below 50 percent in Guannan county when people paid 20 yuan/year per person to join the NRCMS. It seemed, in practice, an average percentage reimbursement was used instead of the scaled structure of reimbursement rates.

Five years into the implementation of the NRCMS, the participating farmers in Guannan had their own health ID cards, called IC. They used their ICs for medical transactions, including payments and reimbursements. The IC helped streamline an otherwise complicated health insurance program into a single operating process. Since the use of health ID cards, some of the procedural problems incurred in the medical and hospital transactions were systematically solved, although the quality of service remained a challenge. Moreover, certain expensive medical devices such as pacemakers and artificial joints and hips were not covered by the NRCMS insurance in 2008, but they were after 2010. Healthcare for women and children remained a serious challenge, as some vaccines for children were not free.

Changshu is a rich city in southern Jiangsu. Since the city government had strong financial recourses to fund the NRCMS, it received no subsidies from the central or provincial government. For the year 2008, the standard premium of NRCMS in Changshu was 300 yuan per person, with the city government and the town government each contributing 110 yuan and the individual 80 yuan. Rural participation in NRCMS was 100 percent. With a higher premium, Changshu city offered higher reimbursement rates. For instance, reimbursement rates for inpatient costs were set as follows: 60 percent for costs below10,000 yuan, 65 percent for 10,001–20,000 yuan, 75 percent for 20,001–30,000 yuan, and 85 percent for above 30,000 yuan.[31] The city government encouraged participants to seek medical treatment at designated town hospitals within the city by providing higher reimbursement rates than for the costs incurred outside the city. Reimbursement rates for inpatient costs below 10,000 yuan at different types of hospitals were set as follows: 60 percent for treatment at designated town hospitals, 50 percent for treatment at specialized or private hospitals, and 45 percent for treatment at hospitals outside of Changshu city. Reimbursement rates for inpatient costs beyond 30,000 yuan were set at much higher levels: 85 percent for treatment at town hospitals, 80 percent for treatment at specialized or private hospitals, and 75 percent for treatment at hospitals outside of Changshu city.[32] It was clear that Changshu city government wished to keep patients within the town administrative boundary, as hospital operations figured into the general economic development of each town administration, contributing to the city as a whole. Data showed that medical reimbursement rates not only were tied to local financial resources but also reflected the level of local economic development.

When getting prescription drugs, the insured patients were asked to remind doctors that they prescribe the medicine on the list provided by the provincial government, called "The List of Basic Medicine for New Rural Cooperative Medical System in Jiangsu Province."[33] The provision of a list of medicine intended to guarantee low-cost drugs but it was also an administrative tactic to prevent doctors from prescribing unnecessarily expensive medicine to make profits. This administrative measure, though meant to prevent the abuse of medical power by doctors and hospitals, sometimes was turned into a bureaucratic headache for patients who truly needed certain expensive medicine to effectively treat their illnesses. As the abuse in prescribing expensive medicine and expensive medical devices for profits is prevalent in China's healthcare system, administrative tactics can only check the abuse to a certain degree if there is little mechanism to hold the abusers accountable.

Who were eligible to enroll in the NRCMS? That was defined by the local government, and it varied from place to place. In Changshu, all registered rural residents were eligible to participate, whereas in Guannan the NRCMS was open to people of various kinds: rural residents, employees of rural enterprises, and individual business persons. Migrant workers who had lived in Guannan county for over one year were also eligible to participate, which led to the tendency for migrant farmers to double dip the system by joining the NRCMS in their hometown and enrolling at their migrated places as well. This phenomenon, no doubt, would cost the government more in both health premiums and the reimbursements. In reality, however, migrant workers were not eligible to enroll in many big cities, nor were they able to use their hometown program in their migrated cities. The central and local governments have continuously increased the premium and the reimbursement rates of NRCMS with increased subsidies over the years. The coverage of insurance also expanded to include more medical services and items to be reimbursed. According to the National Health and Family Planning Commission, 98.9 percent of the rural population nationwide had participated in the NRMCS by the end of 2014.[34]

The NRCMS aims at reducing the financial burden of rural families, but the government has yet to make the healthcare system more accessible and efficient in terms of primary healthcare and prevention of disease. Patterns of disease have shifted in China in the past half century with the decline of infectious diseases and the rise of cancers and heart diseases. Infectious diseases became increasingly less significant as the main cause of death in Chinese society throughout the 1950s–1980s. They became the ninth leading cause of death in China in 1987.[35] In the 1990s, some epidemic infectious diseases returned, due to lax control, human migration, and fast industrialization. Tuberculosis, for instance, has resurged along with rapid industrialization and urbanization, and remains a major public health threat. Rural China suffers more due to less effective medical facilities and health personnel. According to a WHO report, about 80 percent of TB cases occurred among rural migrant workers in 2011 and 75 percent of the TB patients were in their 20s–30s. Especially alarming is the high incidence of multi-drug resistant tuberculosis. The return of old epidemic diseases drains China's health budget and reduces the overall economic productivity. A study shows that in 2001 infectious disease rose up to the seventh cause of death, accounting for about 2.3 percent of all deaths. Neglect of disease prevention was a major reason why old infectious diseases re-emerged while new types of disease posed additional health challenges. Cardiovascular and cerebrovascular diseases have become the leading cause of death, accounting for 32 percent of all deaths in 2001. Cancers or neoplasms have also become a major cause of death, responsible for 29.34 percent of all deaths, compared with 3.24 percent in 1952.[36] Other diseases, such as diabetes, mental illnesses and chronic diseases, have become increasingly significant as health threats in China today.

In response to new disease patterns and health threats, health institutions of disease prevention underwent structural changes in the beginning of the twenty-first century. China re-organized the system of disease prevention institutions and formed the Chinese Center for Disease Control and Prevention (China CDC, 中国疾病预防控制中心) in 2002 after some experiments in cities like Shanghai. The China CDC is clearly modeled after the American CDC and serves as a centralized agency of the Ministry of Health, with corresponding offices in the provincial and local health departments. The China CDC has incorporated the formerly different institutes and centers that were organized around individual diseases or clusters of disease categories into one encompassing organization of disease prevention and research. According to some Chinese scholars, the old institutes and centers of disease prevention were organized with "traditional perspectives of disease etiology and corresponding courses of treatment and prevention" and they responded independently to changes in technology and science in their fields, all of which caused unclear boundaries of disease categories and overlapping and sometimes conflicting mission statements and agency mandates.[37] With the centralization of disease prevention institutions into the CDC system, the old preventive institutes and centers, such as the Institutes of Maternal and Child Health, and the Health and Epidemic Disease Prevention Stations, were either incorporated or gradually lost in the process of forming CDC offices at provincial, municipal, and county levels. The new CDC system intends to modernize prevention and research and to correct the problems of the old system, but it appeared to have conducted limited public health education and service. Health knowledge and disease prevention have increasingly become matters of personal endeavor and peer group influence in China when economic growth dominates government agenda.

The trials and tribulations of piece-meal reforms of the health sector in the past two decades did not solve the fundamental problem that people could not afford to see doctors. The costs of medical care continued to go up and service quality go down, when new problems of fake drugs and various abuse of the system increased. In 2005, the State Council, based on the study by its own research center in partner with WHO, issued a report that the health reforms had so far basically failed and that a new framework of health reform was needed instead. With extensive examination of domestic and foreign experiences and the input of several think-tanks, the State Council hammered out an outline of a comprehensive and long-term health system reform plan in 2009.[38] The plan aims to build an affordable and effective health system to provide everybody with a primary healthcare service. The plan stresses the importance of healthcare in the harmonious development of society and economy and in sustaining social welfare and justice. The government projects to complete the basic structure of the new health system with primary healthcare to all people by 2020. The primary medical and health system (基本医疗卫生制度), as it is called, consists of four major structural components: public health service (公共卫生服务), medical care service (医疗服务), medical insurance and relief (医疗保障), and provision of a pharmaceutical drug supply (药品供应保障). The plan provides details on how to undergo comprehensive reforms in the four major areas.[39]

It is important to note that the public health service has received a renewed attention as a major measure to prevent disease and improve people's health. The public health service pays special attention to the prevention of major diseases, public health disaster relief, maternal and child health, mental health, and surveillance and prevention of infectious, chronic, occupational and endemic diseases, and birth defects. In response to urgent needs of public health and new patterns of disease, the reform plan revitalizes various components of the basic public health service, which includes the establishment of health records for all citizens, health education, coverage for 15 vaccine-preventable diseases, screening of the elderly for major diseases, prevention of major infectious, endemic and chronic diseases, and ensuring births take place at hospitals. The basic public health service is fully funded by the government on an annually increasing scale, which demonstrates the commitment of the government to deepening the health reform to benefit the people. The government subsidized the basic public health service with 15 yuan per capita in 2009 and increased to 25 yuan in 2011 and 40 yuan in 2015.

The important task is to successfully implement the health reform plan in relevant institutions by local governments. A recent study of villages in Hubei and Jiangxi shows the promises and challenges of the basic public health service at local level in rural China.[40] The study found that the local government's handling of public health fund was controversial. For instance, village clinics, which provided the public health service directly to the farmers, received on average only 3 of the government-designated 15 yuan subsidies per capita in 2009–2010, with the rest being shared by the county CDC and township health centers. Village doctors had concerns about the distribution of the public health fund. First, township health centers imposed financial penalties on village doctors for failing to complete public health work. But the township health officials explained that they were subject to the scrutiny of county government and it was not their intention to withhold government subsidies. Second, the town health centers as intermediates in the distribution of fund delayed or prevented village clinics from receiving the subsidies. For instance, some village doctors received no public health service subsidies because of local government financial constraints.[41] The reliance on local government to fund at least part of the subsidies limited the available amount for distribution, especially in poor regions and places where the local governments did not pay the subsidies, which led to sub-standard of public health service. The third major issue was that the public health service took time to complete, which reduced village doctors' time to perform the fees-for-service medical service. Village doctors said they provided a public health service mainly because of policy requirement rather than any other considerations. Out of financial and profit considerations, doctors would spend the daytime on medical service, and only at night (when fewer people came for medical care) did they perform the public health service. Some doctors expressed that public health service was on the low end of their agenda because the work was not valued or recognized. They wanted to do better for public health service if the work was valued and recognized.[42] The study indicates that proper allocation of public health fund and promotion and recognition of good public health work are important to effective implementation of the program.

The problems revealed by the study call for effective supervision and evaluation of local health institutions and governments, particularly those at the town and county levels, in the implementation of public health service program. In fact, effective supervision and evaluation is urgently needed in every aspect of medical and health service at the health institutions such as village clinics, town health centers, county health institutions, and public and private hospitals in general, not only by the authority of immediate superiors but also by doctors and health users. Without the health users' participation in the surveillance and reporting of the quality of public health service, elements of indifference and corruption would take every opportunity to abuse and undermine the health programs.[43] However, citizens have to be fully informed of the health programs to be good monitors and evaluators. As recent as 2014, the *Procuratorial Daily* reported that 90 percent of citizens had little or no idea about the public health service program.[44] The government needs to actively publicize the public health service program and urge citizens to inquire about the service for their own benefits. The absence of public knowledge of the public health service opens up opportunities for local government and health institutions to funnel public health funds for other uses. Equally significant for the implementation of health programs is efficient allocation of government subsidies and public recognition of jobs well done by doctors and health professionals.

Conclusion

Economic reforms have ushered in market forces to structurally change the Chinese economic system. Commercialization and marketization characterized the change of business operation in the past three decades. The government-led market economy encompasses diverse forms of private and state-run enterprises operating on the basis of competition and profitability. In agriculture, the household responsibility system replaced the commune system in the de-collectivization of rural economy. As a result, the rural cooperative medical system collapsed when the economic foundation shifted and the collective-service of barefoot doctors was transformed into the private practice of village doctors. Medical costs rose sharply along with the marketization of the health sector, making medical service increasingly unaffordable for people. The government used piecemeal measures to reform the health sector and to respond to the new challenges such as high costs of medical service and inaccessibility of health protection. But these methods proved ineffective and unsuccessful in solving the serious problems of healthcare. The failure of the piece meal reforms led to new efforts to re-build the NRCMS and the 2009 comprehensive plan to reform the health system with provision of primary healthcare.

Economic reforms unleashed the creative power of Chinese people and dramatically increased the living standards. The economic transformation also brought about profound social changes and challenges. On one hand, national health as a significant expression of modernization and national progress, which served to promote the modernization movement in the early twentieth century and showcase the successful socialist reconstruction in the 1950s–1970s, was largely neglected in the busy pursuit of economic growth in the last 20 years of the twentieth century. On the other hand, industrialization and societal affluence gave rise to new health hazards and diseases. Heart diseases, diabetes, cancers, high blood pressure, and mental illnesses are on the rise in China. Another impact of industrialization and urbanization was the decline of the birth rate. As tens of millions of young farmers migrated to cities, they faced a highly competitive working environment and challenging urban settings to raise children. As a result, a changed pattern of reproduction began to emerge at the turn of the twenty-first century, where couples voluntarily had fewer children especially in rural China.[45] By 2004, the fertility rate had dropped to 1.7 per woman, with 1.3 in urban areas and just under 2.0 in rural areas.[46] China is becoming an aging society, and the government changed the one-child to a two-children policy at the end of 2015.

As the country moves forward, national health plays an important part in the delivery of a good life with social welfare and justice. Moreover, national health cannot be ignored because the well-being of the 1.3 billion Chinese people is the foundation of China's economic and social development. China was and still is searching for a healthcare system that would be feasible under the framework of market economy. Currently, China has three basic medical insurance systems that cover different categories of people: basic medical insurance for urban employees, basic medical insurance for urban residents, and the new rural cooperative medical system for rural residents. In January 2016, the central government publicized the plan to integrate the two health insurance systems for urban and rural residents into one basic health insurance system.[47] If that is done, it will be a significant step towards eliminating the divide of urban and rural residents.

Notes

1 The one-child policy was more effectively carried out in cities than in the countryside where traditional values were strong. See the poster exhibit on Chinese family planning and economic development at http://www.nlm.nih.gov/exhibition/chinesefamilyplanning/. As China is becoming an aging society, the Chinese government started the two-children policy on January 1, 2016.

2 Justin Yifu Lin, "The Household Responsibility System Reform in China: A Peasant's Institutional Choice," *American Journal of Agricultural Economics*, vol. 69, no. 2 (1987), 410–415.

3 http://www.china.org.cn/english/features/Q&A/160352.htm, accessed 3/16/2016.

4 Yue Qianhou and He Puyan, "Shanxi sheng Jishan xian nongcun gonggong weisheng shiye shuping (1949–1984)—Yi Taiyangcun (gongshe) wei zhongdian kaocha duixiang," *Dangdai Zhongguo shi yanjiu* [Contemporary China History Studies], vol. 14, no. 5 (September 2007), 67.

5 For recent development of Huaxi, people can search Huaxicun online.

6 Chen Haifeng, *Zhongguo weisheng baojian shi* (1992), 84.

7 Zhang Kaining, Wen Yiqun and Liang Ping, *Cong chijiao yisheng dao xiangcun yisheng* [From Barefoot Doctors to Village Doctors] (Yunnan renmin chubanshe, 2002), 5. For changes in a local setting, see Sydney D. White, "From Barefoot Doctor to Village Doctor in Tiger Springs Village: A Case Study of Rural Health Care Transformation in Socialist China," *Human Organization*, vol. 57, no. 4 (Winter 1998), 480–490.

8 Chinese official evaluation of the Cultural Revolution was negative with the label of "ten years of disaster." "Barefoot doctors" smacked of the radical tone of that era, although they had served rural health at the forefront with significant contributions to reduction of disease, education and service of family planning, and the general improvement of people's health.

9 Yao Li, "Xinshiqi nongcun hezuo yiliao gaige lunshu [A Review of the Reforms of Rural Cooperative Medical System in the New Era]," *Contemporary China History Studies*, vol. 16, no. 2 (2009), 40.

10 Cai Renhua, *Zhongguo yiliao baozhang zhidu gaige shiyong quanshu* [A Practical Handbook of the Reform of Chinese Health Insurance System] (Beijing: Zhongguo renshi chubanshe, 1997), 356–7.

11 Naisu Zhu, Zhihua Ling, Jie Shen, J. M. Lane and Shanlian Hu, "Factors Associated with the Decline of the Cooperative Medical System and Barefoot Doctors in Rural China," *Bulletin of the World Health Organization*, vol. 67, no. 4 (1989), 431–441.

12 William C. L. Hsiao, "The Chinese Health Care System: Lessons for Other Nations," *Social Science and Medicine*, vol. 41, no. 8 (1995), 1047–1055.

13 Yuanli Liu, "China's Public Health-Care System: Facing the Challenges," *Bulletin of the World Health Organization*, vol. 82, no. 7 (July 2004), 532–38.

14 Major efforts were made to tackle the new health problems by relying on technology in the past two decades. See articles published in the Bulletin of the World Health Organization: Weibing Wang, Qi Zhao, Zhengan Yuan, Yihui Zheng, Yixing Zhang, Liping Lu, Yun Hou, Yue Zhang and Biao Xu, "Tuberculosis-Associated Mortality in Shanghai, China: A Longitudinal Study," vol. 93 (2015), 826–833; and Hsien-Ho Lin, Lixia Wang, Hui Zhang, Yunzhou Ruan, Daniel P Chin and Christopher Dye, "Tuberculosis Control in China: Use of Modelling to Develop Targets and Policies," vol. 93 (2015), 790–798.

15 Ministry of Health of the People's Republic of China, *Reports on the 1998 National Health Service Survey Results* (Beijing: Ministry of Health, 1999).

16 "Fazhan nongcun weisheng shiye shi dangwu zhi ji [The Urgent Task to Develop Rural Healthcare]," *The People's Daily*, January 22, 1991, 8.

17 Ministry of Health, PRC, *National Health Statistics* (Beijing: Ministry of Health, 2002).

18 Yao Li, "Xinshiqi nongcun hezuo yiliao gaige lunshu," 37.

19 The State Council, "To Speed up the Reform and Development of Rural Cooperative Medical System" (Beijing, March 1994).
20 Guy Carrin, Aviva Rona, Yang Hui, Wang Hong, Zhang Tuohong, Zhang Licheng, Zhang Shuo, Ye Yide, Chen Jiaying, Jiang Qicheng, Zhang Zhaoyang, Yu Jun and Li Xuesheng, "The Reform of the Rural Cooperative Medical System in the People's Republic of China: Interim Experience in 14 Pilot Counties," *Social Science and Medicine*, vol. 48 (1999), 963, footnote 8.
21 Ibid., 961–972.
22 Ding Xiaobo, *Nongcun weisheng gaige yu xinxing nongcun hezuo yiliao gongzuo shouce* [Handbook for Rural Health Reforms and New Rural Cooperative Medical System] (Zhongguo caizheng jingji chubanshe, 2005), 26.
23 http://www.gov.cn/zwgk/2005-08/12/content_21850.htm. Accessed 3/22/16.
24 Jiangsu Statistics Bureau, www.jssb.gov.cn. Accessed on September 8, 2008.
25 www.changshu.gov.cn. Accessed on September 7, 2008.
26 Guannan County Office of NRCMS, "Problems in the New Rural Cooperative Medical System and their Solutions" (Guannan County Office of NRCMS, November 2004).
27 Guannan County Office of NRCMS, "Survey Questionnaire on the Implementation of New Rural Cooperative Medical System" (Guannan County Office of NRCMS, 2007).
28 *Collection of Documents* (Guannan County Office of the NRMC Supervision Committee, April 2005).
29 "Notification of the Policy Regarding the New Rural Cooperative Medical System" (Guannan County Office of the NRCMS Supervision Committee, November 15, 2007).
30 "Data of Reimbursements of Medical and Hospital Expenses" (Guannan County NRCMS Office, May 2008).
31 "Collection of Documents on the New Rural Cooperative Medical Insurance in Changshu" (Health Bureau of Changshu City, March 2008), 37.
32 Changshu City NRCMS Management Office, "Rural Medical Health Insurance of Changshu City" (Changshu City NRCMS Management Office and Changshu City Urban Residents Basic Health Insurance Office, 2008).
33 NRMCS Supervision Committee, "Notification of the Policy Regarding the New Rural Cooperative Medical System" (Guannan County, November 15, 2007).
34 http://politics.people.com.cn/n/2015/1105/c1001-27782363.html. The Ministry of Health and the National Population and Family Planning Commission were merged into the National Health and Family Planning Commission in 2013 during the structural re-organization of the central government.
35 Ministry of Health, *Health Statistics Information in China* (Beijing: Ministry of Health, 1991). See also William Hsiao, "The Chinese Health Care System," 1048.
36 Jing Peng, Sheng Nian Zhang, Wei Lu, and Andrew T. L. Chen, "Public Health in China: The Shanghai CDC Perspective," *American Journal of Public Health*, vol. 93, no. 12 (December 2003), 1991–1993.
37 Ibid.
38 Zhu Chen, "Launch of the Health-Care Reform Plan in China," *Lancet*, vol. 373, no. 9672 (April 18, 2009), 1322–1324.
39 The Central Government and the State Council, "Guideline of Deepening the Reform of Medical and Health System) http://finance.people.com.cn/GB/9083061.html. Assessed March 28, 2016.
40 Yan Ding, Helen J. Smith, Yang Fei, Biao Xu, Shaofa Nie, Weirong Yan, Vinod K Diwan, Rainer Sauerborn and Hengjin Dong, "Factors Influencing the Provision of Public Health Service by Village Doctors in Hubei and Jiangxi Provinces, China," *Bulletin of the World Health Organization* vol. 91 (2013), 64–69.
41 Ibid., 65–66.
42 Ibid., 66.
43 There are plenty of news reports on how corrupt officials used different methods to pocket government funds for their own use.

44 Dai Jia, Gao Chuanwei, Zhao Ruichang and Hou Feng, "Where Did the Basic Public Health Service Fund Go? [Jiben gonggong weisheng fuwufei qu nale?]," *Jian Cha Ribao* [Procuratorial Daily], August 15, 2014, http://newspaper.jcrb.com/html/2014-08/15/content_166116.htm. Accessed March 28, 2016.
45 Hong Zhang, "From Resisting to "Embracing?" the One-Child Rule: Understanding New Fertility Trends in a Central China Village," *The China Quarterly*, vol. 192 (2007), 855–875.
46 Therese Hesketh, Li Lu, and Zhu Wei Xing, "The Effect of China's One-Child Family Policy after 25 Years," *The New England Journal of Medicine*, vol. 353, no. 11 (September 2005), 1171–1176, 1172.
47 The State Council, "Guanyu zhenghechengxiang jumin jiben yiliao baoxianzhidu de yijian" [On the integration of the basic health insurance system of urban and rural residents], January 12, 2016, http://www.gov.cn/zhengce/content/2016-01/12/content_10582.htm. Accessed March 10, 2016.

Index